PRACTICAL GUIDE TO
EMERGENCY ULTRASOUND

PRACTICAL GUIDE TO
EMERGENCY ULTRASOUND

KAREN S. COSBY, MD, FACEP

Assistant Professor
Department of Emergency Medicine
Stroger Hospital of Cook County
Rush Medical College
Chicago, Illinois

JOHN L. KENDALL, MD, FACEP

Director, Emergency Ultrasound
Attending Physician
Department of Emergency Medicine
Denver Health Medical Center
Assistant Professor
Division of Emergency Medicine
University of Colorado Health Sciences Center
Denver, Colorado

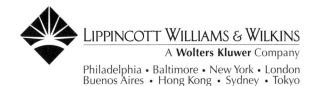

LIPPINCOTT WILLIAMS & WILKINS
A **Wolters Kluwer** Company

Philadelphia • Baltimore • New York • London
Buenos Aires • Hong Kong • Sydney • Tokyo

Acquisitions Editor: Frances DeStefano
Managing Editor: Nicole T. Dernoski
Project Manager: Alicia Jackson
Senior Manufacturing Manager: Benjamin Rivera
Marketing Manager: Angela Panetta
Cover Designer: Larry Didona
Production Service: Schawk Publishing Services
Printer: Edwards Brothers

Library of Congress Cataloging-in-Publication Data
Practical guide to emergency ultrasound / [edited by] Karen S. Cosby, John L. Kendall.
   p. ; cm.
   Includes bibliographical references and index.
   ISBN-13: 978-0-7817-7858-9 (alk. paper)
   ISBN-10: 0-7817-7858-1 (alk. paper)
   1. Ultrasonic imaging. 2. Emergency medicine—Diagnosis.
   [DNLM: 1. Ultrasonography—methods. 2. Emergencies. WN 208 E53 2006]
I. Cosby, Karen S. II. Kendall, John L. III. Title.
RC78.7.U4E64 2006
616.07′543—dc22
                                                    2005022799

Care has been taken to confirm the accuracy of the information presented and to describe
generally accepted practices. However, the authors, editors, and publisher are not responsible
for errors or omissions or for any consequences from application of the information in this
book and make no warranty, expressed or implied, with respect to the currency, completeness, or accuracy of the contents of the publication. Application of the information in a particular situation remains the professional responsibility of the practitioner.

   The authors, editors, and publisher have exerted every effort to ensure that drug selection and dosage set forth in this text are in accordance with current recommendations and
practice at the time of publication. However, in view of ongoing research, changes in govern-
ment regulations, and the constant flow of information relating to drug therapy and drug
reactions, the reader is urged to check the package insert for each drug for any change in indications and dosage and for added warnings and precautions. This is particularly important
when the recommended agent is a new or infrequently employed drug.

   Some drugs and medical devices presented in the publication have Food and Drug Administration (FDA) clearance for limited use in restricted research settings. It is the responsibility of the health care provider to ascertain the FDA status of each drug or device planned
for use in their clinical practice.

   To purchase additional copies of this book, call our customer service department at
(800) 638-3030 or fax orders to (301) 824-7390. International customers should call (301)
714-2324.

   Visit Lippincott Williams & Wilkins on the Internet: at LWW.com. Lippincott Williams
& Wilkins customer service representatives are available from 8:30 am to 6 pm, EST.

10 9 8 7 6 5 4 3 2

To Jeff Schaider and Anne Sydor, who planted the seeds that eventually took root and who gently prodded me into this endeavor.

To those dearest to me, who made daily sacrifices to support and encourage this work.

I dedicate this book to Elizabeth, Matthew, and Hannah, for your understanding, patience, and kindness;

And to Don, for your unselfish commitment, enthusiasm, perseverance, and love.

Karen Cosby

To my fellow authors: Your contributions of time, effort, and insight have helped to bring the spirit of this book to fruition.

To my residents, both current and past: Ultrasound opens a fascinating world of possibility and requires a unique educational approach. I hope you have learned as much from me as I have learned from you.

To my parents: You have always provided a nurturing environment for learning, exploration, and an appreciation for life.

To my wife, Kwai, who both challenges me to be a better man and accepts me as I am, and to my children, Oliver and Maya: This book is dedicated to you. I hope one day you will read it and be as proud of me as I am of you.

John Kendall

TABLE OF CONTENTS

CONTRIBUTORS

Jean Abbott, MD
Associate Professor
Division of Emergency Medicine
University of Colorado School of Medicine
Denver, Colorado

John Bailitz, MD
Assistant Professor
Rush Medical University
Attending Physician
John H. Stroger, Jr. Hospital of Cook
    County
Chicago, Illinois

Aaron E. Bair, MD
Assistant Professor of Emergency Medicine
Department of Emergency Medicine
University of California Davis School of
    Medicine
Sacramento, California

Adam Barkin, MD
Chief Resident
Beth Israel Deaconess Medical Center
Harvard Affiliated Emergency Medicine
    Residency
Boston, Massachusetts

Michael Blaivas, MD, RDMS
Associate Professor
Chief, Section of Emergency Ultrasound
Director, Emergency Medicine Ultrasound
    Fellowship
Department of Emergency Medicine
Medical College of Georgia
Augusta, Georgia

Karen S. Cosby, MD, FACEP
Assistant Professor of Emergency Medicine
Stroger Hospital of Cook County/Rush Medical
    University
Department of Emergency Medicine
Chicago, Illinois

J. Christian Fox, MD, RDMS
Assistant Clinical Professor of Emergency
    Medicine
University of California, Irvine
Irvine, California

Bradley W. Frazee, MD
Assistant Clinical Professor of Medicine
University of California, San Francisco
Attending Physician
Department of Emergency Medicine
Alameda County Medical Center –
    Highland Campus
Oakland, California

Michael Heller, MD
Clinical Professor of Medicine
Temple University School of Medicine
Program Director
Emergency Medicine Residency
St. Luke's Hospital
Bethlehem, Pennsylvania

Stephen R. Hoffenberg, MD, FACEP
Ultrasound Section, Past Chair
American College of Emergency Physicians
Attending Physician
Department of Emergency Medicine
Rose Medical Center
Denver, Colorado

Jeanne Jacoby, MD
Assistant Professor
Temple University School of Medicine
Director, Emergency Ultrasound
Emergency Medicine Residency
St. Luke's Hospital
Bethlehem, Pennsylvania

John L. Kendall, MD, FACEP
Director, Emergency Ultrasound
Attending Physician
Department of Emergency Medicine
Denver Health Medical Center
Assistant Professor
Division of Emergency Medicine
University of Colorado Health Sciences Center
Denver, Colorado

Stephen J. Leech, MD, RDMS
Director, Faculty Ultrasound Education
Emergency Medicine Ultrasound Faculty
Department of Emergency Medicine
Christiana Care Health System
Newark, Delaware

Henry Lin, MD
Assistant Clinical Professor
Columbia University
College of Physicians and Surgeons
New York, New York

Matthew L. Lyon, MD, RDMS
Assistant Professor
Director ED Observation Unit
Associate Director, Section of Emergency
   Ultrasound
Medical College of Georgia
Augusta, Georgia

JoAnne McDonough, MD, MPH
Clinical Instructor
Department of Emergency Medicine
University of California, Irvine
Irvine, California

Jeffrey C. Metzger, MD
Resident Physician
Division of Emergency Medicine
Duke University Medical Center
Durham, North Carolina

Christopher L. Moore, MD, RDMS, RDCS
Assistant Professor
Yale University School of Medicine
New Haven, Connecticut

Kristen Nordenholz, MD
Assistant Professor
Ultrasound Coordinator
Division of Emergency Medicine
University of Colorado School of Medicine
Denver, Colorado

Robert S. Park, MD
Director of Emergency Ultrasound
Assistant Clinical Professor
Division of Emergency Medicine
Duke University Medical Center
Durham, North Carolina

Susan B. Promes, MD, FACEP
Program Director
Associate Clinical Professor
Division of Emergency Medicine
Duke University Medical Center
Durham, North Carolina

John S. Rose, MD
Associate Professor of Emergency Medicine
Department of Emergency Medicine
University of California Davis School of
   Medicine
Sacramento, California

Paul R. Sierzenski, MD, RDMS, FAAEM, FACEP
Director, Emergency Medicine and Trauma
   Ultrasound
Director, Emergency Medicine Ultrasound
   Fellowship
Department of Emergency Medicine
Christiana Care Health System
Newark, Delaware

Vivek S. Tayal, MD, FACEP
Director, Emergency Ultrasound
Carolinas Medical Center, Charlotte,
   North Carolina
Past Chair, ACEP Section on Emergency
   Ultrasound

Carrie Tibbles, MD
Associate Residency Director
Beth Israel Deaconess Medical Center
Harvard Affiliated Emergency Medicine
   Residency
Boston, Massachusetts

Douglas A. E. White, MD
Clinical Instructor, Dept. of Medicine
University of California, San Francisco
Attending Physician
Department of Emergency Medicine
Alameda County Medical Center –
   Highland Campus
Oakland, California

PREFACE

Change comes slowly. The first paper pertaining to emergency ultrasound appeared more than 15 years ago, and while the concept of physicians performing a "limited" ultrasound examination took root and gained favor from clinicians and educators, the growth of this imaging modality has been slower than expected. Formal teaching in ultrasound is now a part of most Emergency Medicine residencies yet, as educators, we find that there is a dramatic drop-off in the application of ultrasound skills once residents leave their academic training grounds and enter practice. There are many barriers that impede the widespread acceptance and use of bedside ultrasound in real-life practice. This book was born from our efforts to identify and understand these difficulties and written with the intent to empower the reader to surmount them.

From an educator's perspective, the ability to incorporate ultrasound into clinical practice requires at least four critical elements. First, the skill must be seen as valuable, one worth learning. Secondly, the skill itself requires specialty knowledge, awareness of ultrasound-relevant anatomy and landmarks. The clinician must have technical knowledge and skill to acquire the image. Lastly, the clinician must be able to take the information and use it in real-time decision making. This text is organized around these four goals. Each chapter begins with indications for ultrasound, then focuses on a review of normal ultrasound anatomy, techniques for acquiring the image, and guidelines for using the information to make clinical decisions.

The emergency physician faces other challenges as well, factors that ultimately may limit their ability to incorporate ultrasound into clinical practice. There are administrative pressures to be efficient. There are financial pressures to optimize billing and reimbursement. There are political pressures within each institution that influence the ability to change clinical practice, especially when it entails interaction with other specialties. We have attempted to address these challenges up front, with guidelines for introducing emergency ultrasound into a new practice, suggestions for quality assurance and credentialing, and practical ideas for making ultrasound efficient and accurate.

As this text enters production, we face an interesting paradox. The widespread integration of ultrasound into clinical practice has occurred relatively slowly, while the technology and potential applications are expanding at a rapid rate. New applications for bedside ultrasound are continually being found, and keeping up with and predicting these trends in a textbook is nearly impossible. Recognizing that limitation, this text includes sections pertaining to many of the applications that are currently considered cutting-edge. Our goal is to narrow the gap between where we stand today and where we hope to be in the next decade of growth. As well, it is becoming increasingly apparent that bedside ultrasound is not an imaging modality specific to emergency medicine, but rather one that is useful to many different clinicians (physicians, nurses, and prehospital personnel) across a variety of specialties (surgeons, intensivists, cardiologists, and internists). While the authors of this textbook are all practicing emergency physicians, the content of this text is applicable to many different practitioners who seek to realize the benefits of bedside ultrasound.

Bedside ultrasound is an evolving standard. In the early years, the use of ultrasound by emergency physicians was viewed as an encroachment into an area that belonged to other specialists. This is no longer the case. Emergency medicine has adopted the technology and developed it for our own purpose, just as other specialties have done. We have contributed significantly to the ultrasound literature. We have developed it for practical bedside applications, applying it to many types of exams not traditionally performed by radiologists. Ultrasound manufacturers have introduced equipment that is designed specifically for bedside use, with increased portability, rapid boot-up times, and improved versatility appropriate for a wide range of applications. Emergency ultrasound can no longer be considered a borrowed skill, nor even an alternative to consultative scans; rather, it has become a discipline in itself.

Change is inevitable. Emergency medicine has a history and philosophy accepting of change and a drive to continually raise the standard of care. We are proud to continue that tradition with this book. Our hope is that this text will help bedside clinicians, regardless of their specialty or level of training, to acquire or improve basic bedside ultrasound skills, enhance their clinical practice, and ultimately raise the standard of care for our patients.

Karen S. Cosby, MD
John L. Kendall, MD

THE HISTORY AND PHILOSOPHY OF EMERGENCY ULTRASOUND

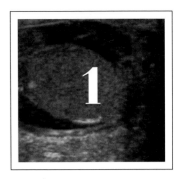

Stephen R. Hoffenberg

INTRODUCTION

Emergency ultrasound is a standard emergency physician skill (1). It is taught in emergency medicine residencies (2,3), tested on board examinations (4,5), and is endorsed by emergency medicine professional societies (1,6). The use of ultrasound performed by the treating emergency physician, interpreting images as they are displayed and simultaneously using them for diagnosis or procedural assistance, differs significantly from the traditional approach of consultative imaging services. Bedside emergency ultrasound has proven to be an appropriate use of technology demonstrated to speed care (7–9), enhance patient safety (10,11), and save lives (12).

THE HISTORY OF EMERGENCY ULTRASOUND

Ultrasound became available for clinical use in the 1960s following more than a decade of investigation. The technology was initially found only in specialized imaging laboratories; however, by the 1970s, ultrasound was being adopted in diverse settings by a variety of clinical specialties. Ultrasound technology and devices improved rapidly, and real-time ultrasound was developed in the early 1980s, which allowed the viewing of ultrasounds without an appreciable delay between signal generation and display of the image. In addition, sufficient images were generated by real-time ultrasound to allow the visualization of continuous motion. Prior to the development of real-time ultrasound, the complexity of acquiring images prevented the practical application of ultrasound for most emergency patients and was an absolute barrier to use at the bedside. Real-time scanning changed how ultrasound is used, who uses ultrasound, and where studies are performed.

Ultrasound devices continued to improve during the 1980s and 1990s. Smaller, faster, and more portable ultrasound equipment was developed in accompaniment with other enhancements such as the transvaginal transducer, multifrequency probes, and color Doppler. These improvements accelerated the movement of technology from the ultrasound suite to the bedside for immediate use in emergency patients.

The growth in clinical applications paralleled technological advancements. As early as 1970, surgeons in Germany were the first to experiment with ultrasound for the detection of free fluid in the abdomen (13,14). In 1976 an American surgeon used ultrasound to describe and grade splenic injuries (15). Emergency physicians began investigating the clinical use of ultrasound in the late 1980s, while the first emergency ultrasound publication appeared in 1988 that addressed the utility of echocardiography performed by emergency physicians (16). Beginning in the late 1980s through the mid 1990s, significant investigation was being done in both the United States and Germany on the detection of hemoperitoneum and hemopericardium in trauma victims. This research ultimately led to the description of the Focused Assessment with Sonography for Trauma (FAST) examination (12,17–21). The FAST examination has essentially replaced diagnostic peritoneal lavage in all but a handful of patients and has been fully integrated into Advanced Trauma Life Support (ATLS) teaching. This examination remains the standard initial ultrasound examination for trauma victims by emergency physicians and trauma surgeons and is often equated with "emergency ultrasonography."

The American College of Emergency Physicians (ACEP) offered its initial course in the emergency applications of ultrasound in 1990. In 1991 both ACEP and the Society of Academic Emergency Medicine (SAEM) published position papers recognizing the utility of ultrasound for emergency patients (22,6). These documents endorsed not only the clinical use of ultrasound, but also ongoing research and education. The SAEM policy added that resident physicians should be trained to perform and interpret emergency ultrasound examinations. In 1994 SAEM published the *Model Curriculum for Physician Training in Emergency Ultrasonography* outlining recommended training standards for emergency medicine residents (23). Shortly following the development of this curriculum, the first textbook dedicated to emergency ultrasound was published in 1995 (24).

In 2001, the ACEP published the *Emergency Ultrasound Guidelines* updating the scope of practice and clinical indications for emergency ultrasonography (25). This policy statement advanced recommendations for credentialing, quality assurance, and the documentation of emergency ultrasounds as well as representing current best practices and standards for ultrasound provided by emergency physicians.

Over the past decade, results of emergency physician–performed ultrasound have been examined for a wide spectrum of clinical conditions, including abdominal aortic aneurysm (26–28), ectopic pregnancy (7,29–32), thoracoabdominal trauma (17–21,33), pericardial effusion (34, 35), determination of cardiac activity (36–38), biliary disease (39–41), renal tract disease (42,43), and procedure guidance (10,11,44–46). Each of these is now considered a primary indication for emergency ultrasound. Ongoing research will likely establish the efficacy of additional emergency applications such as the assessment of undifferentiated hypotension (47,48), the bedside evaluation for deep venous thrombosis (49,9) and a variety of soft tissue and musculoskeletal applications (50–53).

GROWTH OF EMERGENCY ULTRASOUND

A number of factors have driven the development of emergency ultrasound. They include a growing recognition of the utility for ultrasound information, a need for timely access to diagnostic imaging, declining access to consultative services, improved ultrasound technology, and the endorsement of immediate ultrasound by the specialty of emergency medicine.

RECOGNITION OF THE VALUE OF ULTRASOUND

A key factor contributing to the growth of emergency ultrasound is an increased recognition of ultrasound's clinical utility. The primary indications for diagnostic emergency ultrasound are now well established. Where immediate ultrasound is available, it has essentially replaced invasive techniques such as peritoneal lavage and culdocentesis as well as obviating the need for blind pericardiocentesis. Use for procedure guidance, such as central venous access, is an evolving standard of care. Interestingly, the management of cardiac arrest assisted by diagnostic ultrasound (35,36) and the evaluation of patients with nontraumatic hypotension (47,48) are examples of ultrasound usage not contemplated prior to the growth of emergency ultrasound.

TIMELY ACCESS TO IMAGING

For many emergency conditions, ultrasound is needed on an immediate basis. "Immediate" may mean within minutes of patient presentation. Examples include central line placement under ultrasound guidance in the hypotensive patient, and diagnostic scans in hemodynamically unstable patients with suspected aortic aneurysm or blunt trauma. In addition, patients in cardiac arrest, with penetrating chest injuries, or those with undifferentiated hypotension are all candidates for immediate bedside ultrasound. These examinations are extremely time-dependent and typically cannot be supplied in a clinically useful time frame by even the best staffed radiology departments or echocardiography laboratories. For some of these conditions, both diagnostic ultrasound (e.g., abdominal) and echocardiography are required for the same patient, but in most hospitals these studies are supplied by separate consulting services. The ultrasound-trained emergency physician is typically in the best position to utilize immediate ultrasound for a number of emergency conditions.

IMAGING AVAILABILITY

Patients present to the emergency department 24 hours a day, 7 days a week, and a predictable subset require ultrasound evaluation. While recognition of the positive impact of ultrasound imaging on patient care has grown, consulting imaging services have progressively become less available for emergency patients. This is particularly true at night and on weekends. The reasons most often cited for decreasing access includes higher costs incurred by the imaging service for "off-hours" studies and the lack of an adequate number of sonographers to perform these examinations. As a result, emergency physicians may be asked to hold patients who require imaging until the following day, to treat patients prior to diagnostic testing, or to send patients home with potentially life-threatening conditions pending a scheduled outpatient study. Common examples include holding a patient with undiagnosed abdominal pain pending a right upper quadrant study, treating a patient with anticoagulants prior to a deep venous ultrasound exam, or discharging a patient with suspected ectopic pregnancy prior to pelvic imaging.

Delays and decreased access to consultative imaging increase the medical risk to patients, can result in emergency department overcrowding, and may increase medical liability for the emergency physician. Immediate imaging by the emergency physician can provide needed data, significantly decrease requirements for costly consultative studies, and avoid associated delays (7–9,41,54–56).

IMPROVING TECHNOLOGY

Technology improvements in ultrasound devices have made an essential contribution to the development of emergency ultrasound programs. The stationary and operationally complex devices historically associated with ultrasound have been replaced by a variety of highly portable and more intuitive machines. Hardware improvements have been accompanied by software enhancements, resulting in increased speed, flexibility, image quality, and ease of use. These technological advancements have increased the practical utility of ultrasound and have allowed the movement of this technology from the laboratory to the bedside.

SPECIALTY ENDORSEMENT BY EMERGENCY MEDICINE

The use of emergency ultrasound has been endorsed by emergency medicine professional societies, such as ACEP and SAEM (1,6). Assumptions underlying these endorsements are that specialists in emergency medicine are in the best position to recognize the needs of emergency patients and, in addition, have an obligation to utilize available technologies that have been demonstrated to improve patient care. Finally, since ultrasound training has been included in residency education (2,3), emergency specialists now enter practice with the reasonable expectation of utilizing this standard emergency physician skill (1,4,5).

THE PARADIGM OF EMERGENCY ULTRASOUND

The approach to ultrasound performed by the emergency physician differs significantly from that embraced by consultative imaging services. Who performs the study, where the examination is conducted, how quickly it is accomplished, and how study results are communicated all differ. In addition, the scope of the examination and study goals may be quite different. Physician work associated with the examination, the expense of test performance, and how data is integrated into patient care are also unique in each of these approaches. Understanding and communicating the paradigm of emergency ultrasound is an essential step in program implementation.

ULTRASOUND IMAGING BY EMERGENCY PHYSICIANS

The paradigm of emergency ultrasound is reflected in the ACEP policy on *Use of Ultrasound Imaging by Emergency Physicians* (1).

> Ultrasound imaging enhances the physician's ability to evaluate, diagnose, and treat emergency department patients. Because ultrasound imaging is often time-dependent in the acutely ill or injured patient, the emergency physician is in an ideal position to use this technology. Focused ultrasound examinations provide immediate information and can answer specific questions about the patient's physical condition. Such bedside ultrasound imaging is within the scope of practice of emergency physicians.

The paradigm of emergency ultrasound begins with ultrasound performance by the treating physician at the patient's bedside. The examination is contemporaneous with patient care and is performed on an immediate basis. In this context "immediate" means within minutes of an identified need. Interpretation of images is done by the treating physician and occurs as the images are generated and displayed. In this approach, permanent images document what has already been interpreted by the emergency physician, instead of becoming a work product for delayed interpretation by a consultant. Finally, the scope of the examination is focused, or limited, in nature. The treating physician is seeking an answer to a specific question for immediate use that will drive a clinical decision, or is utilized to guide a difficult or high-risk procedure. In this paradigm, the work product is care of the patient that is improved by the appropriate use of ultrasound technology, not the image or a report. It should be emphasized that the focused examinations performed in this paradigm meet the medical needs of the patient without providing unnecessary services.

The paradigm of consultative ultrasound imaging begins when a treating physician requests a study. The patient is usually transported to an ultrasound suite where a sonography technician images the patient. The completed study is presented, or transmitted, to an interpreting physician who documents the study results and communicates these results to the treating physician. The treating physician incorporates reported data into clinical decision making. Ultrasound guidance of emergent procedures is rarely pursued or available under this paradigm. Diagnostic studies are stored as hard copies in file rooms or in a digital format. The consulting physician's work product is an image and a report.

The paradigm of the consulting imaging service represents a complex system that involves multiple providers, movement of the patient, and several steps in a chain of communications. Delays, high costs, and the opportunity for miscommunication are inherent in this approach. For example, one must wait for a sonography technician who may be remotely located in the hospital, completing a study in progress, summoned from home, or not available for emergency studies. All this must occur before the study is obtained, interpreted, or reported for clinical use. Delays associated with this paradigm predictably negate many of the clinical benefits of ultrasound. Finally, consulting studies are usually comprehensive or complete in scope and often seemingly exceed both the treating physician's requirements and criteria for medically necessary services.

The paradigm of emergency ultrasound has been a difficult concept for traditional providers of ultrasound to understand or accept. Emergency ultrasound is not a lesser imitation of comprehensive consulting imaging services, but rather it is a focused and appropriate application of technology that provides essential diagnostic information and guidance of high-risk procedures. Unfortunately, the development of emergency ultrasound has been accompanied by a great deal of misunderstanding. Issues of physician credentialing, the ownership of technology, exclusive contracts, reimbursement, and specialty society advocacy positions have tended to overshadow clinical evidence and the practical experience of improved emergency patient care. Not only does the paradigm of emergency ultrasound offer tangible benefits in patient care, but it also represents a technology that emergency physicians will continue to utilize and refine.

CHARACTERISTICS OF EMERGENCY ULTRASOUND

Indicated emergency ultrasound studies share a common set of characteristics that reflect their clinical utility as well as the practicality of their performance in the emergency department setting. The primary indications for emergency studies address the clinical conditions of thoracoabdominal trauma, ectopic pregnancy, abdominal aortic aneurysm, pericardial effusion, determining cardiac activity, biliary disease, renal tract disease, and procedures that benefit from assistance of ultrasound (1,25). As research, technology, and experience grow, indications and standards for emergency ultrasound will evolve. Characteristics common to effective emergency ultrasound studies include the following:

1. Ultrasound examinations should be performed only for defined emergency indications that meet one or more of the following criteria:
   —A life-threatening or serious medical condition where emergency ultrasound assists in diagnosis or expedites care. An example is a patient with suspected abdominal aortic aneurysm and signs of instability.
   —A condition where an ultrasound examination significantly decreases the cost or time associated with patient evaluation. An example is locating an intrauterine pregnancy in a patient with early pregnancy and vaginal bleeding.
   —A condition in which ultrasound obviates the need for an invasive procedure. An example is echocardiography to rule out pericardial effusion that eliminates the need for pericardiocentesis in a patient with pulseless electrical activity.
   —A condition where ultrasound guidance increases patient safety for a difficult or high-risk procedure. An example is ultrasound guidance for central line placement.

—A condition in which ultrasonography is accepted as the primary diagnostic modality. An example is identifying gallstones in a patient with suspected biliary colic. Note that establishing a diagnosis may often obviate the need for additional testing or acute hospital admission.

2. Emergency physicians conduct focused, not comprehensive, examinations.

   Emergency ultrasound diagnostic studies are goal directed and designed to answer specific questions that guide clinical care. They frequently focus on the presence or absence of a single disease entity or a significant finding such as hemoperitoneum in the blunt-trauma patient. These studies are quite different than the complete examinations typically performed by consulting imaging services. Complete studies evaluate all structures and organs within an anatomic region. They are typically more expensive and time consuming as they may address issues outside of those medically necessary for patient management.

3. Emergency ultrasound studies should demonstrate one or two easily recognizable findings.

   Carefully designed indications result in simple questions, straightforward examinations, and useful answers. For example, free intraperitoneal fluid, a gestational sac, absence of a heartbeat, or the presence of pericardial fluid are all easily recognizable and have clear and immediate clinical utility.

4. Emergency ultrasounds should directly impact clinical decision making.

   Patient care algorithms should be developed for each focused ultrasound indication and the result of the study should be used to determine subsequent care. Any exam that will not reasonably be expected to change clinical decision making should be performed on an elective basis.

5. Emergency ultrasounds should be easily learned.

   Some findings, such as the presence or absence of an intrauterine pregnancy with an endovaginal transducer, are relatively easy to learn. Other evaluations such as evaluation for focal myocardial wall motion abnormalities in ischemic heart disease are more difficult to learn. A body of evidence that has been accumulated by emergency physicians identifies studies that are most reasonably learned and result in reliable clinical data (57–61).

6. Emergency physicians should conduct ultrasound studies that are relatively quick to perform.

   Emergency physicians have limited time with each patient and they generally have responsibility for the safety of many patients in the department at any given time. Ultrasound procedures selected by emergency physicians should be completed in a reasonable amount of time. Selecting focused examinations that are more quickly performed does not diminish the value of the data, intensity of the service, or the positive impact on patient care. For example, an echocardiography performed in the presence of penetrating cardiac injury may be quickly performed, yet it provides potentially life-saving information that cannot be obtained by physical examination.

7. Emergency departments should have the capacity to perform ultrasound examinations at the bedside on an immediate basis for the unstable patient and in a timely fashion for the stable patient.

   This requires that the emergency physician be prepared to conduct and interpret emergency ultrasound examinations and that equipment is available for immediate use. ACEP policy recommends that optimal patient care is provided when dedicated ultrasound equipment is located within the emergency department (1).

CORE DOCUMENTS

An understanding of emergency ultrasound includes a review of policy statements and clinical guidelines addressing the use of ultrasound. These documents should be utilized not only in formulating a program but should also be referenced in discussions with members of the medical staff and with hospital administration as well as being used to establish guidelines and standards for training, credentialing, and quality improvement.

ACEP AND SAEM POLICY STATEMENTS ON EMERGENCY ULTRASOUND

In 1991 the ACEP policy on *Ultrasound Use for Emergency Patients* stressed the clinical need for the immediate availability of diagnostic ultrasound on a 24-hour basis (22). In addition, the policy called for the training and credentialing of physicians who provide these services and encouraged research for the optimal use of emergency ultrasound. This position was endorsed by the SAEM policy in the same year (6). SAEM added language to their policy that encouraged research to determine optimal training requirements for performance of emergency ultrasound and suggested that specific training should be included during residency.

The ACEP policy was updated in 1997 and again in 2001. The most recent version of the policy, *Ultrasound Use by Emergency Physicians* (1), is a statement of current thinking within the specialty of emergency medicine (Table 1.1). This policy articulates the value of emergency ultrasound, outlines the primary diagnostic and procedural uses of ultrasound, and recognizes ultrasound as a standard emergency physician skill. In addition, it states that residents should be trained in ultrasound, emergency departments should be equipped with dedicated ultrasound equipment, and that emergency physicians should be reimbursed for the added work of ultrasound performance. Finally, the policy states that ultrasound is within the scope of practice of emergency physicians and that the hospital's medical staff should grant privileges based upon training standards developed by each physician's respective specialty.

ACEP EMERGENCY ULTRASOUND GUIDELINES

The 2001 ACEP *Emergency Ultrasound Guidelines* describes the scope of practice for emergency ultrasound as well as providing recommendations for training and proficiency, specialty-specific credentialing, quality improvement, and documentation criteria for emergency ultrasound (25). This document is comprehensive as well as being regarded as the clearest statement addressing emergency medicine's approach to diagnostic and procedural ultrasound. In addition, these guidelines articulate ultrasound standards that are broadly accepted by the specialty of emergency medicine. The *Emergency Ultrasound Guidelines* is an authoritative resource and should be referenced when formulating an ultrasound program or providing informational materials to credentials committee, hospital administration, or interested specialists.

THE CORE CONTENT AND THE MODEL OF THE CLINICAL PRACTICE OF EMERGENCY MEDICINE

In 1997 a joint policy statement was published by ACEP, the American Board of Emergency Medicine (ABEM), and SAEM titled the *Core Content for Emergency Medicine* (4). The purpose of this joint policy was to represent the breadth of the practice of emergency medicine, to outline the content of emergency medicine at risk for board examinations, and to develop graduate and continuing medical education programs for the practice of emergency medicine. Bedside ultrasonography was included in the procedure and skills section for cardiac, abdominal, traumatic, and pelvic indications.

In 2001 this document was updated and published as *The Model of the Clinical Practice of Emergency Medicine* (5). This publication includes bedside ultrasound in the list of procedures and skills integral to the practice of emergency medicine. These two documents are often used to establish core privileges for emergency physicians.

MODEL CURRICULUM FOR PHYSICIAN TRAINING IN EMERGENCY ULTRASONOGRAPHY

In 1994 the SAEM Ultrasound Task Force published the *Model Curriculum for Physician Training in Emergency Ultrasonography (Model Curriculum)* outlining resource materials as well as recommended hours of didactic and hands-on education (23). The model was

Table 1.1: Ultrasound Use by Emergency Physicians. Reprinted with permission from the American College of Emergency Physicians.

Ultrasound Use by Emergency Physicians

Ultrasound imaging enhances the physician's ability to evaluate, diagnose, and treat emergency department (ED) patients. Because ultrasound imaging is often time-dependent in the acutely ill or injured patient, the emergency physician is in an ideal position to use this technology. Focused ultrasound examinations provide immediate information and can answer specific questions about the patient's physical condition. Such bedside ultrasound imaging is within the scope of practice of emergency physicians.

Therefore, the American College of Emergency Physicians (ACEP) endorses the following principles.

- Bedside ultrasound evaluation, including examination, interpretation, and equipment, should be immediately available 24 hours a day for ED patients.
- Emergency physicians providing emergency ultrasound services should possess appropriate training and hands-on experience to perform and interpret limited bedside ultrasound imaging.
- The use of ultrasound imaging by emergency physicians is appropriate in clinical situations that include, but are not limited to: thoracoabdominal trauma, ectopic pregnancy, abdominal aortic aneurysm, pericardial effusion, determining cardiac activity, biliary disease, renal tract disease, and procedures that would benefit from assistance of ultrasound.
- Emergency ultrasound procedures and interpretations are standard emergency physician skills that should be delineated in emergency physician privileges.
- Dedicated ultrasound equipment within the ED should be considered optimal for patient care.
- Each hospital medical staff should review and approve criteria for granting ultrasound privileges based on background and training for the use of ultrasound technology and ensure that these criteria are in accordance with recommended training and education standards developed by each physician's respective specialty.
- Training in performing and interpreting ultrasound imaging studies should be included in emergency medicine residency curricula.
- Continued research in the area of ultrasound should be encouraged.
- Emergency physicians should be appropriately reimbursed for providing emergency ultrasound procedures in the ED.

This policy statement was prepared by the Emergency Medicine Practice Committee. It was approved by the ACEP Board of Directors June 2001. It replaces one by the same title approved by the ACEP Board of Directors June 1997. The original policy statement titled "Use of Ultrasound for Emergency Department Patients" was approved by the ACEP Board of Directors January 1991.

constructed primarily for residents in training; however, it did address the practicing emergency physician by stating that instruction, covering topics that follow the task force outline, and a total of 150 examinations would constitute training in emergency medicine ultrasonography. The *Model Curriculum* was comprehensive and has proven invaluable in guiding the development of residency training programs as well as the initial training and continuing education for the practicing emergency physician.

THE AMERICAN MEDICAL ASSOCIATION APPROACH TO ULTRASOUND PRIVILEGING

The American Medical Association (AMA) developed policy in 1999 on *Privileging for Ultrasound Imaging* (62). This policy recognizes the diverse uses of ultrasound imaging in the practice of medicine. Furthermore, the AMA recommended that training and educational standards be developed by each physician's respective specialty and that those standards should serve as the basis for hospital privileging. The AMA policy is in full agreement with

ACEP policy and affirms the use of ultrasound by a variety of physician specialties rather than restricting ownership of the technology of ultrasound.

While the AMA and ACEP's approach may seem rational, experience in hospital credentialing has demonstrated opposition to the concept of individual specialties developing training and education standards for their use of ultrasound. Providers of consultative ultrasound services, most notably radiology and cardiology, have been quite active in developing policy that recommends training standards for practitioners outside their own specialties and these publications have been used in debates regarding hospital credentialing as well as third-party reimbursement (63–65).

ADDITIONAL POSITIONS: AMERICAN COLLEGE OF RADIOLOGY, AMERICAN SOCIETY OF ECHOCARDIOGRAPHY, AND AMERICAN INSTITUTE OF ULTRASOUND IN MEDICINE

Policy statements regarding physician qualifications and ultrasound training standards have been published by other organizations such as the American College of Radiology (ACR), the American Society of Echocardiography (ASE), and the American Institute of Ultrasound Medicine (AIUM). These policies differ substantially from those adopted by the specialty of emergency medicine. In discussions regarding ultrasound, the emergency physician should be prepared to address these advocacy positions, as they may be cited as published, and authoritative standards that apply to all practitioners using ultrasound.

The *ACR Standard for Performing and Interpreting Diagnostic Ultrasound Examinations* requires that physicians who have not completed a radiology residency must have interpreted and reported 500 supervised ultrasound examinations during the previous 36 months and within the subspecialty they practice (63). The ASE position, *Echocardiography in Emergency Medicine: A Policy Statement by the American Society of Echocardiography and the American College of Cardiology*, directly addresses the SAEM Model Curriculum as being inadequate (65). Under this policy the highest level of competence achievable by an emergency physician is termed an "echocardiographic laboratory extender." Requirements for this status would include 3 months of training and 150 supervised examinations. Even with this training, emergency physicians could use echocardiography for clinical decision making only in "unusual circumstances and for life-threatening conditions." As well, all of these emergency examinations would require an over-read by a cardiology "competent reader," such as an echocardiography panel member.

A third policy is the AIUM *Training Guidelines for Physicians Who Evaluate and Interpret Diagnostic Ultrasound Examinations* (66). The AIUM differs from the ACR and ASE in that it is a multidisciplinary organization, rather than a specialty society, and includes various physician specialties, sonographers, scientists, engineers, and equipment manufacturers. The AIUM training standards require either completion of a residency that includes 3 months of ultrasound training plus 300 supervised examinations, or 100 hours of continuing medical education dedicated to ultrasound plus 300 supervised examinations. This training would apply to only a single subspecialty area and if more than one subspecialty area was contemplated, such as heart and abdomen, then 500 supervised examinations would be required.

These policies have several themes in common. They are all designed with the assumption that physicians will be interpreting comprehensive studies and as such, the focused ultrasound examinations utilized by emergency physicians have not been contemplated. In addition, the numbers of studies these policies require far exceed training standards accepted, and recently affirmed, by emergency medicine authorities including ABEM, ACEP, SAEM, the Council of Emergency Medicine Residency Directors (CORD) and the Residency Review Committee for Emergency Medicine (RRC-EM) (67). While specific numbers of studies for each of the emergency indications have not been established, available data do support the emergency medicine approach to focused examination education (57–61). Finally, these policies are not in agreement with ACEP and AMA recommendations that hospital privileging be determined in accordance with the recommended training and education standards developed by each physician's respective specialty (1,62).

AN EVOLVING STANDARD OF CARE

A frequently asked question is, "What is the standard of care for ultrasound?" Is the standard of care the study performed by a consultative imaging service or is it the immediate use of ultrasound at the bedside for indications demonstrated to improve patient outcomes? How does a standard of care relate to a "best practice"? Would the failure of an emergency physician to utilize ultrasound constitute substandard care?

The simplest definition of a standard of care is how a similarly qualified practitioner would manage a patient's care under the same or similar circumstances. Standards are based in peer-reviewed literature and in consensus opinion regarding clinical judgment. They are national in scope rather than based on community norms and are tested in a court of law where they are generally established by expert witness testimony.

A best practice is a technique that through experience and research has proven to reliably lead to a desired outcome. A best practice is based in evidence and represents a commitment to using all the knowledge and technology at one's disposal to ensure improved patient care. As best practices become more broadly adopted, they eventually become recognized as standards of care. Substantial peer-reviewed evidence has demonstrated that emergency physician–performed ultrasound is reliable for each of the primary indications of emergency ultrasound and would therefore be regarded by the specialty of emergency medicine as best practices.

Central venous catheter placement facilitated by ultrasound is an interesting example. Ultrasound guidance has been found to reduce the number of needle passes, the time to catheter placement, and to decrease the complication rate for central venous access (10,11). Peer-reviewed literature has demonstrated the effectiveness of this technique in the emergency department where the treatment of critically ill and injured patients often requires immediate central vascular access (44–46). The Agency for Healthcare Research and Quality report *Making Health Care Safer: A Critical Analysis of Patient Safety Practices* cited the use of real-time ultrasound guidance during central line insertion to reduce complications as "one of the most highly rated patient safety practices based upon potential impact of the practice and the strength of supporting evidence (10)." This is a best practice that has been adopted by a growing number of emergency physicians and it represents an evolving standard of care.

CONCLUSION

Improvements in technology have allowed the movement of ultrasound from the imaging laboratory to the patient's bedside. Technology enhancements have been accompanied by an evidence-based recognition of the value of immediate ultrasound in a variety of clinical conditions encountered in the emergency department. The demonstrated value of emergency ultrasound has led to endorsement by emergency medicine professional organizations, inclusion into emergency medicine residency training, and integration into clinical practice. The focused use of emergency ultrasound and the characteristics of these examinations have been well described, yet they are frequently misunderstood, mischaracterized, or undervalued, and clinical issues have often been confused with hospital politics and physician economics. In this context an understanding of a variety of policy statements by emergency medicine professional societies and by other professional societies is helpful in discussions surrounding the use of ultrasound by emergency physicians. Most importantly, the use of ultrasound by the treating emergency physician represents an advance in the care of emergency patients, an appropriate use of technology, a clinical best practice, and an evolving standard of care.

REFERENCES

1. American College of Emergency Physicians. Use of ultrasound imaging by emergency physicians [policy #40121]. Ann Emerg Med 2001;38:469–470.
2. Moore CL, Gregg S, Lambert M. Performance, training, quality assurance, and reimbursement of emergency physician-performed ultrasonography at academic medical centers. J Ultrasound Med 2004;23:459–466.
3. The Accreditation Council for Graduate Medical Education (ACGME); Emergency Medicine Residency Review Committee; Program Requirements; Guidelines; Procedures and Resuscitations; Bedside ultrasound. 2002. Available at: http://www.acgme.org. Accessed Nov. 3, 2004.
4. Allison EJ Jr, Aghababian RV, Barsan WG, et al. Core content for emergency medicine. Task Force on the Core Content for Emergency Medicine Revision. Ann Emerg Med 1997;29: 792–811.
5. Hockberger RS, Binder LS, Graber MA, et al. The model of the clinical practice of emergency medicine. Ann Emerg Med 2001;37:745–770.
6. SAEM Ultrasound Position Statement, 1991. Society for Academic Emergency Medicine Web site. Available at: http://www.saem.org/publicat/ultrasou.htm. Accessed Nov. 3, 2004.
7. Shih CH. Effect of emergency physician-performed pelvic sonography on length of stay in the emergency department. Ann Emerg Med 1997; 29:348–351.
8. Blaivas M, Harwood RA, Lambert MJ. Decreasing length of stay with emergency ultrasound examination of the gallbladder. Acad Emerg Med 1999; 6:1020–1023.
9. Theodoro D, Blaivas M, Duggal S, et al. Real-time B-mode ultrasound in the ED saves time in the diagnosis of deep vein thrombosis (DVT). Am J Emerg Med 2004;22:197–200.
10. Agency for Healthcare Research and Quality. Ultrasound guidance of central vein catheterization. In: Making health care safer: a critical analysis of patient safety practices; Chapter 21. Available at: http://www.ahcpr.gov/clinic/ptsftinv/chap21.htm. Accessed Nov. 3, 2004.
11. Hind D, Calvert N, McWilliams R, et al. Ultrasonic locating devices for central venous cannulation: meta-analysis. BMJ 2003;327:361.
12. Plummer D, Brunette D, Asinger R, et al. Emergency department echocardiography improves outcome in penetrating cardiac injury. Ann Emerg Med 1992;21:709–712.
13. Goldberg BB, Goodman GA, Clearfield HR. Evaluation of ascites by ultrasound. Radiology 1970;96:15–22.
14. Kristensen JK, Buemann B, Kuhl E. Ultrasonic scanning in the diagnosis of splenic haematomas. Acta Chir Scand 1971;137:653–657.
15. Asher WM, Parvin S, Virgillo RW, et al. Echographic evaluation of splenic injury after blunt trauma. Radiology 1976;118:411–415.
16. Mayron R, Gaudio FE, Plummer D, et al. Echocardiography performed by emergency physicians: impact on diagnosis and therapy. Ann Emerg Med 1988;17:150–154.
17. Tiling T, Bouillon B, Schmid A, et al. Ultrasound in Blunt Abdominothoracic Trauma. In: Border J, Algoewer M, Reudi T, eds. Blunt Multiple Trauma. New York:Marcel Dekker Inc, 1990:415–433.
18. Tso P, Rodriguez A, Cooper C, et al. Sonography in blunt abdominal trauma: a preliminary progress report. J Trauma 1992;33:39–43.
19. Rozycki GS, Ochsner MG, Jaffin JH, et al. Prospective evaluation of surgeons' use of ultrasound in the evaluation of trauma patients. J Trauma 1993; 34:516–526.
20. Ma OJ, Mateer JR, Ogata M, et al. Prospective analysis of a rapid trauma ultrasound examination performed by emergency physicians. J Trauma 1995; 38:879–885.
21. McKenney MG, Martin L, Lentz K, et al. 1,000 consecutive ultrasounds for blunt abdominal trauma. J Trauma 1996; 40:607–610.
22. ACEP Policy Statement. Use of Ultrasound for Emergency Department Patients. June 1991. Updated 1997 and 2001 as: Use of ultrasound imaging by emergency physicians. American College of Emergency Physicians Web site. Available at: http://www.acep.org/1,684,0.html. Accessed Nov. 3, 2004.
23. Mateer J, Plummer D, Heller M, et al. Model curriculum for physician training in emergency ultrasonography. Ann Emerg Med 1994;23:95–102.

24. Heller M, Jehle D, eds. Ultrasound in Emergency Medicine. 1st Ed. Philadelphia: WB Saunders, 1995.

25. ACEP Policy Statement. ACEP emergency ultrasound guidelines. 2001. American College of Emergency Physicians Web site. Available at: http://www.acep.org/library/pdf/ultrasound_guidelines.pdf. Accessed Nov. 3, 2004.

26. Kuhn M, Bonnin RL, Davey MJ, et al. Emergency department ultrasound scanning for abdominal aortic aneurysm: accessible, accurate, and advantageous. Ann Emerg Med 2000;36:219–223.

27. Knaut AL, Kendall JL, Dobbins J, et al. Ultrasonographic measurement of abdominal aortic diameter by emergency physicians approximates results obtained by computed tomography [abstract]. Acad Emerg Med 2000;7:493.

28. Tayal VS, Graf CD, Gibbs MA. Prospective study of accuracy and outcome of emergency ultrasound for abdominal aortic aneurysm over two years. Acad Emerg Med 2003;10:867–871.

29. Mateer JR, Aiman EJ, Brown MH, et al. Ultrasonographic examination by emergency physicians of patients at risk for ectopic pregnancy. Acad Emerg Med 1995;2:867–873.

30. Durham B, Lane B, Burbridge L, et al. Pelvic ultrasound performed by emergency physicians for the detection of ectopic pregnancy in complicated first-trimester pregnancies. Ann Emerg Med 1997;29:338–347.

31. Burgher SW, Tandy TK, Dawdy MR. Transvaginal ultrasonography by emergency physicians decreases patient time in the emergency department. Acad Emerg Med 1998;5:802–807.

32. Dart RG. Role of pelvic ultrasonography in evaluation of symptomatic first-trimester pregnancy. Ann Emerg Med 1999;33:310–320.

33. Tayal VS, Beatty MA, Marx JA, et al. FAST (focused assessment with sonography in trauma) accurate for cardiac and intraperitoneal injury in penetrating anterior chest trauma. J Ultrasound Med 2004;23:467–472.

34. Mandavia DP, Hoffner RJ, Mahaney K, et al. Bedside echocardiography by emergency physicians. Ann Emerg Med 2001;38:377–382.

35. Tayal VS, Kline JA. Emergency echocardiography to detect pericardial effusion in patients in PEA and near-PEA states. Resuscitation 2003;59:315–318.

36. Blaivas M, Fox J. Outcome in cardiac arrest patients found to have cardiac standstill on the bedside emergency department echocardiogram. Acad Emerg Med 2001;8:616–621.

37. Salen P, O'Connor R, Sierzenski P, et al. Can cardiac sonography and capnography be used independently and in combination to predict resuscitation outcomes? Acad Emerg Med 2001;8:610–615.

38. Moore CL, Rose GA, Tayal VS, et al. Determination of left ventricular function by emergency physician echocardiography of hypotensive patients. Acad Emerg Med 2002;9:186–193.

39. Rosen CL, Brown DF, Chang Y, et al. Ultrasonography by emergency physicians in patients with suspected cholecystitis. Am J Emerg Med 2001;19:32–36.

40. Kendall JL, Shimp RJ. Performance and interpretation of focused right upper quadrant ultrasound by emergency physicians. J Emerg Med 2001;21:7–13.

41. Durston W, Carl ML, Guerra W, et al. Comparison of quality and cost-effectiveness in the evaluation of symptomatic cholelithiasis with different approaches to ultrasound availability in the ED. Am J Emerg Med 2001;19:260–269.

42. Henderson SO, Hoffner RJ, Aragona JL, et al. Bedside emergency department ultrasonsography plus radiography of the kidneys, ureters, and bladder vs intravenous pyelography in the evaluation of suspected ureteral colic. Acad Emerg Med 1998;5:666–671.

43. Rosen CL, Brown DF, Sagarin MJ, et al. Ultrasonography by emergency physicians in patients with suspected ureteral colic. J Emerg Med 1998;16:865–870.

44. Hilty WM, Hudson PA, Levitt MA, et al. Real-time ultrasound-guided femoral vein catheterization during cardiopulmonary resuscitation. Ann Emerg Med 1997; 29:331–336; discussion 337.

45. Hudson PA, Rose JS. Real-time ultrasound guided internal jugular vein catheterization in the emergency department. Am J Emerg Med 1997;15:79–82.

46. Miller AH, Roth BA, Mills TJ, et al. Ultrasound guidance versus the landmark technique for the placement of central venous catheters in the emergency department. Acad Emerg Med 2002;9:800–805.

47. Rose JS, Bair AE, Mandavia D, et al. The UHP ultrasound protocol: a novel ultrasound approach to the empiric evaluation of the undifferentiated hypotensive patient. Am J Emerg Med. 2001;19:299–302.

48. Jones AE, Tayal VS, Sullivan DM, et al. Randomized, controlled trial of immediate versus delayed goal-directed ultrasound to identify the cause of nontraumatic hypotension in emergency department patients. Crit Care Med 2004;32:1703–1708.

49. Blaivas M, Lambert MJ, Harwood RA, et al. Lower-extremity Doppler for deep venous thrombosis—can emergency physicians be accurate and fast? Acad Emerg Med 2000;7:120–126.

50. Valley VT, Stahmer SA. Targeted musculoarticular sonography in the detection of joint effusions. Acad Emerg Med 2001;8:361–367.

51. Blaivas M, Theodoro D, Sierzenski PR. A study of bedside ocular ultrasonography in the emergency department. Acad Emerg Med 2002;9:791–799.

52. Blaivas M, Theodoro D, Duggal S. Ultrasound-guided drainage of peritonsillar abscess by the emergency physician. Am J Emerg Med 2003;21:155–158.

53. Blaivas M, Sierzenski P, Lambert M. Emergency evaluation of patients presenting with acute scrotum using bedside ultrasonography. Acad Emerg Med 2001;8:90–93.

54. Branney SW, Moore EE, Cantrill SV, et al. Ultrasound based key clinical pathway reduces the use of hospital resources for the evaluation of blunt abdominal trauma. J Trauma 1997;42:1086–1090.

55. Frezza EE, Ferone T, Martin M. Surgical residents and ultrasound technician accuracy and cost-effectiveness of ultrasound in trauma. Am Surg 1999;65:289–291.

56. Durston WE, Carl ML, Guerra W, et al. Ultrasound availability in the evaluation of ectopic pregnancy in the ED: comparison of quality and cost-effectiveness with different approaches. Am J Emerg Med 2000;18:408–417.

57. Lanoix R, Baker WE, Mele JM, et al. Evaluation of an instructional model for emergency ultrasonography. Acad Emerg Med 1998;5:58–63.

58. Mandavia DP, Aragona J, Chan L, et al. Ultrasound training for emergency physicians—a prospective study. Acad Emerg Med 2000;7:1008–1014.

59. Jones AE, Tayal VS, Kline JA. Focused training of emergency medicine residents in goal-directed echocardiography: a prospective study. Acad Emerg Med 2003;10:1054–1058.

60. Smith RS, Kern SJ, Fry WR, et al. Institutional learning curve of surgeon-performed trauma ultrasound. Arch Surg 1998;133:530–535; discussion 535–536.

61. McCarter FD, Luchette FA, Molloy M, et al. Institutional and individual learning curves for focused abdominal ultrasound for trauma: cumulative sum analysis. Ann Surg 2000;231:689–700.

62. American Medical Association House of Delegates. H-230.960 Privileging for Ultrasound Imaging. American Medical Association Web site. Available at: http://www.ama-assn.org/apps/pf_new/pf_online?f_n=browse&doc=policyfiles/HnE/H-230.960.HTM. Accessed Nov. 3, 2004.

63. American College of Radiology. ACR practice guideline for performing and interpreting diagnostic ultrasound examinations. 2001. American College of Radiology Web site. Available at: http://www.acr.org/s_acr/bin.asp?TrackID=&SID=1&DID=12267&CID=539&VID=2&DOC=File.PDF. Accessed Nov. 3, 2004.

64. Quinones MA, Douglas PS, Foster E, et al. ACC/AHA clinical competence statement on echocardiography: a report of the American College of Cardiology/American Heart Association/American College of Physicians-American Society of Internal Medicine Task Force on Clinical Competence. J Am Coll Cardiol 2003;41:687–708.

65. Stewart WJ, Douglas PS, Sagar K, et al. Echocardiography in emergency medicine: a policy statement by the American Society of Echocardiography and the American College of Cardiology. Task Force on Echocardiography in Emergency Medicine of the American Society of Echocardiography and the Echocardiography and Technology and Practice Executive Committees of the American College of Cardiology. J Am Coll Cardiol 1999;33:586–588.

66. American Institute of Ultrasound in Medicine. Training guidelines for physicians who evaluate and interpret diagnostic ultrasound examinations. 2000. American Institute of Ultrasound Medicine Web site. Available at: http://www.aium.org/accreditation/practice/eight.asp. Accessed Nov. 3, 2004.

67. Heller MB, Mandavia D, Tayal VS, et al. Residency training in emergency ultrasound: fulfilling the mandate. Acad Emerg Med 2002;9:835–839.

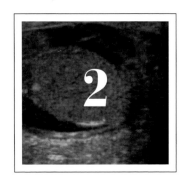

EMERGENCY ULTRASOUND PROGRAM DEVELOPMENT

Stephen R. Hoffenberg

PROGRAM DEVELOPMENT

Starting an ultrasound program is both a clinical and administrative challenge. It begins with the determination that ultrasound will improve the care of your patients, that you have physician support within your group for a single standard of care that incorporates emergency ultrasound, and that adding clinician-performed ultrasound is achievable in the political environment of your hospital. The decision has become easier as emergency ultrasound has evolved from an investigational technique to an evidence-based best practice and ultrasound education has become a required element of emergency medicine training (1).

There are a number of tasks that must be addressed when starting an ultrasound program, such as identifying a program leader and entering into discussions with other departments and hospital administration. The staff must be trained in the clinical techniques and decision-making processes specific to the use of ultrasound. The group must also develop credentialing criteria, establish a quality assurance program, select equipment, and devise a compliant approach to reimbursement (2–4).

LEADERSHIP

A consistent indicator for success in ultrasound implementation is a dedicated ultrasound program leader. The role of this leader is to explore the medical literature, to define the scope of the program, and to identify needed resources. In addition to developing documents and addressing program design and credentialing, the leader must also serve as a liaison with medical staff regarding emergency ultrasound. Probably the most important task of an ultrasound program leader is overseeing the quality of emergency ultrasounds. Successful programs have dedicated leadership that sustains the effort required to implement bedside ultrasound.

RELATIONS WITH OTHER SPECIALTIES AND DEPARTMENTS

Emergency ultrasound has been welcomed by many members of the medical staff as the addition of a clinically useful technology. The effort to create an emergency ultrasound program has been understood by those specialties that have similarly added clinician-performed ultrasound. Obstetrician-gynecologists routinely utilize ultrasound on the labor deck, as do many family practitioners. Critical care physicians and trauma surgeons have progressively adopted diagnostic ultrasound as well as procedure guidance with ultrasound (5–8). Vascular surgeons, urologists, perinatologists, and retina surgeons, among others, have found advantage in adding ultrasound to their practices. These specialists are often supportive of the use of ultrasound by emergency physicians. This is particularly true when the emergency department has communicated the current status of emergency ultrasound education and research and has explained how ultrasound will be introduced, used, and monitored. Finally, when medical staff politics are an issue, it is advisable to seek input and to develop support from those members of the medical staff and departments that are most likely to understand and endorse the addition of emergency ultrasound.

Radiology and cardiology represent traditional providers of consultative ultrasound services. While individual radiologists or cardiologists may be supportive of emergency ultrasound, both specialties have organized themselves to resist the credentialing of emergency practitioner ultrasound. These specialties have rejected the training standards developed by emergency medicine and the concept that training standards should be developed by a physician's specialty or used as a basis for hospital credentialing. Both groups have adopted the position that standards developed by their own specialty organizations should apply to all practitioners of ultrasound and they seek to regulate physicians outside of their own specialties. The standards they promote are often not appropriate to the paradigm of emergency ultrasound and cannot reasonably be achieved by emergency physicians. They address standards for comprehensive examinations, rather than for focused studies, and are designed for practitioners primarily engaged in referral imaging rather than for those who would use ultrasound in the direct care of their patients (9–11).

Cardiology adopted the use of ultrasound technology early and established the value of echocardiography, whereas radiologists have not traditionally performed this service. Cardiologists have pursued a consultative laboratory model for cardiac ultrasound but, interestingly, the development of compact and highly portable ultrasound devices has changed the perspective of many cardiologists. It has become clear that portable echocardiography devices are more accurate than physical examination in the detection of pericardial effusion, valvular lesions, and depressed myocardial contractility (12–15). An increasing number of cardiologists are utilizing compact ultrasound devices, and some are adopting a new attitude toward the utility of bedside ultrasound. Unfortunately, the training standards and policies published by the American College of Cardiology (ACC) and the American Society of Echocardiography (ASE) exclude emergency physicians from being eligible to independently perform or interpret emergency echocardiography (10,11). These policies rely primarily on expert opinion and seemingly overlook evidence regarding the efficacy of echocardiography performed by emergency physicians (16–22).

In practice, few emergency physicians have experienced resistance from staff cardiologists regarding the evaluation of patients by echocardiography for pericardial fluid, cardiac activity, or unexplained hypotension. When medical staff cardiologists are presented with the focused objectives of emergency echocardiography, the positive impact on patient care is often appreciated and supported.

Relationships with the specialty of radiology have remained the most difficult for developing emergency ultrasound programs. While at some institutions emergency ultrasound has been supported by radiologists interested in patient access to care or radiologists who may recognize the role of focused applications, such situations remain the exception rather than the rule. Radiologists are the largest providers of consultative ultrasound services. They have developed the paradigm for consultative services and have a vested interest in the control of ultrasound imaging. They have argued that the quality of studies, qualifications of providers, and the paradigm of emergency ultrasound do not meet standards established by their specialty. Often there is a lack of understanding as to what emergency ultrasound is and what is needed for the management of an emergency patient or an emergency department. Furthermore, radiologists routinely promote their right to provide services on an exclusive basis but often restrict services to certain times of day, days of the week, or type of examination (23). As with cardiology, the value of focused studies has not been recognized by radiology leadership, and published standards address physician qualifications to interpret comprehensive consultative studies (9).

When implementing an emergency ultrasound program, the emergency physician should be direct and open with the department of radiology. Keep in mind that a consensus may never be reached with radiology and while open discussion is positive, endless discussion will not improve patient care. Your goal should be to educate the medical staff and hospital administration as to the proven value of immediate ultrasound that includes enhanced patient throughput, decreased medical risk, and improved outcomes. In an era of emergency department overcrowding, limited radiology resources, an adverse medical-legal environment, and concerns regarding patient safety, ultrasound is a technology offering advantages that cannot be ignored in deference to the interests of other specialties.

RELATIONS WITH HOSPITAL ADMINISTRATION

Hospital administration has several goals surrounding emergency ultrasound. Its central goal is to offer the highest quality of care to emergency patients. Additional goals include improving patient satisfaction, enhancing patient safety, and decreasing the costs of providing medical care. At the same time, administration wants to preserve needed revenues and maintain collegial relationships between departments. When proposing an emergency medicine ultrasound program, all of these issues should be discussed with hospital administration.

Patient satisfaction has been correlated with emergency department throughput times and increased throughput has been demonstrated to improve with the addition of emergency ultrasound (24,25). Patient safety has been enhanced (26,27) and the cost of providing emergency ultrasound is less than the cost of a consulting imaging service (28–31). Most savings are realized in decreased personnel costs, particularly for sonographer "on-call" expenses during nights and weekends (29–31). Additional benefits may accrue in instances when sonographers are unavailable or object to providing 24-hour coverage 7 days a week. The impact of emergency ultrasound on hospital revenues is complex and will vary based on the total number of studies performed, the mix of complete versus limited studies billed by the hospital, and the emergency department patient financial mix. Finally, find out when capital budget item requests should be submitted, as securing funding for equipment in the middle of a budget year is often difficult for hospital administration. A well prepared "white paper" outlining supporting documents and including credentialing standards, quality improvement plans, equipment requirements, and a full explanation of the advantages of immediate ultrasound will be of great help to administration.

PHYSICIAN TRAINING

The majority of emergency medicine residents are being taught ultrasound and will meet emergency medicine training standards by completion of their training. Residency-trained physicians should be granted emergency ultrasound privileges when joining a medical staff that recognizes emergency ultrasound privileges (2). In many instances these privileges will simply be a part of emergency medicine core privileges. In other instances, additional evidence of competency may be required, such as confirmation by the physician's residency director of a sufficient number of cases with demonstrated quality. Candidates for recruitment who have been trained in ultrasound often view the use of ultrasound by a practice as an indicator of quality.

Most practicing emergency physicians did not receive ultrasound training during residency. Others were in training when ultrasound was being introduced and have had exposure without sufficient structured education to meet emergency ultrasound training guidelines. This situation is not unusual, as physicians practicing in all specialties add new skills on an ongoing basis. Emergency physicians trained prior to the incorporation of ultrasound must acquire necessary training through continuing medical education in order to maintain a quality practice and meet evolving standards of care.

The best choice for training depends on the goals of the practitioner or the goals of the practice. Is this an individual wanting to explore the utility of ultrasound on behalf of his or her group, or is this a practitioner wanting to enhance specific skills, such as ultrasound-guided procedures? Is this an individual wanting special expertise in order to administer an ultrasound program? Or, is this a practice that has made the decision to train the entire group for the incorporation of bedside ultrasound? Each of these educational goals requires a different approach.

For those exploring the utility of ultrasound on behalf of their practice, or for those seeking a specific skill, national or regional educational meetings are the best options. Such meetings are frequently sponsored by professional emergency medicine societies or academic emergency medicine programs. These meetings may incorporate ultrasound education within their curriculum, offer dedicated ultrasound educational programs, or present "add on" courses associated with other educational forums. National meetings are less practical for group practices wanting to add ultrasound because it is difficult to send an entire group to a national meeting without staggering the education over months or years and at great expense.

Groups that have decided to pursue ultrasound as a practice standard are often best served by bringing a course to their location. A number of commercial courses are available and are taught by emergency physicians or by a combination of emergency physicians and sonographers. These courses should be specific to emergency medicine, cover the primary emergency indications, and meet the didactic and cognitive requirements for initial training as published in the *Emergency Ultrasound Guidelines* (2). They are generally two days in length and provide 16 hours of category-I credit for continuing medical education. The advantage of these courses is that they travel to the practice location, are minimally disruptive to clinical scheduling, simultaneously educate a maximum number of practitioners, and minimize costs to the practice.

Many introductory ultrasound courses offer information on the administrative aspects of an ultrasound practice. This includes credentialing, quality control, documentation, professional relationships, and reimbursement. The ultrasound section of the American College of Emergency Physicians (ACEP) is a reliable resource for current information on these administrative subjects. Finally, those with a special interest in emergency ultrasound including research, specialized applications, the education of residents, or advanced program administration may explore one of the emergency ultrasound fellowships.

CREDENTIALING

Physician credentialing and privileging are responsibilities of the hospital board and are undertaken with recommendations from the medical staff. "Credentialing" refers to application for medical staff membership, whereas "privileging" refers to the delineation of specific clinical procedures allowed by the practitioner. Physician privileges have historically been requested as a list of individual procedures and practitioners have documented the numbers of each procedure they have performed. More recently core privilege sets have been requested and granted in blocks that include the skills basic to the physician's specialty, and privileging has been accomplished without the burden of cataloging numbers for each routine procedure. Specialized procedures may be separately privileged in addition to core privileges and are those felt to require added evidence of competency, such as advanced training or the tracking of activity levels.

Bedside ultrasound is now viewed as a core skill of emergency practice and may not require separate privileging if documents such as the *Core Content for Emergency Medicine* (32) or *The Model of the Clinical Practice of Emergency Medicine* (33) are referenced as the basis for core privileges. However, because there are many emergency physicians trained prior to the teaching of this skill, emergency ultrasound will often be viewed as a privilege that is separately granted and one requiring additional documentation.

The process of establishing new clinical privileges begins with the organization and review of information relevant to the procedure within a department and compliance with any hospital policies addressing how new privileges are granted. Recommendations of the department are forwarded to the credentials committee. The credentials committee is generally experienced in evaluating criteria for privileging and has often dealt with multiple specialties performing similar procedures. Examples include family practitioners performing deliveries or cardiologists seeking privileges for angioplasty outside of the heart. Most meaningful debate will occur at this level; it frequently involves input from a broad range of practitioners, and should be a main focus of your organizational efforts. The recommendations of the credentials committee are generally accepted by the medical executive committee and they are then forwarded to the hospital board where approval can be anticipated.

Currently accepted criteria for emergency ultrasound credentialing are outlined in the *Emergency Ultrasound Guidelines* (2) and they should be presented as standards developed and endorsed by the specialty of emergency medicine. The *Emergency Ultrasound Guidelines* describe two generally accepted pathways for credentialing. The first is by residency training in emergency ultrasound with verification of satisfactory performance by the graduate's residency director. The second path entails completion of an introductory course in emergency ultrasound that is compliant with the ACEP training guidelines followed by a provisional period of performing training examinations. During the provisional period, 100% of the studies should be reviewed. Training examinations continue until 25–50 studies of satisfactory quality are recorded for each of the primary indications, or until 150 total studies are completed. Up to one-half of the training examinations may occur in the midst of a training course, or they may be nonclinical examinations of volunteers. At least half of these training examinations should be clinically indicated and include some percentage of abnormal findings. Confirmation of each study should be obtained whenever possible and may include direct supervision, an over-read of studies, confirmatory data such as a consultative ultrasound, computed tomography (CT), surgery, or clinical outcome. Following satisfactory completion of training examinations during the provisional period, full privileging should be granted.

Most examination results are not used for clinical decision making during the provisional period. It should be noted that this approach is not always possible and clearly normal or clearly abnormal findings in the context of the clinician's judgment may drive patient-care decisions. For example, when used during penetrating cardiac trauma, the clear delineation of pericardial fluid in a hypotensive patient should prompt immediate surgical intervention rather than a confirmatory imaging study.

Keep several things in mind surrounding credentialing discussions. First, privileges for ultrasound are not granted by radiology or cardiology, rather they are granted by the hospital board and should be based upon the best interests of patient care. Furthermore, immediate ultrasound performed by the treating physician is not a poor substitute for consultative imaging as it may be portrayed. It represents an evidence-based advance in patient care that has been adopted by multiple physician specialties in a variety of clinical settings. Second, the credentials committee will often be faced with discussion surrounding the conflicting policy statements of multiple specialty societies. You should be familiar with the relevant policies of ACEP, the Society for Academic Emergency Medicine (SAEM), the American Board of Emergency Medicine (ABEM) and the American Medical Association (AMA), as well as policies of the American College of Radiology (ACR), the American College of Cardiology (ACC), the American Society of Echocardiography (ASE), and the American Institute of Ultrasound in Medicine (AIUM) (9–11,32–37). Be prepared to discuss these policies in the context of quality, risk management, patient safety, access to care, the paradigm of emergency ultrasound, and the current medical literature. It is advised that you recommend the ACEP and AMA principle that training and education standards should be developed by each physician's respective specialty and those standards should serve as the basis for hospital privileging.

Finally, the issue of exclusive contracts is often brought into credentialing discussions. Exclusive contracts are put into place when they improve patient care, assure access to care through needed physician coverage, and are approved by the hospital board. Exclusive contracts are most appropriate in the context of managing consultative and referral services and are less appropriate when applied to medically indicated and immediate services provided by a treating physician. Exclusive contracts should not be used as an argument that results in limiting patient access to needed services, hindering quality improvements within other specialties, or controlling necessary patient care services for economic gain.

Quality Assurance

Implementing an emergency ultrasound program is a major quality improvement effort and may be one of the more significant long-term contributions to patient care within the emergency department. A well-considered quality program will contribute to gaining the support of your medical staff and hospital administration in addition to monitoring ultrasound quality. There are two aspects of an emergency ultrasound quality program. The first addresses the basic competencies surrounding ultrasound techniques and involves initial education, performance of training studies, and documentation of examinations. This component is closely related to credentialing, the exercise of provisional privileges, and demonstrating quality for advancement to full ultrasound privileges (2). The second component addresses utilizing ultrasound competencies to achieve defined quality objectives in patient care or quality improvement.

In developing a quality program you should begin by outlining long-term quality objectives as well as identifying specific opportunities to improve patient care. Several aspects of care that can be improved through the application of immediate ultrasound include the timeliness of care, the optimal diagnostic management of specific disease states, enhanced patient safety, and the appropriateness of therapeutic interventions. Corresponding opportunities to improve on these aspects of care might include decreasing delays that accompany the diagnosis of ectopic pregnancy, the accurate and early diagnosing of aortic aneurysm, decreasing complication rates of central venous access, and limiting unnecessary pericardiocentesis performed during cardiac resuscitation. Each of these goals is relevant to your practice and represents an opportunity to evaluate the effectiveness of your ultrasound program. To evaluate basic ultrasound skills, each practice should develop indicators of performance that includes parameters such as adherence to predefined indications for ultrasound studies, documentation of studies in the chart or in a quality log, accuracy of interpretation based on comparative data, and the technical quality of the study. Often a scoring system is used that assigns each indicator a range of points. When scores are placed into a database, performance can be analyzed by individual indicators or in aggregate by the type of study, practitioner, or physician group. Data can be used to guide education or for credentialing purposes, and trends can easily be demonstrated with this type of quantifiable data.

During program startup, quality review for both individuals and the group should be conducted on 100% of studies. Once the quality committee determines that appropriate quality has been achieved, the review process may shift from a 100% review phase to an ongoing quality assurance phase. The ongoing phase should be similar to most other quality assessment processes in the emergency department and may include periodic focused reviews, a sampling methodology, and the review of adverse outcomes.

One of the practical problems facing a startup program is determining who should review these emergency studies. Most programs develop a subcommittee of the department's quality committee to oversee the implementation process and review ultrasound studies. In a facility with one or more emergency physicians credentialed or experienced in ultrasound, these physicians should lead review of these studies. When no experienced emergency physicians are available, then outside assistance should be sought from an experienced emergency physician in the region who can be recruited for review purposes. If that physician is not on your medical staff, their assistance will require an invitation as an outside reviewer and a confidentiality agreement to maintain peer review protection.

Alternatively, if relationships are good with other physicians on your medical staff credentialed to perform ultrasound, such as obstetrics-gynecology, surgery, family medicine, critical care, or radiology, then invite one or more of these physicians to join your subcommittee for review purposes. It is not advisable, however, to turn the responsibility for quality assurance over to another department. This should remain under the leadership of your own department as would any other emergency medicine quality effort. In addition, any assisting physician from outside of your department must understand the paradigm of emergency ultrasound evaluations and criteria appropriate for clinician-performed emergency studies, and you must be assured there is no conflict of interest for reviewers who provide consultative imaging services.

Finally, the term "quality assurance" has a second meaning associated with ultrasound that relates to device function and maintenance. Equipment quality assurance includes periodic checks of electrical and mechanical safety, calibration, and image quality as well as tracking device cleaning and adherence to infection control policies. Assistance in device quality assurance should be secured from the equipment manufacturer and hospital biomedical engineering.

EQUIPMENT SELECTION

Ultrasound devices continue to improve in capability and suitability for the bedside performance of ultrasound as well as in cost. There are no best devices; there are many choices and physician preferences vary. The essential features include portability, display and image quality, transducer selection, a rapid startup time, a recording device, durability, and a service contract. Given the rapid improvements in equipment any specific recommendations would soon be out of date.

The first requirement for the bedside ultrasound device is portability. Some physicians prefer compact devices that can be carried by hand and others prefer cart-based portable devices with larger displays. What is important is that the device can be easily moved and negotiate emergency department hallways, as well as fit into the sometimes cramped spaces found in patient care rooms. Image and display quality are key elements because emergency ultrasounds are interpreted as they are generated and displayed. When comparing devices, side-by-side performance gives the best assessment of display and image quality.

The full spectrum of emergency studies requires the purchase of three to four transducers. If limited examination types are contemplated (such as trauma scans only), one may need only a single transducer. Multifrequency transducers are desirable and are supported by most ultrasound devices. A basic set of transducers includes a curvilinear probe, generally 3.5 to 5.0 MHz, for abdominal scanning and subxiphoid cardiac views. A smaller footprint curvilinear 3.5 MHz or multifrequency probe is optimal if separate cardiac and abdominal probes are not purchased. An endovaginal transducer is essential if first-trimester pelvic examinations are contemplated. A high-frequency linear transducer should be purchased for central line placement under ultrasound guidance. Finally, a dedicated cardiac transducer completes the selection of transducers.

Devices with a rapid boot-up time are desirable. Unlike ultrasound units in a radiology department that are often powered up and stationary throughout the day, emergency department devices are moved from room to room, often many times an hour. Some ultrasound machines may take 3 to 4 minutes to start up before you can scan, and an equal amount of time to shut down. When sequentially scanning multiple patients in different rooms, such as in the case of a multivictim motor vehicle collision, long boot-up times are tremendously problematic. Choose a device that is quick to boot-up or one with a non-interruptible power supply that can be unplugged, moved, and plugged in again without a shutdown and startup.

A method for recording such as a thermal printer or disc storage is essential. Emergency ultrasound performance requires one or more representative images available for study documentation, quality review, and reimbursement purposes. At present, emergency ultrasound studies are not typically managed in PACS systems (picture archiving and communication systems) and DICOM interface capabilities (specialized digital imaging and communications in medicine) are not a device requirement. Video recording devices are excellent for teaching purposes and, while standard for complete echocardiograms, they are rarely purchased or used in the clinical practice of emergency ultrasound.

Finally, durability and equipment service are essential. Few environments are rougher on equipment than the emergency department. The constant movement of the unit, the potential for damage to transducers, and body fluids on exposed controls can all lead to device failure. Find out how you can obtain service, what is the anticipated down-time for required service, and include a service contract with any device purchase contract.

REIMBURSEMENT

The focused ultrasound procedures performed by emergency physicians represent physician work that is separate and distinct from the work included in the evaluation and management codes (E&M codes). When medically indicated and properly documented, these ultrasound studies meet Current Procedural Terminology (CPT) service descriptions and should be reimbursed (4,34,38). Compliant reimbursement is complex, changes frequently, and is impacted by specific payer policies and by negotiated contractual relationships. Ultrasound reimbursement requires an understanding of the basic concepts of CPT coding, ICD-9 coding (International Classification of Diseases, 9th revision), and medical necessity in addition to medical record and image documentation. Emergency billing companies and emergency practice managers may not be familiar with the codes or requirements for billing these services and should be referred to the informational paper, *Emergency Ultrasound Coding and Reimbursement,* available on the ACEP website (4).

CPT codes
CPT codes describe the service performed and CPT code modifiers provide added information about the service provided. For example, a limited ultrasound of the abdomen is coded as 76705. This is normally modified with a −26 modifier indicating that only the professional component and not the complete code, which includes the facility component, is being used. There are CPT codes that accurately describe each of the primary ultrasound studies. The one exception is the focused assessment with sonography in trauma (FAST) examination, which is not described by a unique code. Rather, it is a clinical approach combining limited echocardiography with a limited abdominal study. Interestingly, the CPT codes for diagnostic ultrasound reimburse the physician for the interpretation of the study, but not for performance of the study. Performance of an ultrasound is currently reimbursed to the hospital as part of the technical component of the CPT code.

ICD-9 codes and medical necessity
ICD-9 codes generally describe diagnoses, signs, symptoms, or abnormal diagnostic tests. These codes are less familiar to physicians than are CPT codes and are usually applied by professional coders either at the hospital or professional billing office rather than by physician providers. Third-party payers use ICD-9 codes to determine if an ultrasound was medically necessary and accuracy in ICD-9 coding is important because payers frequently compare the ultrasound CPT code to a list of preauthorized ICD-9 codes in an effort to edit out, or deny, services that they believe are unnecessary.

Payer policy

Payers have their own rule sets regarding which services are covered, what constitutes a medically necessary service, and what coding combinations are permissible. When physicians agree to contract with a payer, they are agreeing to the payer's payment policies. Medicare's payer policy can vary by region and private payers may have dramatically different approaches for reimbursement. Even when a service is well described by CPT, a payer may put into place special rules that exclude emergency ultrasounds simply by creating a policy that denies payment for ultrasound services provided by emergency physicians. These issues may become more important as emergency ultrasound use grows and payers fear an increase in claims from physicians who have historically not conducted these procedures or utilized these codes.

DOCUMENTATION

Ultrasound documentation refers to the ultrasound interpretation, or report, in the medical record as well as to the archiving of images. Proper documentation of ultrasound interpretations requires a written report signed by the physician and included in the medical record. The report may be a templated note, a handwritten note, or it may be dictated. A report may be included in the patient encounter note with a proper heading or it may be separately recorded. Documentation should indicate the medical necessity of the study, identify the structures or organs studied, and supply an interpretation of the findings. Image documentation, or archiving, is necessary for all diagnostic studies as well as for vascular access; however images are not a requirement for the other procedural guidance ultrasounds. Standards directing how images are stored, on what recording media they are captured, where they are kept, the number of images per study, or other specific requirements are not addressed by CPT and are usually regulated by departmental or hospital policy.

CONCLUSION

The addition of ultrasound to the practice of emergency medicine has presented multiple challenges for the emergency physician. These have included the clinical challenges of adapting ultrasound technology to the unique environment of the emergency department, of accumulating evidence supporting a variety of emergency applications, and of implementing effective training for physician practitioners. Emergency physicians have addressed administrative challenges surrounding ultrasound program design as well as the development of hospital credentialing criteria and quality assurance programs. In addition, emergency physicians have confronted political challenges that have centered on often difficult professional relationships with providers of consulting ultrasound services, efforts to regulate the practice of emergency ultrasound, and the demands of communicating the unfamiliar paradigm of emergency ultrasound.

Despite these challenges, ultrasound has been integrated into the training of emergency physicians and into the practice of emergency medicine. Emergency patients and emergency physicians have been rewarded with tangible benefits that include enhanced efficiency of emergency care, increased accuracy of diagnosis, and improved emergency patient outcomes.

REFERENCES

1. The Accreditation Council for Graduate Medical Education (ACGME); Emergency Medicine Residency Review Committee; Program Requirements; Guidelines; Procedures and Resuscitations; Bedside ultrasound. 2002, Available at: http://www.acgme.org. Accessed Nov. 3, 2004.
2. ACEP Policy Statement. ACEP emergency ultrasound guidelines. 2001. American College of Emergency Physicians Web site. Available at: http://www.acep.org/library/pdf/ultrasound_guidelines.pdf. Accessed Nov. 3, 2004.

3. Tandy TK 3rd, Hoffenberg S. Emergency department ultrasound services by emergency physicians: model for gaining hospital approval. Ann Emerg Med 1997;29:367–374.

4. Hoffenberg SR, Tayal V, Dean A, et al. Emergency ultrasound coding and reimbursement. Ultrasound Section, ACEP. Available at: http://www.acep.org/1,4953,0.html. Accessed Nov. 3, 2004.

5. Fry WR, Clagett GC, O'Rourke PT. Ultrasound-guided central venous access. Arch Surg 1999;134:738–740; discussion 741.

6. Rozycki GS, Pennington SD, Feliciano DV. Surgeon-performed ultrasound in the critical care setting: its use as an extension of the physical examination to detect pleural effusion. J Trauma 2001;50:636–642.

7. Osranek M, Bursi F, O'Leary PW, et al. Hand-carried ultrasound-guided pericardiocentesis and thoracentesis. J Am Soc Echocardiogr 2003;16:480–484.

8. Mayo PH, Goltz HR, Tafreshi M, et al. Safety of ultrasound-guided thoracentesis in patients receiving mechanical ventilation. Chest 2004;125:1059–1062.

9. American College of Radiology. ACR practice guideline for performing and interpreting diagnostic ultrasound examinations. 2001. American College of Radiology Web site. Available at: http://www.acr.org/s_acr/bin.asp?TrackID=&SID=1&DID=12267&CID=539&VID=2&DOC=File.PDF. Accessed Nov. 3, 2004.

10. Quinones MA, Douglas PS, Foster E, et al. ACC/AHA clinical competence statement on echocardiography: a report of the American College of Cardiology/American Heart Association/American College of Physicians-American Society of Internal Medicine Task Force on Clinical Competence. J Am Coll Cardiol 2003;41:687–708.

11. Stewart WJ, Douglas PS, Sagar K, et al. Echocardiography in emergency medicine: a policy statement by the American Society of Echocardiography and the American College of Cardiology. Task Force on Echocardiography in Emergency Medicine of the American Society of Echocardiography and the Echocardiography and Technology and Practice Executive Committees of the American College of Cardiology. J Am Coll Cardiol 1999;33:586–588.

12. Kimura BJ, Pezeshki B, Frack SA, et al. Feasibility of "limited" echo imaging: characterization of incidental findings. J Am Soc Echocardiogr 1998;11:746–750.

13. Galasko GI, Lahiri A, Senior R. Portable echocardiography: an innovative tool in screening for cardiac abnormalities in the community. Eur J Echocardiogr 2003;4:119–127.

14. DeCara JM, Lang RM, Spencer KT. The hand-carried echocardiographic device as an aid to the physical examination. Echocardiography 2003;20:477–485.

15. Kirkpatrick JN, Davis A, Decara JM, et al. Hand-carried cardiac ultrasound as a tool to screen for important cardiovascular disease in an underserved minority health care clinic. J Am Soc Echocardiogr 2004;17:399–403.

16. Plummer D, Brunette D, Asinger R, et al. Emergency department echocardiography improves outcome in penetrating cardiac injury. Ann Emerg Med 1992;21:709–712.

17. Tayal VS, Beatty MA, Marx JA, et al. FAST (focused assessment with sonography in trauma) accurate for cardiac and intraperitoneal injury in penetrating anterior chest trauma. J Ultrasound Med 2004;23:467–472.

18. Mandavia DP, Hoffner RJ, Mahaney K, et al. Bedside echocardiography by emergency physicians. Ann Emerg Med 2001;38:377–382.

19. Tayal VS, Kline JA. Emergency echocardiography to detect pericardial effusion in patients in PEA and near-PEA states. Resuscitation 2003;59:315–318.

20. Blaivas M, Fox J. Outcome in cardiac arrest patients found to have cardiac standstill on the bedside emergency department echocardiogram. Acad Emerg Med 2001;8:616–621.

21. Salen P, O'Connor R, Sierzenski P, et al. Can cardiac sonography and capnography be used independently and in combination to predict resuscitation outcomes? Acad Emerg Med 2001;8:610–615.

22. Moore CL, Rose GA, Tayal VS, et al. Determination of left ventricular function by emergency physician echocardiography of hypotensive patients. Acad Emerg Med 2002;9:186–193.

23. American College of Radiology. ACR practice guideline for radiologist coverage of imaging performed in hospital emergency departments. 2003. American College of Radiology Web site. Available at: http://www.acr.org/s_acr/bin.asp?TrackID=&SID=1&DID=12231&CID=541&VID=2&DOC=File.PDF. Accessed Nov. 3, 2004.

24. Shih CH. Effect of emergency physician-performed pelvic sonography on length of stay in the emergency department. Ann Emerg Med 1997;29:348–351.

25. Blaivas M, Harwood RA, Lambert MJ. Decreasing length of stay with emergency ultrasound examination of the gallbladder. Acad Emerg Med 1999;6:1020–1023.

26. Agency for Healthcare Research and Quality. Ultrasound guidance of central vein catheterization. In: Making health care safer: a critical analysis of patient safety practices; Chapter 21: Available at: http://www.ahcpr.gov/clinic/ptsftinv/chap21.htm. Accessed Nov. 3, 2004.

27. Hind D, Calvert N, McWilliams R, et al. Ultrasonic locating devices for central venous cannulation: meta-analysis. BMJ 2003:327:361.

28. Branney SW, Moore EE, Cantrill SV, et al. Ultrasound based key clinical pathway reduces the use of hospital resources for the evaluation of blunt abdominal trauma. J Trauma 1997;42:1086–1090.

29. Frezza EE, Ferone T, Martin M. Surgical residents and ultrasound technician accuracy and cost-effectiveness of ultrasound in trauma. Am Surg 1999;65:289–291.

30. Durston WE, Carl ML, Guerra W, et al. Ultrasound availability in the evaluation of ectopic pregnancy in the ED: comparison of quality and cost-effectiveness with different approaches. Am J Emerg Med 2000;18:408–417.

31. Durston W, Carl ML, Guerra W, et al. Comparison of quality and cost-effectiveness in the evaluation of symptomatic cholelithiasis with different approaches to ultrasound availability in the ED. Am J Emerg Med 2001;19:260–269.

32. Allison EJ Jr., Aghababian RV, Barsan WG, et al. Core content for emergency medicine. Task Force on the Core Content for Emergency Medicine Revision. Ann Emerg Med 1997;29:792–811.

33. Hockberger RS, Binder LS, Graber MA, et al. The model of the clinical practice of emergency medicine. Ann Emerg Med 2001;37:745–770.

34. American College of Emergency Physicians. Use of ultrasound imaging by emergency physicians [policy #40121]. Ann Emerg Med 2001;38:469–470.

35. SAEM Ultrasound Position Statement, 1991. Society for Academic Emergency Medicine Web site. Available at: http://www.saem.org/publicat/ultrasou.htm. Accessed Nov. 3, 2004.

36. American Medical Association House of Delegates. H-230.960 Privileging for Ultrasound Imaging. American Medical Association Web site. Available at: http://www.ama-assn.org/apps/pf_new/pf_online?f_n=browse&doc=policyfiles/HnE/H-230.960.HTM. Accessed Nov. 3, 2004.

37. American Institute of Ultrasound in Medicine. Training guidelines for physicians who evaluate and interpret diagnostic ultrasound examinations. 2000. American Institute of Ultrasound Medicine Web site. Available at: http://www.aium.org/accreditation/practice/eight.asp. Accessed Nov. 3, 2004.

38. American College of Emergency Physicians. Interpretation of diagnostic studies. Policy #400109. Ann Emerg Med 1997;29:572–573.

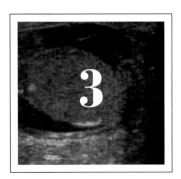

Fundamentals of Ultrasound

John S. Rose
Aaron E. Bair

Introduction

Any textbook on ultrasound has a chapter entitled "Physics," or "Knobology" as it is euphemistically known. In this practical guide to ultrasound, it is important that the fundamentals of ultrasound transmission and image production be covered, because bedside ultrasound is one of the few technologies in clinical practice where the provider both acquires and interprets the image. One must understand the pitfalls and techniques in image acquisition to accurately use ultrasound. This chapter will review the basics of ultrasound transmission, cover the basics of ultrasound equipment, and review basic principles of image acquisition.

Ultrasound Physics

One of the first principles one must understand is that medical ultrasound uses sound energy. Therefore, all of the laws that govern sound transmission apply when using ultrasound. Basic fundamentals of physics can be used to understand and optimize scanning technique. Sound is measured in Hertz (Hz) with human hearing detecting sound in the frequency range of 20 Hz to 20,000 Hz. Diagnostic ultrasound is in the frequency range of 2.5 MHz to 12 MHz. Although ultrasound is well outside the range of human hearing, it behaves no differently than any other sound wave and is subject to all of the effects of mechanical energy.

As sound waves travel through a medium, they cause molecules to vibrate. The molecules vibrate at a given frequency depending on the frequency of the sound. The sound wave then propagates through the medium (tissue) at that frequency. The frequency of these wavelengths determines how they penetrate tissue and affect image detail. The energy of a sound wave is affected by many factors. The spatial pulse length (SPL) is the basic unit of imaging. The SPL is a sound wave packet that is emitted from the transducer. Much like sonar, where the sound wave is sent out at a given frequency and then bounces off an object to localize it, diagnostic ultrasound can use sound waves to generate an anatomic picture. In essence, the sound waves "interrogate" the tissues to create an image. By adjusting various parameters of the sound wave and its production, the ultrasound wave can be used to relay information.

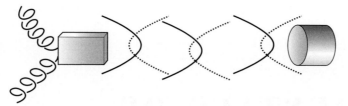

Figure 3.1. *Piezoelectric effect.* Notice that if a current is applied to the crystal on the left a signal is generated. As sound waves return and hit the crystal it will vibrate and generate a current.

The working component of any ultrasound machine that generates the sound wave is the piezoelectric element. Piezoelectric elements are unique crystals that vibrate at a given frequency when alternating current is applied. Similarly, if an ultrasonic wave hits a piezoelectric crystal, it will vibrate and generate an electric current across the dipole (Fig. 3.1). The unique aspects of these crystals enable them to be both a speaker and a microphone. In medical ultrasound, piezoelectric crystals are placed in a sealed container, called a transducer, that comes in contact with the patient to generate an ultrasound image.

IMPEDANCE

Once a sound wave leaves the transducer, the work begins. As the sound wave travels through tissue, several things occur that affect the generation of an image. As a sound wave travels through a medium of one density and crosses into a medium of another density, it encounters impedance at the interface between the two media. Impedance is the resistance to propagation of sound. Reflection of the sound occurs at this interface (Fig. 3.2). The amount of reflection is proportional to the difference in the acoustic impedance between the two media. In general, objects that have very high acoustic impedance, such as bone, reflect much of the signal. In contrast, liquid has much lower impedance and therefore, reflects very little. Liver has moderate impedance, so a portion of the sound is reflected back to the transducer and the remainder is transmitted to deeper structures. An image is generated from the signal that is reflected back to the transducer. If the body had only one uniform density with tissues of similar or identical impedance, then no image could be generated because no reflection would occur. The fact that different tissues have differing impedance allows detailed imaging by ultrasound. For tissue with greater impedance, the reflected signal that returns to the transducer is greater and therefore produces a brighter (more echogenic) image on the monitor. For tissues with lower impedance, more of the signal continues unchanged and less is returned, generating less of a reflected signal and creating a darker, grayer image. If no reflection occurs, a black (echo-free) image is seen on the monitor.

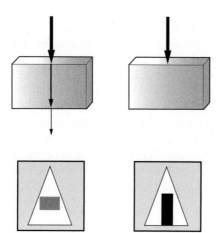

Figure 3.2. *Impedance.* The illustration on the left demonstrates that as the sound waves hit an object, impedance causes some signal to return to the transducer and some to continue. The continuing signal is attenuated. The amount of reflected signal depends on the impedance of the object. In the illustration on the right, if the object is very dense, the entire signal is attenuated and there is acoustic silence or an anechoic signal on the monitor. The top images illustrate a sound wave striking an object. The bottom figures illustrate the image generated on the monitor.

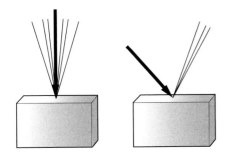

Figure 3.3. Perpendicular scanning. The figure on the left demonstrates good perpendicular scanning. The entire signal is returning to the transducer. The signal on the right is hitting the object of interest at an angle causing poor signal return, resulting in a less sharp image.

ATTENUATION

Attenuation is the loss of signal energy as it passes through tissue. Higher impedance generally causes more attenuation. Attenuation is partly a function of the intrinsic impedance of the tissues; it is also affected by scanning technique. Only sound that returns to the transducer produces an image. The initial sound signal sent out from the transducer can be returned as an echo and register as a signal; however, some sound waves may be reflected away from the transducer (scatter). Scatter can by caused by a variety of factors. Gas, skin density, and scanning angle all contribute to scatter. To help minimize scatter, it is important to keep the ultrasound beam as perpendicular as possible to the object of interest (Fig. 3.3). Scanning at an angle can cause sound to bounce off an object and not return to the transducer. You will notice that when you scan at a more acute angle, the image appears less sharp. The more perpendicular to the object of interest the beam is, the sharper the image. *It is very important that you try to scan perpendicular to the object of interest to optimize the ultrasound image.*

RESOLUTION

"Resolution" refers to the ability of the sound waves to discriminate between two different objects and generate a separate image for each. There are two types of resolution. "Axial resolution" is the ability to resolve objects that are parallel to the ultrasound beam (Fig. 3.4A). The size of the wavelength is the major determinant of axial resolution. High frequency wavelengths are better able to resolve objects close together and provide good axial resolution. High frequency waves, though, are more subject to attenuation and therefore lack tissue penetration. Lower frequency signals have lower axial resolution, but deeper tissue penetration. The second type of resolution is lateral resolution. Lateral

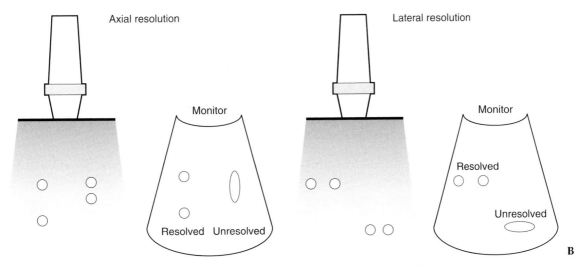

Figure 3.4. Resolution. Examples of axial and lateral resolution. Axial resolution is in line with the scanning plane (**A**). Lateral resolution is perpendicular to the scanning plane (**B**). (Redrawn from Simon and Snoey, eds. *Ultrasound in Emergency and Ambulatory Medicine.* St. Louis, MO: Mosby-Year Book, Inc., 1997.

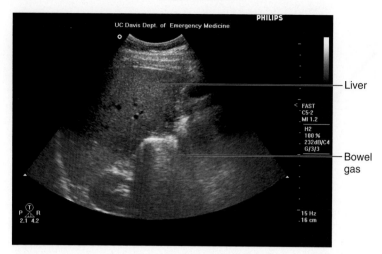

Figure 3.5. *Liver and bowel gas.* Note the well-defined liver but poorly defined bowel gas. Bowel gas causes scattering of the signal and loss of resolution.

resolution is the ability of sound waves to discriminate between objects that are perpendicular to the ultrasound beam. Lateral resolution is a function of beam width. Beam width is a function of the focus control on the ultrasound machine (Fig. 3.4B).

ULTRASOUND AND TISSUE

As sound travels through different media, it interacts in different ways. The ultrasound wave travels through tissue causing molecules to vibrate. The density of the tissue affects the transmission of the sound waves. Tissue that has molecules that are organized and relatively close together transmit better than those that are disorganized or farther apart. In looking at different tissue, this relationship can be seen.

Solid parenchymal organs provide good ultrasound images since they are compact and have some fluid density. The liver is a good example of an organ with excellent transmission properties. A uniform density makes it a superior organ for scanning. Notice how sharp and defined the image of the liver is in Figure 3.5 compared to the surrounding structures that are less defined.

Fluid densities are ideal for imaging with ultrasound because the molecules have some uniformity. The bladder is an excellent object to scan. In Figure 3.6, the bladder is clearly seen

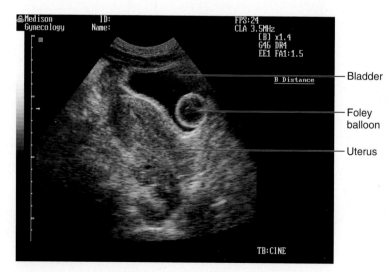

Figure 3.6. *Acoustic window.* The bladder displaces bowel gas and gives a clear acoustic window to the uterus. (Note the inflated Foley balloon in the bladder.)

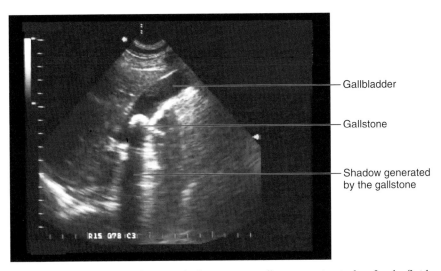

Figure 3.7. *Gallbladder with stone.* The liver is an excellent acoustic window for the fluid-filled gallbladder. The large gallstone creates a dark shadow. In addition, the tissue behind the gallbladder is more echogenic than surrounding tissue. This is enhancement artifact.

but the surrounding bowel is less defined. Notice that objects far field to the bladder are also clear. A fluid-filled structure allows for the uniform transmission of sound waves to deeper tissue. This is one example of an acoustic window. In an acoustic window an object is used as an acoustic filter for a deeper object. The bladder is often used in scanning to provide an acoustic window; it provides a uniform tissue that allows most of the signal to penetrate deeper tissue and also displaces the bowel allowing for the clearer visualization of the uterus that lies deeper. Fluid-filled organs surrounded by solid organs are also examples of acoustic windows and excellent scanning mediums. The gallbladder is another good example (Fig. 3.7). The liver parenchyma acts as an acoustic window for the fluid-filled gallbladder.

If the structure is too dense it may interfere with the transmission of sound waves. Structures that lie deep to bone cannot easily be imaged because most of the signal is reflected and is not able to penetrate deeper. Scanning over a rib produces a shadow or anechoic space beyond the rib (Fig. 3.8). Adjusting the transducer to move away from the rib allows for the signal to reach deeper structures. However, just because bone is dense doesn't mean it is excluded from all clinical applications for ultrasound. In musculoskeletal ultrasound, the near field cortex can be visualized in order to find a joint space for arthrocentesis.

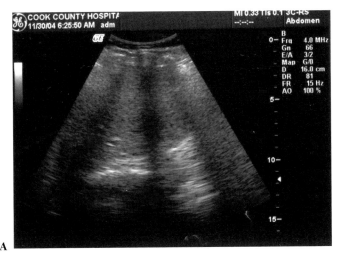
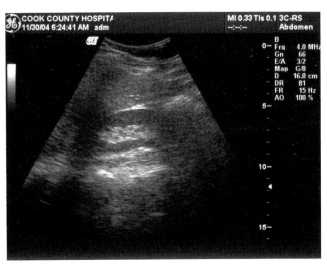

A   **B**

Figure 3.8. *Rib shadow.* Ribs cause the complete attenuation of signal and generate a shadow. Rib shadows interfere with scanning through an intercostal approach for the liver (**A**). Ribs commonly interfere with imaging the kidneys (**B**).

Gas gives a different problem. Molecules in gas (air) are randomly placed. Sound waves disperse in air, reflecting the signal in different directions. When gas is scanned, the image is ill-defined because the transducer sees a random array of signals. Consequently, ultrasound protocols avoid gas-filled areas such as bowel and lung. In fact, in ultrasound, *air is your enemy*. Excessive bowel gas, subcutaneous air, and lung fields are all impediments to effective scanning. Acoustic windows take advantage of good scanning locations that avoid air or gas.

ARTIFACTS

Artifacts are commonly generated from tissue interfaces. Many artifacts are just an annoyance but some are used diagnostically. The following section lists commonly encountered artifacts.

REVERBERATION

Reverberation is an artifact created when an object is imaged more than once from repeated reflections by an interface near the transducer. Reverberation gives numerous horizontal lines on the monitor (Fig. 3.9). Reverberation can be limited by changing the angle of the transducer.

MIRROR

Mirror artifact is produced when an object is located in front of a very strong reflector. In essence, a second representation of the object is placed at the incorrect location behind the strong reflector in the image. If a sonographic structure has a curved appearance, it may focus and reflect the sound like a mirror. This commonly occurs at the diaphragm (Fig. 3.10).

RING DOWN

Ring down is an image artifact created when an object vibrates at a characteristic resonance frequency. This artifact resembles a comet tail artifact without the specific banding seen with the comet tail. The terms *comet tail* and *ring down* are used interchangeably even though they are technically different. Ring down is commonly seen from bowel gas, especially just after a meal. One can take advantage of ring down artifact to locate a needle when doing an ultrasound-guided procedure (Fig. 3.11).

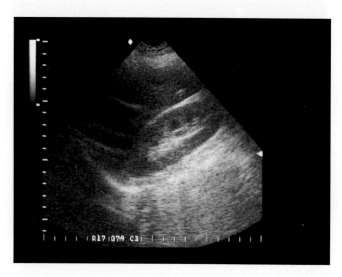

Figure 3.9. *Reverberation.* Note the lines on the left of the image. This is a reverberation artifact.

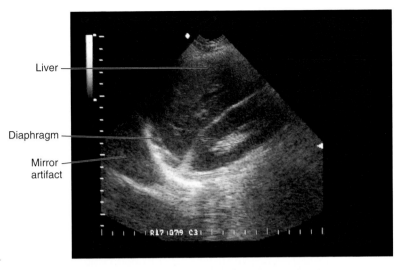

Liver

Diaphragm

Mirror
artifact

A

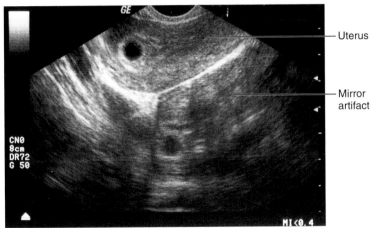

Uterus

Mirror
artifact

B

Figure 3.10. Mirror artifact. In A, there appears to be liver parenchyma on both sides of the diaphragm. This represents a mirror artifact caused by reflected signal. In B, identical images of the uterus are seen side by side. Image B courtesy of Karen Cosby, MD.

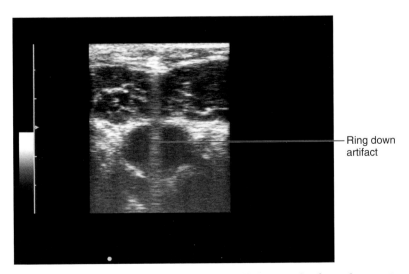

Ring down
artifact

Figure 3.11. Ring down artifact. This is an excellent example of ring down artifact from a needle during central line cannulation.

SHADOWING

Shadowing is an anechoic signal caused by failure of the sound beam to pass through an object. This blockage is caused by reflection or absorption of the sound and may be partial or complete. For example, air bubbles in the duodenum allow poor transmission of the sound beam because most of the sound is reflected. In addition, a calcified gallstone does not allow any sound to pass through and shadowing is pronounced. Shadowing like this is used to help diagnose gallstones (Fig. 3.7).

ENHANCEMENT

Enhancement is commonly seen as a hyperechoic or bright area on the far side of a cystic structure. It is caused because sound traveling through a fluid-filled structure is barely attenuated; the structures distal to a cystic lesion appear to have more echoes than neighboring areas. The back wall of a cystic structure will appear thicker and brighter (more echogenic) than the anterior wall; this is known as *posterior* wall enhancement. The tissue behind a cystic structure appears more echogenic than other surrounding tissue; this is also referred to as "increased through transmission" (Fig. 3.7). These properties are especially noticeable when an echogenic structure, such as a gallstone, is imaged in a cystic structure, such as the gallbladder. The echogenic gallstone is especially noticeable in the echo-free space of the gallbladder lumen. In addition, the echo-free shadow produced by the stone is sharply contrasted to the surrounding area behind the gallbladder that is enhanced by increased through transmission.

EDGE ARTIFACT

Sound waves travel in straight lines. When they encounter a rounded or curved structure, the sound wave is refracted away from the original line of propagation, leaving an acoustically silent space. This generates a shadow. This distorted image is commonly seen along the sides of cystic structures (Fig. 3.12).

SIDE LOBE

Side lobe artifact is generated from secondary intensity lobes displaced from the main ultrasound beam that are created by interference. Side lobe artifact can be seen especially around the bladder. Side lobes can misrepresent interface locations in the image.

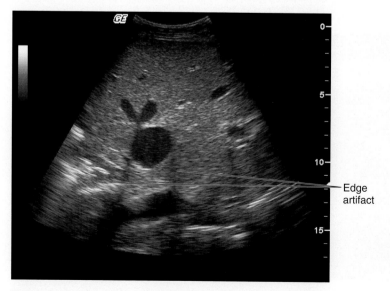

Figure 3.12. Edge artifact. Shadows are seen along the curved sides of cystic structures, caused by refraction of the sound wave along the curved interface. In this image, an oblique view of the inferior vena cava is seen.

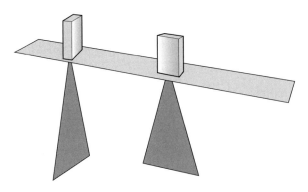

Figure 3.13. *Two dimensional planes of imaging.* This figure illustrates the 2-D signal that comes out of the transducer. Note that the transducer needs to be rotated to visualize the object in two planes perpendicular to each other.

ULTRASOUND AND 2-D

When sound is sent out from the transducer, it is important to conceptualize the form the sound takes. The sound travels from the transducer in flat two-dimensional (2-D) planes (Fig. 3.13). At any one moment objects are only visualized in one plane. The transducer can be "fanned" or tilted from side to side to better visualize an object (Fig. 3.14). Scanning in two planes perpendicular to each other and fanning through an object allows for more of a three-dimensional (3-D) conceptualization. This can be difficult to see from a two-dimensional textbook page.

In order to keep our relationships consistent, reference tools are used. Each transducer has a position marker (indicator) that corresponds with the position marker on the ultrasound monitor. This is a guide to help remind the sonographer to which orientation the transducer is positioned. Scanning protocols are not just random images; rather they are accepted views of a particular anatomic area.

If possible, the object of interest should be scanned in two planes perpendicular to each other to give the best 3-D representation available. Images can be referenced in one of two ways. Some organs have an orientation conveniently imaged in reference to the major axis of the body. A longitudinal orientation refers to a cephalad-caudad (or sagittal) view (Fig. 3.15A). A transverse orientation refers to a cross-sectional view similar to that produced by conventional computed tomography (CT). If an object lies in an oblique plane relative to the body (e.g., kidney), it is best referenced by its own axis. These objects are typically imaged in their long and short axes. When a longitudinal orientation is desired, by convention, the transducer indicator is positioned toward the patient's head (Fig. 3.15A). The

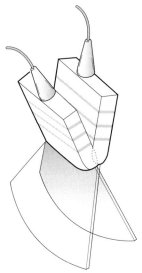

Transducer movement

Figure 3.14. *Fanning.* Rocking or fanning the transducer produces a 3-D perspective of the object of interest. (Redrawn from Simon and Snoey, eds. *Ultrasound in Emergency and Ambulatory Medicine.* St. Louis, MO: Mosby-Year Book, Inc., 1997.)

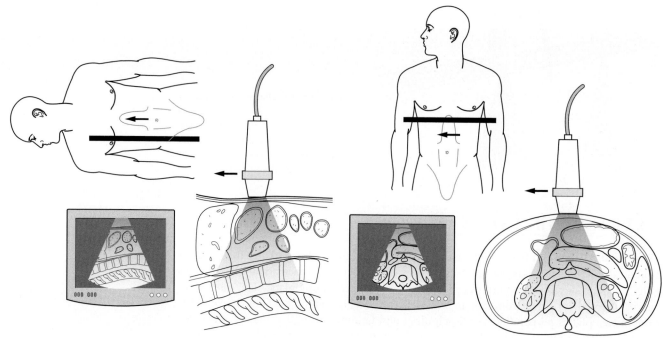

Figure 3.15A *Longitudinal axis.* Long axis scanning with the position marker (indicator) towards the patient's head. The arrow notes the indicator position.

Figure 3.15B *Transverse axis.* Short axis scanning with the position marker (indicator) towards the patient's right side. (Redrawn from Heller and Jehle, eds. *Ultrasound in Emergency Medicine.* Philadelphia, PA: W.B. Saunders, 1995.)

ultrasound monitor projects the image closest to the patient's head on the left side of the ultrasound monitor; the image closest to the patient's feet toward the right. When a transverse orientation is desired, the transducer indicator is placed toward the patient's right side (Fig. 3.15B). In this position the ultrasound monitor projects the patient's right side to the left of the monitor, the image closest to the patient's left side toward the right. Clinicians will recognize this view because it is the same orientation provided on traditional CT cuts. In most common applications the position marker on the monitor is on the left side. This differs from classic echocardiography orientation where it is placed on the right side of the image. The guides help develop a better image when scanning in two dimensions.

PRIMER ON EQUIPMENT

All ultrasound units share some common features. Although each manufacturer will have certain specific components, all machines have some basic knobs and features. The following section explores the basics of each of these features and describes variations and the practical nature of each.

TRANSDUCERS

The transducer is the scanning device where the piezoelectric crystals are stored and emit and receive sound. There are four main types of transducers available on the market. Each type has its advantages and disadvantages. Generally, most transducers today are sealed and have limited serviceability. In addition, many manufacturers claim their transducers are multifrequency. A transducer may have a range or effective frequency (i.e., 3.5–5.0 MHz).

Mechanical transducer

In a mechanical transducer the piezoelectric crystals are physically oscillated back and forth to produce the scanning field. The transducer has a slight vibration. The advantage to this type of transducer is that it can be designed to have a very small footprint. A footprint is the actual

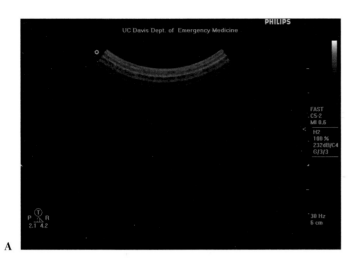
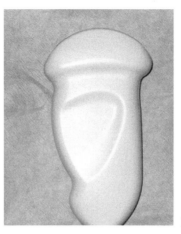

Figure 3.16. Curvilinear array transducer. Image A illustrates the image footprint generated by a curvilinear transducer. Note the curved image at the top of the screen.

transducer surface that comes in contact with the patient. Small footprint transducers allow for scanning through intercostal spaces with limited shadowing. In addition, they tend to be less expensive compared to electronic transducers. Their primary disadvantage is that the mechanism can be easily broken with any blunt force against the transducer. This is generally a disadvantage in a busy emergency department where objects can inadvertently hit a transducer. Mechanical transducers can be a good value and give excellent scanning resolution.

Array or electronic transducers

The vast majority of transducers on the market are of the array or electronic type. In these transducers, the crystals are fixed in an array and fire electronically to generate the field of view. There are different arrays available. Array transducers are described based on the positioning of the crystals. Most array transducers have the crystals in a line and are thus called linear arrays. The face of the transducer can be curved to give a wider field of view. This type is termed a curvilinear array transducer (Fig. 3.16). The array may be in a straight line for a more perpendicular field. These are termed straight linear arrays (Fig. 3.17). In both types of linear arrays, the crystals are fired sequentially to produce the field of view.

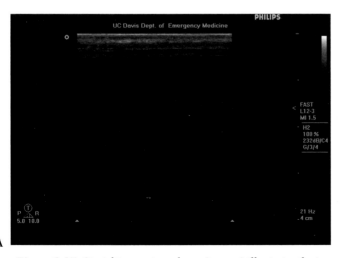
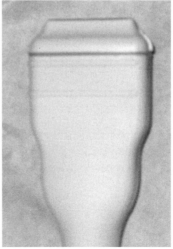

Figure 3.17. Straight array transducer. Image A illustrates the image footprint generated by a straight array transducer. Note the straight image at the top of the screen.

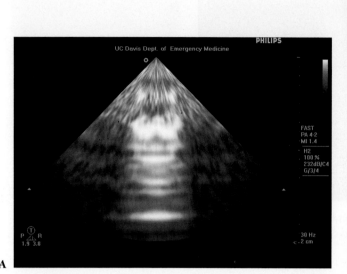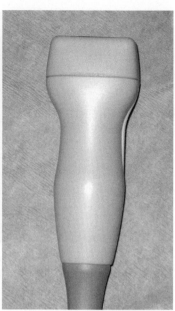

A   B

Figure 3.18. *Phased array transducer.* Note the small footprint and very small image footprint on the screen.

A more sophisticated array is the phased, or sector array, transducer (Fig. 3.18). In this type of array, the crystals are not in a line, they are layered in a staggered fashion. This allows for a very small footprint. The computer in the ultrasound machine then fires the crystals in phase to electronically oscillate the ultrasound and generate a wide field of view. These types of transducers tend to be more expensive. They are commonly used in echocardiography where a small footprint transducer is required.

Gain

The gain control adjusts the signal that returns to the unit. It can be compared to the volume knob on a stereo system. The intensity of the reflected sound wave is amplified to produce a visual image. As the volume is turned up on a stereo, the music becomes clearer until it is too loud and there is too much signal to noise. Similarly, as gain is increased, the amount of signal processed is increased and the image becomes brighter until there is too much signal and the image is washed out. Novice operators commonly run the gain too high. Experienced sonographers tend to run just enough to give a clear image but not wash out the image (Fig. 3.19).

Time Gain Compensation (TGC)

TGC is similar to gain. The TGC controls the gain at different levels of the ultrasound image. TGC is controlled by slider controls on most ultrasound units. The top control adjusts the near field gain; the bottom control adjusts the far field gain. The TGC controls allow attenuated signals to be boosted at specific levels rather than overall. The TGC controls can be compared with the equalizer on a stereo. Generally the TGC is not adjusted very much once it has been set (Fig. 3.20).

Focus

Focus controls the lateral resolution of the scanning beam. The focus is generally set for each application, although it may need to be adjusted for specific scanning situations. Adjustments in focus won't be dramatic so don't expect the focus to be the difference between making a diagnosis and not making a diagnosis.

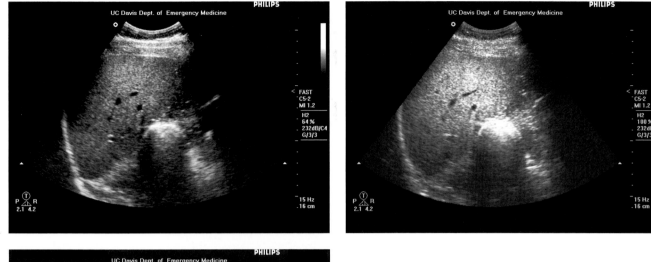

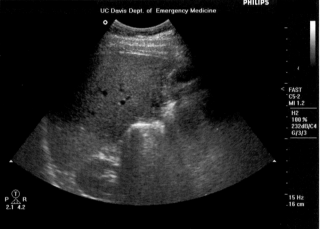

Figure 3.19. *Optimizing gain.* In A, the gain is too low and the image is too dark. In **B**, the image has too much gain and the image is washed out. In **C**, gain is optimal, resulting in excellent contrast.

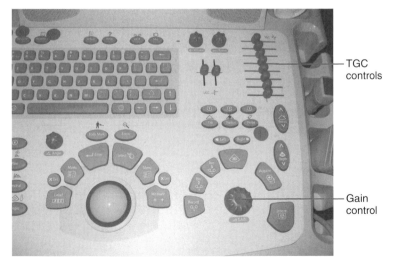

Figure 3.20. *Gain and time gain compensation (TGC).* Note the gain knob in the lower right. The TGC levers are in the upper right of the keyboard.

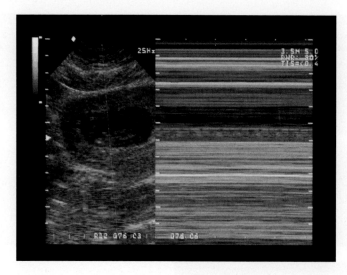

Figure 3.21. *B- and M-mode image.* A B-mode scan of an 8-week fetus is seen on the left. The reference channel cursor is aligned with the fetal heart rate. This single channel is plotted over time giving the M-mode screen on the right.

FREEZE

A selected image in the real-time acquisition is designated for continuous display until this mode is turned off. The freeze button holds an image still and allows printing, measuring, and manipulation.

CALIPERS

These markers are available to measure distances. Some ultrasound units add a feature for ellipsoid measurement. This feature provides a dotted line that can be drawn around the outline of a structure to calculate either the circumference or the area.

B-MODE

This is termed "brightness mode scanning"; it modulates the brightness of a dot to indicate the amplitude of the signal displayed at the location of the interface. B-mode is the 2-D scanning customarily done for diagnostic ultrasound.

M-MODE

If a series of B-mode dots are displayed on a moving time base, the motion of the mobile structures can be observed. One piezoelectric channel is plotted over time. This gives a real-time representation of a moving object such as the heart (Fig. 3.21).

IMAGE ACQUISITION

It is important to understand a few basic principles to optimize image acquisition. If these are adhered to then the quality of your scanning will be excellent. Each of these principles highlights topics covered in the previous sections. One can see these as the "take home" points.

1. Use accepted scanning locations and acoustic windows. Although ultrasound images may appear random at the beginning, each protocol has standard images that need to be acquired. Just as an electrocardiogram has standard lead placement, ultrasound images

for a given application are standardized so that those reviewing the images can make an accurate interpretation. Most accepted applications take advantage of acoustic windows such as a full bladder, liver, or spleen.

2. Scan perpendicular to the object of interest. Only sound that returns to the transducer is processed. A scan perpendicular to an object provides the best return of signal and optimizes detail. It is important to recognize that a transducer that is placed perpendicular to a deeper tissue object may not necessarily be perpendicular to the skin surface.

3. Obtain at least two views perpendicular to each other through any object of interest. Looking at an object in two perpendicular planes is critical for proper ultrasound interrogation. A few studies will not fully allow this practice, such as the critically injured trauma patient, but most applications will. Do not come to any conclusions until you have scanned in at least two planes. Sometimes what appears to be edge artifact in one plane can be a clear gallstone in another plane.

4. Scan through an object of study to give a 3-D view. This is important clinically to avoid misinterpreting the artifact. Fanning the transducer through the object of study will give the best 3-D detail.

This chapter briefly covers some basics in ultrasound fundamentals. As one scans, more details will become clear. Ultrasound is unique because the image acquisition component is as important as the interpretation. Take time to understand the components of your particular machine and enjoy scanning!

RECOMMENDED READING

1. Brant WE. *Ultrasound: The Core Curriculum*. Philadelphia: Lippincott Williams & Wilkins, 2001.
2. Curry RA, Tempkin BB. *Ultrasonography: An Introduction to Normal Structure and Functional Anatomy*. 1st ed. Philadelphia: WB Saunders, 1995.
3. Goldstein A. Overview of the physics of US. Radiographics 1993;13:701–704.
4. Hedrick WR, Hykes DL, Starchman DE. *Ultrasound Physics and Instrumentation*. 3rd ed. St. Louis: Mosby, 1995.
5. Higashi Y, Mizushima A, Matsumoto H. *Introduction to Abdominal Ultrasonography*. 1st ed. New York: Springer-Verlag New York, 1991.
6. Kremkau FW. *Diagnostic Ultrasound: Principles, Instruments, and Exercises*. 3rd ed. Philadelphia: WB Saunders, 1989.
7. Kremkau FW, Taylor KJW. Artifacts in ultrasound imaging. J Ultrasound Med 1986;5:227–237.
8. Noce JP. Fundamentals of diagnostic ultrasonography. Biomed Instrum Technol 1990;24: 456–459.
9. Report of the Ultrasonography Task Force. Council on Scientific Affairs. Medical diagnostic ultrasound instrumentation and clinical interpretation. JAMA 1991;265:1155–1159.
10. Rumack CM, Wilson SR, Charboneau JW. *Diagnostic Ultrasound*. 1st ed. St. Louis: Mosby, 1991.
11. Scanlan KA. Sonographic artifacts and their origins. AJR Am J Roentgenol 1991;156:1267–1272.

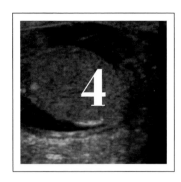

TRAUMA

Vivek S. Tayal
John L. Kendall

INTRODUCTION

For many, "trauma ultrasound" is synonymous with "emergency ultrasound." The use of ultrasound in the evaluation of the traumatically injured patient originated in the 1970s when trauma surgeons in Europe and Japan first described sonography for rapid detection of life-threatening hemorrhage. While the original studies set conservative goals of determining whether ultrasound could in fact detect peritoneal fluid (1–3), they shortly evolved to a point where ultrasound was lauded as a replacement for diagnostic peritoneal lavage (DPL) (4–8). This rapid ascension was fueled by evidence that ultrasound could not only accurately detect free fluid in body cavities, but also do it quickly, noninvasively, at the bedside, and without exposing the patient to radiation. The experience of physicians in the United States with ultrasound in the setting of trauma came to publication in the early 1990s as a number of papers reported similar results to those out of Europe and Japan (9). From these studies came the first description of the exam being performed as the "Focused Abdominal Sonography for Trauma," or the FAST exam (10). Later this terminology was changed to "Focused Assessment with Sonography for Trauma" (11), but the goal remained the same: the evaluation of trauma patients with the aid of ultrasound.

Beyond a purely historical perspective, trauma ultrasound is also equated with emergency ultrasound due to its widespread acceptance in Emergency Departments (ED). Ultrasound proved to be such a practical and valuable bedside resource for trauma that it received approval by the American College of Surgeons and was incorporated into standard teaching of the Advanced Trauma Life Support curriculum. With this endorsement, the use of ultrasound became a new standard for trauma centers throughout the world. In fact in many trauma centers bedside ultrasound has become the initial imaging modality used to evaluate the abdomen and chest in patients who present with blunt and penetrating trauma to the torso. As emergency physicians gained basic ultrasound skills for trauma, it became only natural to expand those skills to other applications. For many, ultrasound introduced a resource that greatly expanded the ability to assess and treat all patients.

CLINICAL APPLICATIONS

The primary goal of the FAST exam in its original description was the noninvasive detection of fluid (blood) within the peritoneal and pericardial spaces. Ultrasound provides a method to detect quantities of fluid within certain spaces that are either undetectable by the physical exam or without the use of other invasive (DPL), expensive [computed tomography (CT)], or potentially delayed (clinical observation) methods. As experience has been gained, trauma ultrasound has been expanded to include assessment for specific solid organ injury and the detection of pleural effusions (hemothorax) and pneumothorax. The clinical scenarios where this information becomes exceedingly useful are in the evaluation of patients presenting with blunt or penetrating trauma to the chest or abdomen. This chapter will discuss the clinical applications, techniques, and use of the standard FAST exam, as well as expanded applications for those with more advanced skills.

IMAGE ACQUISITION

EQUIPMENT

Most trauma ultrasound is performed with compact or cart-based systems using a 3.5 MHz transducer. While the exam can be done with a curvilinear abdominal transducer, the tighter the radius of the probe and the smaller the footprint, the easier it is to perform the upper quadrant, cardiac, and thoracic views of trauma ultrasound. A smaller footprint can facilitate imaging between and around the ribs.

A single general-purpose transducer used for most abdominal scanning is sufficient for the FAST exam. Most machines sold today have multifrequency transducers with frequency and depth controls that allow adjustment for a variety of applications and body habitus. Adjustments can optimize imaging. For instance, in larger adults, a lower frequency (2 MHz) may be optimal, whereas in children and smaller statured adults, a higher frequency (5 MHz) may provide better imaging (12). Some physicians prefer a phased array transducer for cardiac imaging and a linear probe (with better near field resolution), if available, for the detection of pneumothorax and for sonographic procedural guidance.

TIMING AND SPEED

The acronym "FAST" suggests a quick survey of the peritoneal and pericardial spaces. Usually the exam can be completed in 3 to 5 minutes and is done simultaneously with resuscitation, or as part of the secondary survey in the stable patient. Though the study should be done relatively quickly, this does not mean that the ultrasound exam should be done haphazardly (13). Biplanar views of each window with angling of the transducer, rotation to a 90 degree angle, and further manipulation should be done to survey the entirety of the potential space. Usually a static image of a representative window is frozen, and printed to paper, disc, or even film. Serial sonographic examinations have been proposed but very few studies have shown the utility of such an approach (14).

BASIC EXAM

The basic FAST exam includes 4 views (Fig 4.1) (11):

1. Perihepatic (right upper quadrant)
2. Perisplenic (left upper quadrant)
3. Pelvic (Pouch of Douglas or retrovesicular)
4. Pericardial (cardiac)

Perihepatic

The right upper quadrant view, also known as the Morison's pouch or perihepatic view, is commonly viewed as the classic image of trauma ultrasound. It allows for visualization of free fluid in the potential space between the liver and right kidney. In addition, fluid above

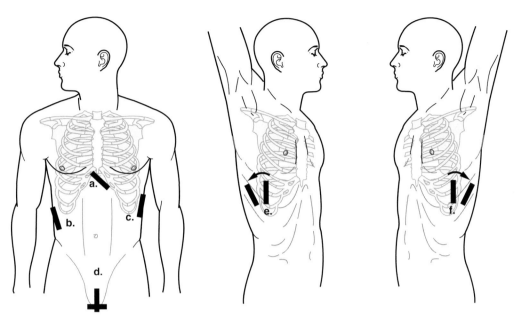

Figure 4.1. Transducer placement for views of the FAST exam. (a) subxihoid; (b) perihepatic; (c) perisplenic; (d) pelvic; (e and f) extended thoracic views.

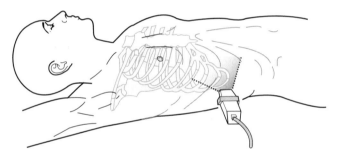

Figure 4.2. Right upper quadrant transducer positioning for the FAST exam.

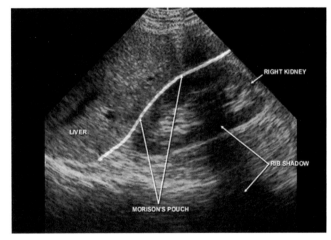

Figure 4.3. Ultrasound image demonstrating normal appearance of Morison's pouch.

and below the diaphragm in the costophrenic angle or subdiaphragmatic space can be seen. The transducer is initially placed in a coronal orientation in the midaxillary line over an intercostal space of one of the lower ribs (Fig. 4.2). The indicator on the transducer should be directed toward the patient's head. Once Morison's pouch is visualized (Fig. 4.3), the transducer should be angled in all directions to fully visualize the potential spaces of the right upper quadrant. Angling anteriorly and posteriorly will allow for the complete interrogation of Morison's pouch. The sonographer will need to manipulate the transducer to minimize artifact from the ribs. The real-time image can be optimized by gently rocking the transducer to create a mental three-dimensional view of the space. In addition, the transducer can be directed cephalad to visualize the pleural and subdiaphragmatic space (Fig. 4.4). Moving the transducer caudad brings the inferior pole of the kidney and the superior aspect of the right paracolic gutter into view (Fig. 4.5).

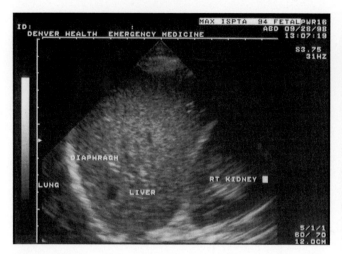

Figure 4.4. Normal ultrasound anatomy of the right subdiaphragmatic space.

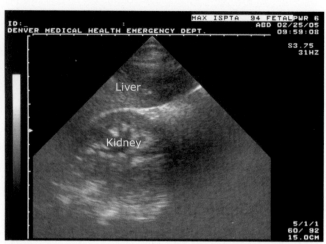

Figure 4.5. Normal inferior pole of the right kidney and the paracolic gutter.

Perisplenic

The left upper quadrant view is also known as the perisplenic or, less accurately, the splenorenal view. It can be challenging to obtain because the spleen does not provide as large a sonographic window as the liver, and the examiner frequently needs to reach across the patient in order to access the left upper quadrant. In contrast to the perihepatic view, ideal placement of the transducer in the left upper quadrant is generally more cephalad and posterior. A good starting point is the posterior axillary line in the 9th and 10th intercostal space (Fig. 4.6). The indicator should be directed toward the patient's head. If the splenorenal space is not visualized, it is typically because the transducer is not posterior or superior enough, so movement in either or both of these directions will improve the image. The transducer should be angled to see the anterior, posterior, superior, and inferior portions of the perisplenic space. Important landmarks to visualize include the spleen-kidney space (Fig. 4.7), the spleen-diaphragm interface (Fig. 4.8), and the inferior pole of the kidney-paracolic gutter transition (Fig. 4.9).

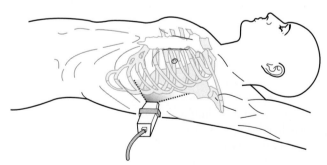

Figure 4.6. Left upper quadrant transducer positioning for the FAST exam.

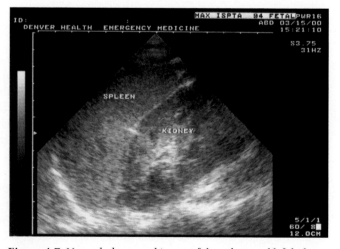

Figure 4.7. Normal ultrasound image of the spleen and left kidney.

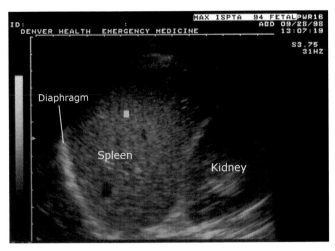

Figure 4.8. Normal sonographic anatomy visualized in the left subdiaphragmatic space.

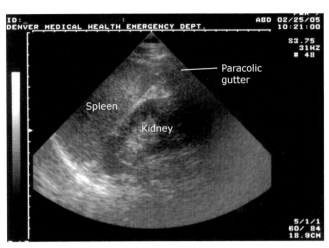

Figure 4.9. Normal appearance of the inferior pole of the left kidney and the paracolic gutter.

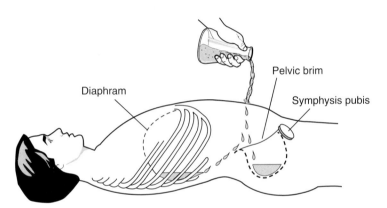

Figure 4.10. Locations of the dependent areas of the peritoneal cavity.

Pelvic

The pelvic view is an important and potentially underappreciated window for detecting free peritoneal fluid. Since it is one of the most dependent and easily visualized portions of the peritoneal cavity, fluid collections may be seen here before being detected in other areas (Fig. 4.10). As well, it is away from the chest and upper abdomen, so images can be obtained simultaneously with the evaluation and resuscitation of the trauma patient. The key to the pelvic view is scanning through a moderately full bladder to facilitate visualization of the underlying and adjacent structures, so imaging should be done before placement of a Foley catheter or spontaneous voiding. The transducer is initially placed just superior to the symphysis pubis in a transverse orientation with the indicator directed to the patient's right (Fig. 4.11 **a**, **b**). From here the transducer can be angled cephalad, caudad, and side to side to fully visualize the perivesicular area. It is also important to image the bladder in a sagittal orientation. To obtain this view, the transducer should be rotated clockwise so that the indicator is directed towards the patient's head (Fig. 4.11). The transducer can then be angled side to side, superiorly, and inferiorly to gain a full appreciation of the retrovesicular space (Fig. 4.11 c).

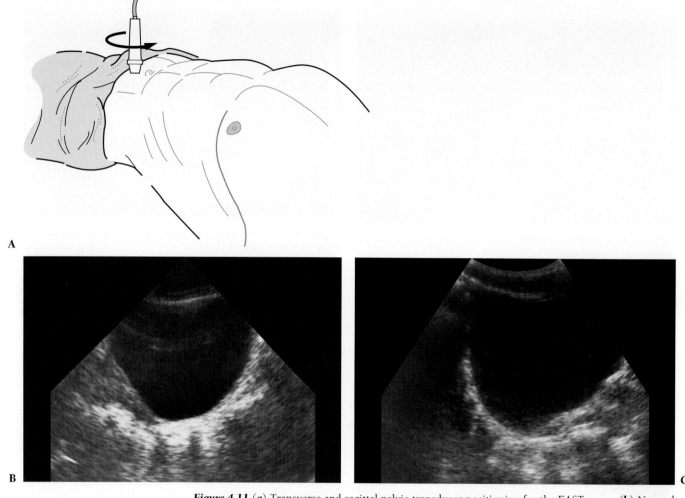

Figure 4.11 (***a***) Transverse and sagittal pelvic transducer positioning for the FAST exam. (***b***) Normal transverse transabdominal anatomy of a male bladder. (***c***) Normal sagittal transabdominal anatomy of a male bladder.

Pericardial

The subxiphoid approach is the most commonly used and convenient way to visualize cardiac structures and the pericardial space. The four-chamber subxiphoid view is performed with the transducer oriented transversely in the subcostal region and the indicator directed to the patient's right. The transducer should be held almost parallel to the skin of the anterior torso as it is pointed to a location just to the left of the sternum toward the patient's head (Fig. 4.12 **a**, **b**). Gas in the stomach frequently obscures views of the heart, but this can be minimized by using the left lobe of the liver as an acoustic window. This is accomplished by moving the transducer further to the patient's right. The liver should come into view as well as the interface between the liver and the right side of the heart (Fig. 4.13). The subxiphoid view may not be obtainable in all patients, so other cardiac views should be obtained to rule out traumatic pericardial effusion, especially in those with anterior pericardial fat pads (15). The approach to obtaining alternative cardiac views can be found in the echochardiography chapter (Chapter 5).

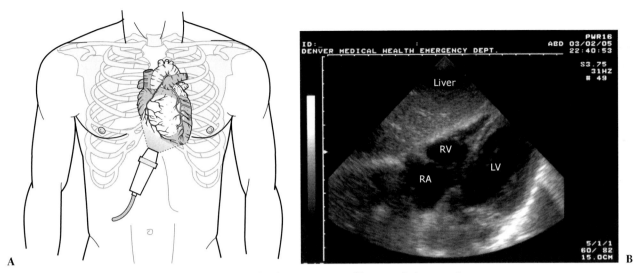

Figure 4.12 (***a***) Subxiphoid transducer position for the FAST exam. (***b***) Normal ultrasound anatomy visualized from the subxiphoid transducer position (RV, right ventricle; RA, right atrium; LV, left ventricle).

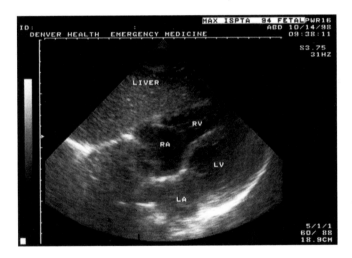

Figure 4.13. Ultrasound image demonstrating the liver as an acoustic window to the heart from the subxiphoid transducer position (RV, right ventricle; RA, right atrium; LV, left ventricle; LA, left atrium).

EXTENDED VIEWS

Paracolic gutters
The paracolic gutters are additional sonographic views that may increase the sensitivity of the standard FAST exam for the detection of peritoneal fluid. They are obtained by placing the transducer in either upper quadrant in a coronal plane and then sliding it caudally from the inferior pole of the kidney (Fig. 4.14 **a, b**). Alternatively, the transducer can be placed in a transverse orientation medial to the iliac crests. It can be angled inferiorly and superiorly to assess for the presence of loops of bowel outlined by peritoneal fluid.

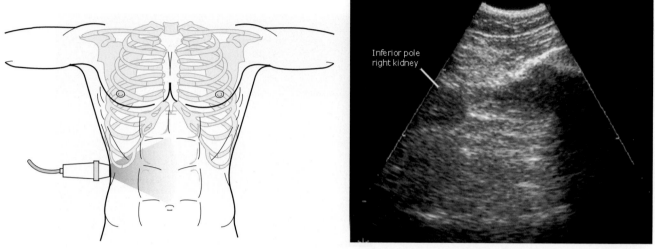

Figure 4.14 (*a*) Right paracolic gutter transducer position for the FAST exam. (*b*) Typical ultrasound appearance of the paracolic gutter.

Costrophrenic angle or pleural base

The sonographic evaluation of the pleural space for fluid is an adaptation of the right and left upper quadrant views described in the standard FAST exam. The transducer is initially placed in position to obtain a right or left upper quadrant view. It is then angled or moved superiorly to visualize the diaphragm and pleural space (Fig. 4.15 **a, b**). The region immediately above the diaphragm should be imaged to detect fluid. In the normal patient, air from lung tissue will scatter the signal and create shadowing and artifact. When pleural fluid is present, an anechoic space appears above the diaphragm. Visualization can be improved if the liver or spleen is used as an acoustic window to the pleural space (Fig. 4.16), but even with optimal transducer placement, only a small portion of the pleural space is typically accessible in patients without pathology.

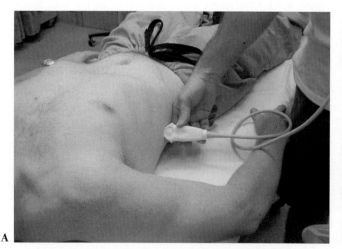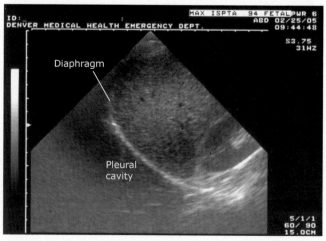

Figure 4.15 (*a*) Pleural base transducer position for the FAST exam. (*b*) Sonographic appearance of the inferior aspect of a normal pleural cavity.

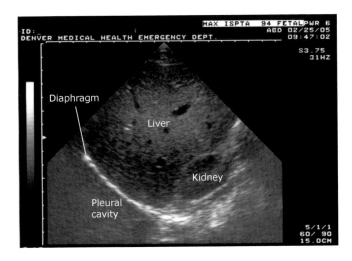

Figure 4.16. Ultrasound image of the liver acting as an acoustic window to the costophrenic angle. Note how the scan plane uses as much of the liver tissue as possible to view the pleural base.

Anterior thorax (pneumothorax)

Interrogation of the anterior pleura for the presence of pneumothorax can be done with a number of transducers, although it is preferable to use a high-frequency, linear model that is set to a shallow depth of penetration (4 to 6 cm). The transducer is placed longitudinally in the midclavicular line over the third or fourth intercostal space (Fig. 4.17).

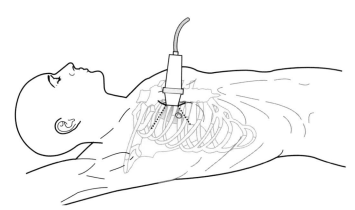

Figure 4.17. Anterior thorax transducer placement for the evaluation of pneumothorax.

ORDER

While there is no current standard for the order in which the views of the FAST exam are obtained, arguments have been made for starting with certain windows. For instance, the right upper quadrant view is a common starting point because it is one of the most sensitive and specific locations for detecting hemoperitoneum and many physicians routinely scan from the patient's right side (16–18). Alternatively the pelvic view may be the first view obtained, as it is one of the most dependent portions of the peritoneal cavity so smaller fluid collections may detected here before other locations (16). As well, placement of a urinary catheter to decompress the bladder essentially eliminates the sonographic window to the pelvis, so there is a priority in obtaining this window before the Foley is placed. Another approach is to scan the left upper quadrant first, but this is usually advocated by institutions that have a protocol of scanning from the patient's left side. Finally, the subxiphoid approach is often proposed as a starting point for the FAST exam so that potentially life-threatening cardiac injuries can be quickly identified. As well, intracardiac blood can be used as a reference point of an anechoic fluid collection to facilitate adjustment of the overall gain and time gain compensation (TGC). All in all, there is no standard order for performing the FAST exam and in many instances the order will be dictated by the patient's clinical presentation and institutional preferences.

Normal Ultrasound Anatomy

Peritoneal Space

The basic FAST exam requires the sonographer to be familiar with the sonographic appearance of the major abdominal solid viscera (liver, spleen, uterus), to have the ability to recognize fluid collections in potential spaces, and to have the technical ability to acquire 4 to 6 standard FAST exam views. The most important skill for trauma ultrasound is the ability to detect free fluid in the potential recesses within the peritoneal cavity (Fig. 4.18). These include Morison's pouch, the perisplenic space, and views of the pelvis and the pericardium. Free intraperitoneal fluid appears as anechoic signals that outline other structures or fills potential spaces.

Liver and Gallbladder

The normal liver has a homogeneous, medium-level echogenicity (Fig. 4.19). Glissen's capsule outlines the liver with an echogenic, defined border. The liver parenchyma is punctuated by a variety of vascular and biliary vessels that appear as anechoic linear structures. A detailed knowledge of the hepatic architecture is helpful but not necessary because the FAST exam relies only on recognizing normal homogenous hepatic architecture from a disrupted or inhomogenous pattern of a traumatized liver.

The gallbladder is a round or oval cystic structure within the liver. It is located on the medial, inferior surface of the liver and will commonly be seen during scanning of the peri-

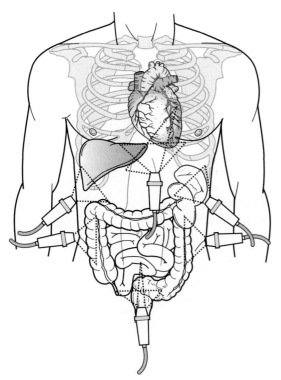

Figure 4.18. Typical transducer positions used to evaluate potential spaces within the peritoneal cavity.

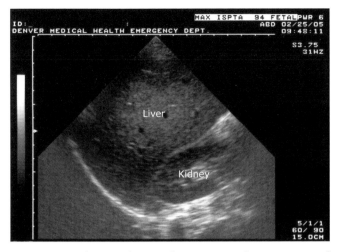

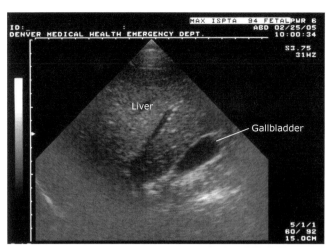

Figure 4.19. Ultrasound image demonstrating the appearance of normal liver tissue.

Figure 4.20. Sonographic appearance of the gallbladder while scanning in the perihepatic region.

hepatic area if the transducer is angled anteriorly from Morison's pouch (Fig. 4.20). It is not necessary to identify the gallbladder during the FAST exam, although the gallbladder may be seen to float or bob around in the face of free fluid and may be sonographically enhanced by surrounding fluid.

SPLEEN

The spleen is a solid organ with a homogenous cortex and echogenic capsule and hilum (Fig. 4.21). It has a medium-gray echotexture similar to that of the liver, but is smaller in size. The vessels within the parenchyma are less apparent than those in the liver. Since the spleen occupies a posterior-lateral location, it may be difficult to assess the entirety of the parenchyma using a single transducer location and multiple planes may be needed to visualize the whole organ.

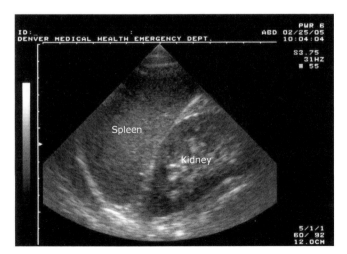

Figure 4.21. Ultrasound image demonstrating the appearance of normal splenic parenchyma.

BOWEL

The bowel can have a number of different sonographic appearances depending upon its contents. Air within the lumen of the bowel creates gray shadows that distort the view of surrounding structures. This distortion often makes it difficult to achieve a fine resolution of the image. When the bowel is filled with fluid or solid matter, it can appear to be cystic or solid. However, with simple and brief observation, the image will typically change with visible peristaltic waves. When free fluid is present, anechoic spaces may separate loops of bowel and mesentery, creating a confusing pattern to the novice eye. Loops of bowel may bob about with percussion of the abdomen or movement of the ultrasound transducer.

KIDNEYS

The kidneys are paired retroperitoneal organs that have a distinct sonographic appearance. They are visualized immediately inferior to the liver and spleen. Their surface (Gerota's fascia) is characterized by a bright echogenic line that outlines the renal cortex. The cortex itself has a medium-gray echotexture that is slightly hypoechoic compared to the hepatic and splenic parenchyma (Fig. 4.22). The central renal sinus is typically echogenic, unless there is a component of hydronephrosis, which, depending on the degree of obstruction, will appear anechoic (Fig. 4.23).

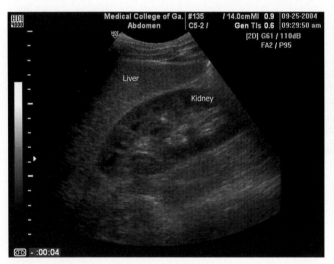

Figure 4.22. Ultrasound image demonstrating the appearance of normal renal parenchyma. (Courtesy of Mike Blaivas.)

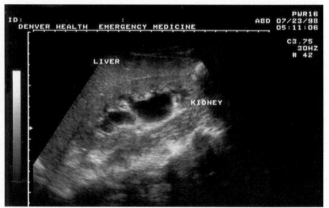

Figure 4.23. Ultrasound taken from a patient with moderate hydronephrosis.

UTERUS

The uterus is the major identifiable organ within the female pelvis. It is situated just above the bladder and has a pear-shaped appearance when viewed in its long axis in the sagittal orientation (Fig. 4.24). The lower uterine segment and cervix define the cul-de-sac, the most dependent peritoneal space where free fluid is likely to accumulate (Fig. 4.25).

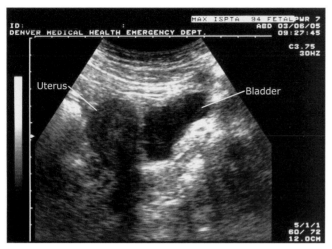

Figure 4.24. Sagittal orientation of the female pelvis showing the relationship of a normal uterus and bladder.

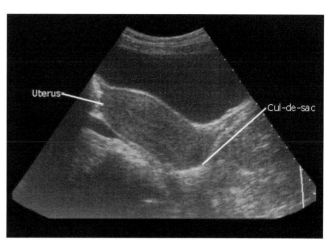

Figure 4.25. Transabdomonal ultrasound image demonstrating the cervix and pelvic cul-de-sac.

BLADDER

The bladder is a retroperitoneal organ that is the most sonographically visible portion of the lower urinary tract. It occupies the midline in the lower pelvis, typically at or below the pubic symphysis. When the bladder is empty, the transducer may need to be directly below the pubic ramus to visualize it. When full, the distended bladder provides an excellent acoustic window to pelvic structures (Fig. 4.26). It is important to distinguish between fluid in the bladder and free intraperitoneal fluid.

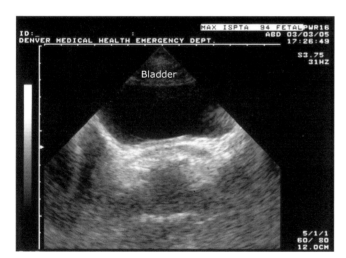

Figure 4.26. Transabdominal pelvic ultrasound of a full bladder in the transverse orientation.

THORAX

Pericardium

The pericardium is usually seen as a white echogenic line surrounding the heart. When pericardial fluid is absent, the parietal pericardium and the visceral pericardium are usually indistinguishable and are seen as a single echogenic line. On occasion the space between the parietal pericardium and visceral pericardium will have a small amount of epicardial fat or may contain up to 10 ml of serous physiologic fluid (Fig. 4.27).

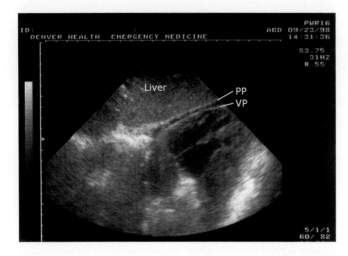

Figure 4.27. Subxiphoid orientation of the heart demonstrating separation of the layers of the pericardium by a small amount of pericardial fluid (VP, visceral pericardium; PP, parietal pericardium).

Cardiac chambers

The chambers of the heart have very distinct locations and appearances. The base of the heart, which includes the atria and major valves, is to the right and slightly posterior, while the apex of the heart points to the left, anteriorly and inferiorly. The right-sided chambers have thin walls that can collapse when pressure within the pericardial space is elevated, as in the case of a pericardial effusion. The left ventricle has a thicker wall and is usually larger than its counterpart on the right (Fig. 4.28). Although a number of approaches can be used to examine the heart and pericardium, the FAST exam typically uses a subxiphoid approach.

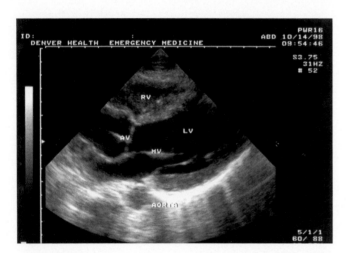

Figure 4.28. The chambers of the heart visualized from the long axis parasternal transducer position. Note that this view uses the emergency medicine orientation; see Chapter 5 (RV, right ventricle; LV, left ventricle; MV, mitral valve; AV, aortic valve).

Pleural cavity

The sonographic assessment of the normal pleural base anatomy is rarely clear, since the scatter and reflection from the lung precludes significant sound penetration. As the transducer is angled or moved to visualize the costophrenic angle, views of the liver, spleen, and diaphragm will give way to scatter artifact that looks like the screen has become dirty: this is the appearance of normal lung. On the other hand, elucidating normal sonographic anatomy of the anterior thorax is extremely useful. The most visible and superficial finding is the acoustic shadowing from the ribs (Fig. 4.29). The pleural space is just deep to the posterior aspect of the ribs. It can be recognized as an echogenic line that has the appearance of to-and-fro sliding (Fig. 4.30). This is termed the "sliding sign," and if it is seen the

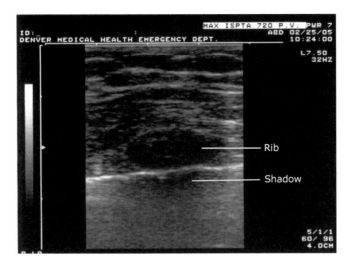

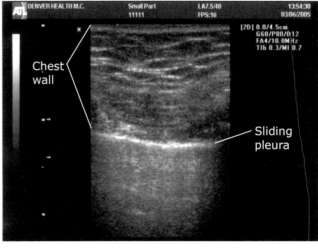

Figure 4.29. Anterior thorax transducer position demonstrating the appearance of rib shadow.

Figure 4.30. Ultrasound anatomy visualized during scanning to assess for the presence of a "sliding sign."

exam is considered negative for a pneumothorax, because the visceral and parietal pleura are in proximity. Additional sensitivity for visualizing these structures may be achieved by using power color Doppler (19). Using the "power slide" technique, normal lung anatomy is easily noted by the presence of color signal enhancement.

PATHOLOGY

FREE PERITONEAL FLUID

Fluid (blood) in the trauma patient is usually detected in the dependent areas of the peritoneal cavity including the hepatorenal space (Morison's pouch), the perisplenic space, the pelvis, and the paracolic gutters. In general, free fluid appears anechoic (black) and is defined by the borders of the potential spaces it occupies (Fig. 4.31). As an example, free fluid in Morison's pouch will be bounded by Glisson's capsule or the liver anterolaterally and Gerota's fascia or the kidney posteromedially. There are a number of variables that affect the appearance and location of fluid within the peritoneal cavity. These include the site of origin of the bleeding, the rate of accumulation, time since the injury, and movement of fluid within the peritoneal cavity.

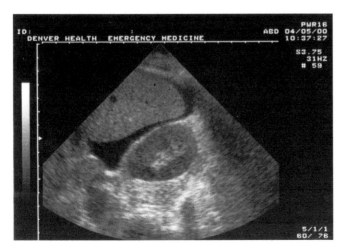

Figure 4.31. Peritoneal fluid visualized in the perihepatic region.

Minimum amount of fluid

The ability to detect free intraperitoneal fluid by ultrasound was first illustrated in a cadaver study in 1970 that demonstrated that as little as 100 cc of instilled peritoneal fluid was detectable by ultrasound when the body was placed in a hand-knee position and scanned from the abdomen (1). Additional studies have been done since, including one finding that as little as 10 mL of fluid could be consistently visualized in the pouch of Douglas (20). The minimal amount of fluid detected by ultrasound depends on a number of factors, most notably, the location of the fluid and the positioning of the patient. Most studies that have assessed the ability of ultrasound to detect minimal volumes of peritoneal fluid have focused on Morison's pouch using a saline infusion model (20–23). In one study using DPL as a model for intraperitoneal fluid, the mean volume detected in Morison's pouch was 619 mL (standard deviation, 173 mL). Only 10% of the sonographers could detect fluid volumes of 400 mL or less (21). Using a similar DPL model, another study assessed the minimum volume detected using the pelvic view (24). They determined that the average minimum detectable volume was 157 mL by one participant and 129 mL by an independent reviewer, thus suggesting that the pelvic view may be more sensitive than Morison's pouch for small volumes of peritoneal fluid.

Patient positioning has also been studied as a factor in detecting peritoneal fluid. For instance one study found that the optimal positions for detecting minimal volumes of fluid in a cadaver model were right lateral decubitus or facing downward while being supported on both hands and knees (1). Since neither of these positions is practical for scanning the trauma patient, other positioning has been investigated. For example, a small amount (5 degrees) of Trendelenburg positioning has been shown to statistically increase the sensitivity for detecting peritoneal fluid in the right upper quadrant (25).

Finally, attempts have been made to correlate the width of the fluid stripe in Morison's pouch with intraperitoneal fluid volumes. In a DPL model, a mean stripe width of 1.1 cm was found after 1 L of saline had been instilled (22). Other studies have proposed that fluid can be seen at similar or even smaller volumes (26,27), but how the authors of these studies derived their results is largely unknown and, therefore, their conclusions are unsubstantiated.

Fluid flow patterns

Fluid in the peritoneal cavity can collect and subsequently spread in a predictable manner, which can aid in its detection. One study found that in the supine position, the

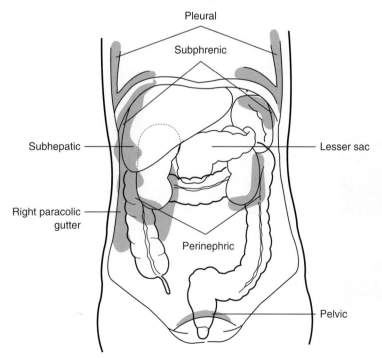

Figure 4.32. Potential spaces within the torso where fluid can collect.

pelvis is the most dependent portion of the peritoneal cavity and the right paracolic gutter is the main communication between the upper and lower abdominal compartments (Fig. 4.32) (28). Measured flow patterns have shown that fluid tracking up the right paracolic gutter preferentially collects in Morison's pouch before progressing to the right subphrenic space. Interestingly, the phrenicocolic ligament restricts similar flow between the left paracolic gutter to the left upper quadrant, so fluid in the supramesocolic space actually spreads across the midline into the right upper quadrant. Clinical studies support these findings as the majority of peritoneal fluid collections are detected in the perihepatic region (16,29).

Perihepatic fluid

Fluid can accumulate and be found in a variety of perihepatic locations. Most commonly it will be detected in the hepatorenal space or Morison's pouch. It appears as an anechoic fluid collection with well-defined edges that are bordered by Glisson's capsule of the liver and Gerota's fascia of the right kidney (Fig. 4.33). Fluid can also collect in the subphrenic space and will appear as a crescent-shaped anechoic collection that is bordered by the diaphragm superiorly and the liver inferiorly (Fig. 4.34). Other less common areas where fluid may be detected are at the superior pole of the kidney in Morison's pouch (Fig. 4.35) or at the tip of the liver (Fig. 4.36).

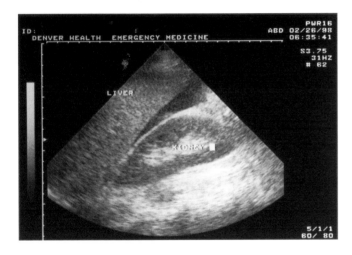

Figure 4.33. Ultrasound appearance of free fluid in Morison's pouch.

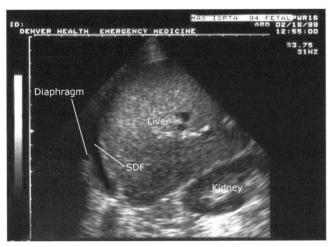

A

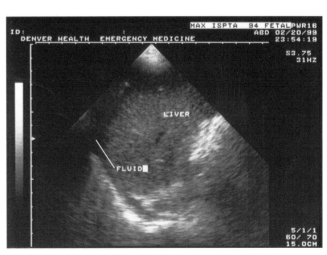

B

Figure 4.34 a, b. Images of fluid visualized in the right subdiaphragmatic space (SDF, subdiaphragmatic).

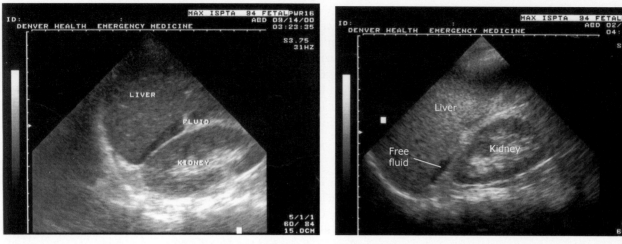

Figure 4.35 a, b. Examples of the appearance of peritoneal fluid collecting at the superior pole of the right kidney.

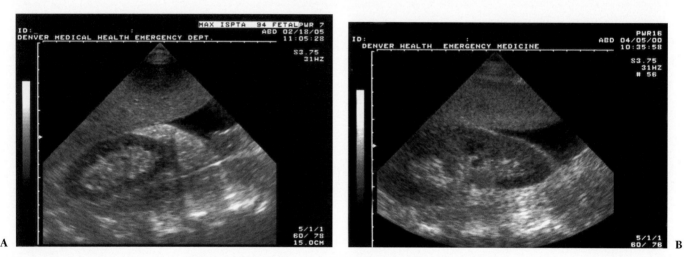

Figure 4.36. Examples of peritoneal fluid visualized at the tip of the liver.

Perisplenic fluid

Free fluid in the left upper quadrant collects differently than in the perihepatic area, primarily because the phrenicocolic ligament restricts fluid from filling the splenorenal interface. Consequently, fluid is most commonly detected in the subphrenic space and appears as a crescent-shaped, anechoic fluid collection that is bordered superiorly by the diaphragm and inferiorly by the spleen (Fig. 4.37). Alternatively, fluid may be seen at the tip of the spleen (Fig. 4.38). On rare occasions when large amounts of fluid are present, fluid can be found between the spleen and the kidney (Fig. 4.39).

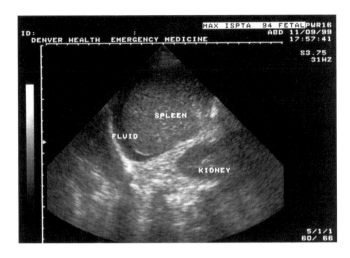

Figure 4.37. Peritoneal fluid detected in the left subdiaphragmatic space.

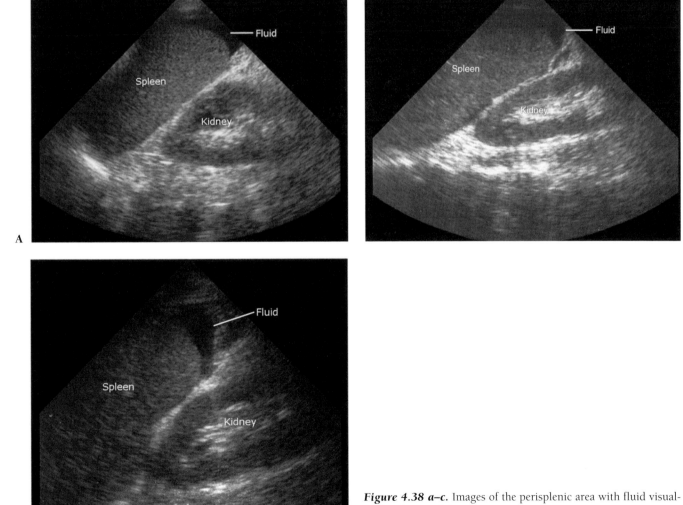

Figure 4.38 a–c. Images of the perisplenic area with fluid visualized at the tip of the spleen.

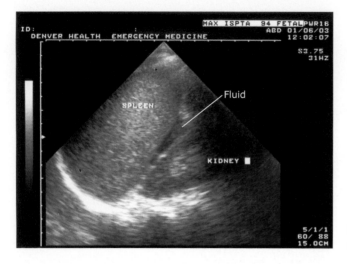

Figure 4.39. Ultrasound image of the left upper quadrant demonstrating fluid in the interface between the spleen and kidney.

Pelvic fluid

Free fluid in the pelvis has a variety of appearances depending on patient gender and transducer orientation. In the transverse plane, fluid in a male pelvis can be seen in the retrovesicular space as an anechoic fluid collection that outlines the posterior wall of the bladder (Fig. 4.40 **a**, **b**). In the transverse orientation of the female pelvis, fluid will collect posterior to the uterus (Fig. 4.41) or, if enough fluid is present, between the body of the uterus and the bladder. When viewing the pelvis in the sagittal orientation, fluid will collect in the same places as in the transverse orientation, but it will appear differently. For instance, in the male pelvis, the fluid will collect posterior to the bladder, but it is represented by an anechoic space between the dome of the bladder and the bowel wall (Fig. 4.42 **a**, **b**, **c**). It has a similar appearance in the female patient except that it collects in the space between the uterus and bowel (Fig. 4.43 **a**, **b**). As with all scanning applications, both transverse and sagittal planes are critical to fully evaluate the pelvis for fluid, as there are many imaging artifacts and confusing structures that can confound the exam.

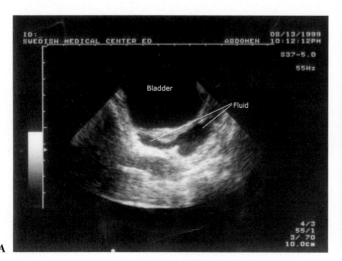

A

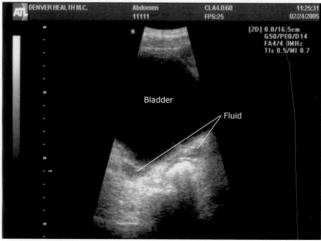

B

Figure 4.40 a, b. Sonographic appearance of fluid collecting posterior to the bladder in male patients with the transducer in the transverse orientation.

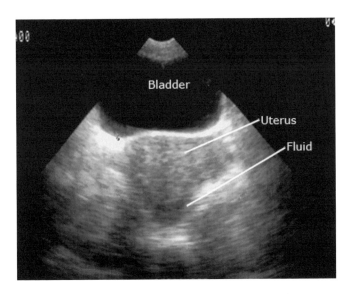

Figure 4.41. Ultrasound image of free fluid located posterior to the uterus with the transducer in the transverse orientation.

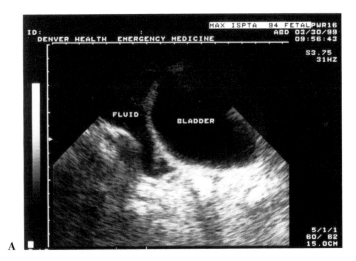

A

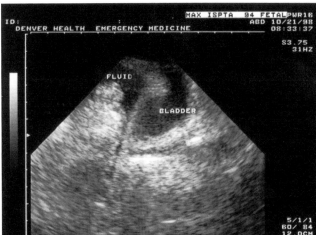

B

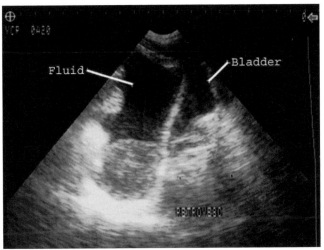

C

Figures 4.42 a–c. Sagittal orientation of male pelvis demonstrating fluid at the superior aspect of the bladder.

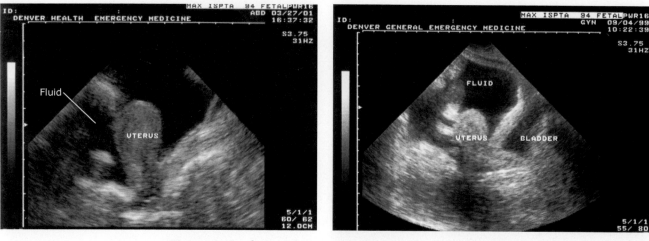

Figures 4.43 a, b. Sagittal orientation of female pelvis demonstrating fluid at the superior aspect of the bladder and uterus.

Paracolic gutter fluid

Fluid in the paracolic gutter has a specific appearance as it forms an anechoic, sharp-edged border to loops of bowel in the area (Fig. 4.44 **a, b**). The fluid pockets will vary in size and the space between loops of bowel will change with peristalsis.

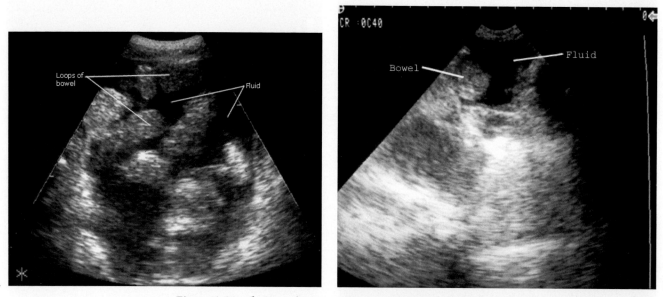

Figure 4.44 a, b. Paracolic gutter ultrasound images with fluid outlining loops of bowel.

Echogenic hemorrhage and clot

Most fresh peritoneal hemorrhage will appear anechoic, however, as clot forms and organizes, it becomes more echogenic. Clotted blood has a midlevel echo pattern that has some sonographic similarities to tissue, such as the spleen or liver parenchyma (Fig. 4.45). Col-

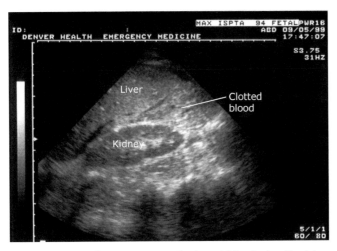

Figure 4.45. Perihepatic view with clotted blood visualized between the liver and the kidney. Note the similar echo pattern between the clotted blood and the liver tissue.

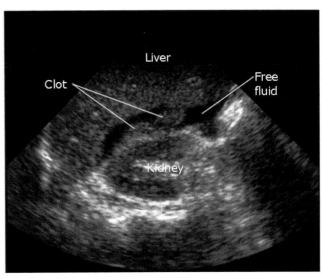

Figure 4.46. A positive Morison's pouch view with free fluid outlining clotted blood.

lections of clotted blood can be found in patients with long transport times or large volumes of peritoneal bleeding. The ability to differentiate clotted peritoneal blood from normal parenchyma can at times be difficult, but in most cases, thorough inspection of the area in question will demonstrate that an anechoic stripe, representing free peritoneal fluid, borders the clotted blood (Fig 4.46).

Solid Organ Injury

The sonographic appearance of specific organ injury varies. The ultrasound appearance of parenchymal damage in the liver can appear as anechoic or echogenic distortion of the normal architecture (Fig 4.47 **a–c**), and manifestations of injury can include subcapsular fluid collections and intraperitoneal fluid (30–34). The most common pattern of parenchymal liver injury identified by ultrasonography in patients with blunt abdominal trauma is a discrete region of increased echoes followed by a diffuse hyperechoic pattern (Fig. 4.48 **a–c**).

Spleen injuries, much like liver injuries, can have a variety of appearances. The most sensitive finding is either hemoperitoneum or a subcapsular fluid collection, whereas the most specific finding is an alteration in the normal homogenous architecture of the parenchyma (35–37). Sonographic patterns of splenic parenchymal injury include (most commonly) a diffuse heterogeneous appearance (Fig. 4.49), hyperechoic and hypoechoic splenic crescents (Fig. 4.50), and discrete hyperechoic or hypoechoic regions within the spleen (Fig. 4.51).

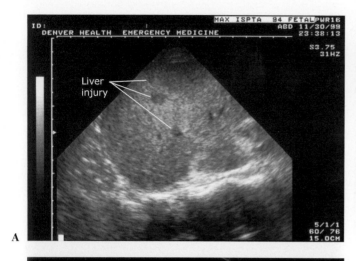

A

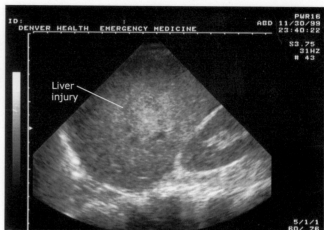

B

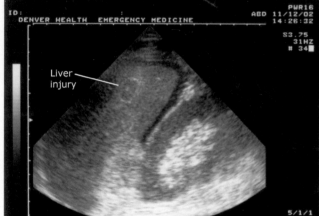

C

Figures 4.47 a–c. Examples of liver injuries visualized as a distortion of the normal tissue anatomy.

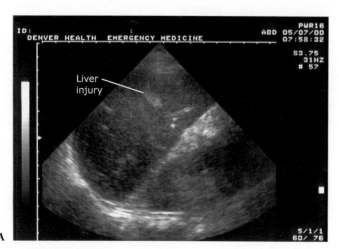

A

Figure 4.48 a–c. Liver injury manifesting sonographically as hyperechoic lesions within the parenchyma.

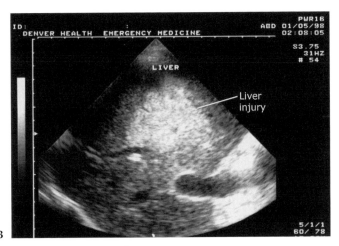

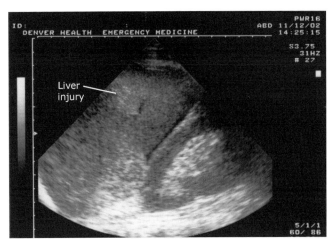

B   **C**

Figure 4.48 (continued)

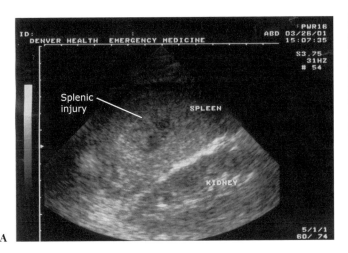

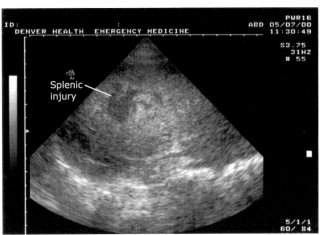

A   **B**

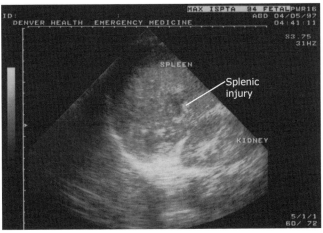

C

Figure 4.49 a–c. Injury seen by ultrasound as a heterogeneous appearance to the splenic tissue.

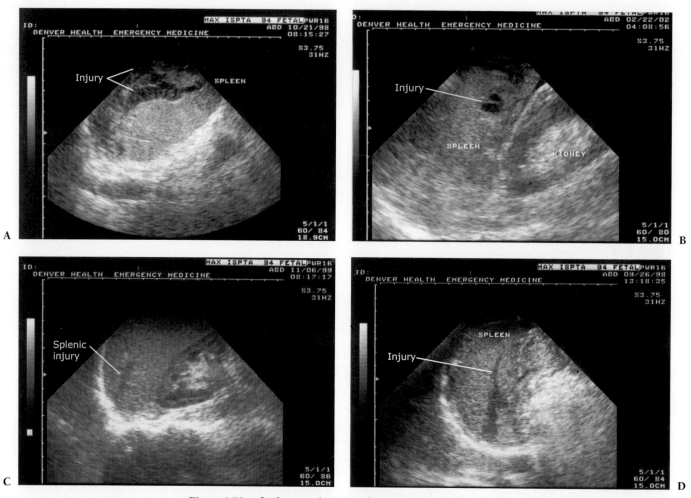

Figure 4.50 a–d. Ultrasound images of splenic injuries seen as hypoechoic cresent-shaped lesions.

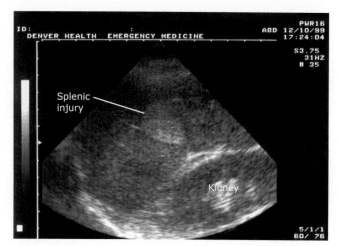

Figure 4.51. Hyperechoic lesion within the spleen representing parenchymal injury.

PERICARDIAL EFFUSION

Hemorrhage can accumulate quickly in the potential space between the visceral and parietal pericardium and create hypotension due to a cascade of increasing intrapericardial pressure leading to a lack of right heart filling followed by decreased left ventricular stroke volume. Fluid in the pericardial space appears as an anechoic stripe that conforms to the outline of the cardiac structures. In most cases, the fluid should have the same anechoic character as blood within the cardiac chambers. From the subxiphoid orientation, fluid will initially be seen between the right side of the heart and the liver, which is the most dependent area visualized (Fig. 4.52). In the parasternal orientation, fluid may also be seen anteriorly superior to the right ventricle or posteriorly as it outlines the free wall of the left atria and ventricle (Fig. 4.53). The descending aorta is an important landmark for the posterior pericardial sac. Pericardial fluid will often collect just anterior to the descending aorta (Fig. 4.54).

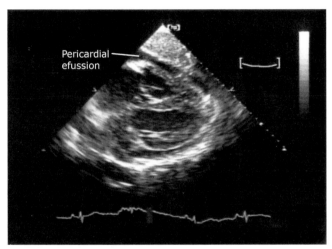

Figure 4.52. Ultrasound image taken from the subxiphoid transducer position demonstrating fluid in the pericardial space.

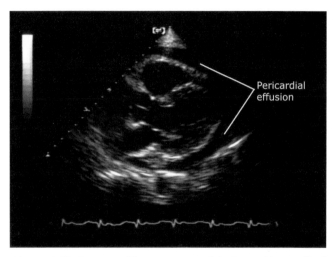

Figure 4.53. Parasternal long axis view of the heart showing fluid in the pericardial space.

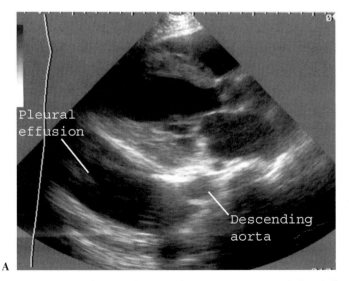

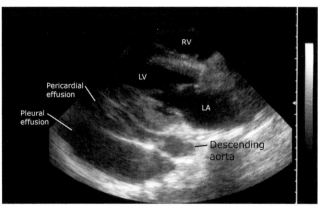

Figure 4.54. Ultrasound images demonstrating pericardial and pleural effusions from the long axis parasternal transducer position. (*a*) Note that the descending aorta is the structure that delineates pericardial from pleural fluid (*b*) (RV = right ventricle, LV = left ventricle, LA = left atrium).

Circumferential effusion

Various methods have been suggested for quantifying pericardial effusions viewed by ultrasound. One of the most straightforward methods is to determine whether the effusion is circumferential. Those that are circumferential but less than a centimeter in width are considered moderate-sized collections, whereas those greater than one centimeter in width are classified as large (Fig. 4.55). It is important to note that even small pericardial effusions can cause tamponade, so quantifying the amount of fluid within the pericardial space is secondary to assessing the patient's hemodynamic status.

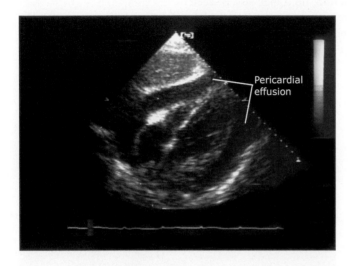

Figure 4.55. Ultrasound image demonstrating a circumferential pericardial effusion viewed from the subxiphoid transducer position.

Echogenic effusions

Effusions that are echogenic present a diagnostic challenge. Echogenic effusions may occur if blood clots are present, but may be due to preexisting pathology such as infection (pus), inflammation (fibrinous material), or malignancy. Instead of an anechoic appearance to the effusion, the fluid may have a similar echogenic character to surrounding structures such as the liver or ventricular tissue (Fig. 4.56 a–c). This isoechoic character can make the assessment for pericardial effusion challenging.

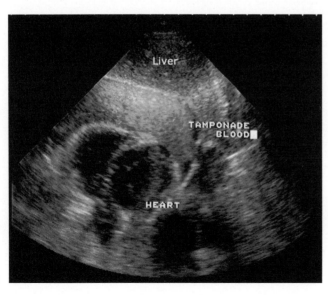

A

Figure 4.56 a–c. Images demonstrating clotted hemopericardium.

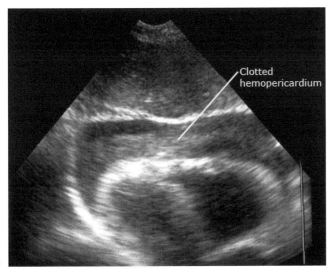

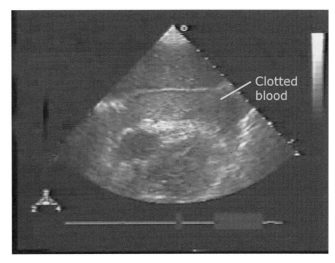

B

C

Figures 4.56 (continued)

Cardiac tamponade
After determining that a pericardial effusion is present, the next step is to determine whether there is sonographic evidence of cardiac tamponade. The pathophysiology of tamponade is characterized by increasing pericardial pressure that eventually exceeds atrial and ventricular pressures, thus inhibiting cardiac filling. As pericardial pressure increases, there is sequential collapse of the right atrium and subsequently the right ventricle (Fig. 4.57). Although the right atrial collapse occurs sooner than right ventricular collapse, this finding is less specific for diagnosing tamponade (38). Another potentially helpful sonographic finding is bowing of the interventricular septum into the left ventricle. This late finding is very specific for tamponade (39).

An additional means of assessing for elevated central venous pressure is to image the inferior vena cava. One method is the "sniff test," in which the patient is instructed to inhale quickly through his or her nose while the examiner simultaneously visualizes the inferior vena cava. Two studies have shown that incomplete collapse (< 40%) of the inferior vena cava correlates well with elevated central venous pressure measurements (Fig. 4.58 **a, b**) (40,41).

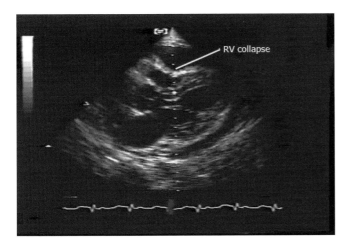

Figure 4.57. Long axis parasternal ultrasound image demonstrating collapse of the right ventricle in a patient with cardiac tamponade.

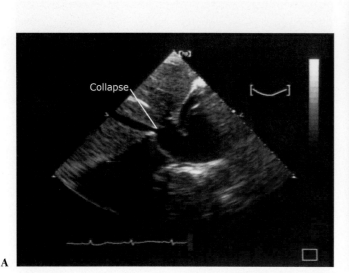

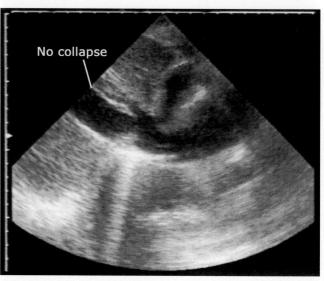

Figure 4.58 a. Image taken of a patient with a moderate-sized pericardial effusion. Note how the vena cava collapses with respiration. *b.* Image taken of another patient with a moderate sized pericardial effusion. In this case, note how there is no evidence of collapse of the vena cava with respiration. This patient had cardiac tamponade.

PLEURAL ABNORMALITIES

Pleural fluid

The sonographic appearance of hemothorax is an anechoic fluid collection localized to the costophrenic angle (Fig. 4.59). While it is imperative to visualize the diaphragm in order to be assured that the fluid is contained within the pleural cavity, other structures will frequently be seen, such as the lung. It appears as a triangular structure superior to the diaphragm that will exhibit wave-like movement that corresponds with the patient's respirations (Fig. 4.60).

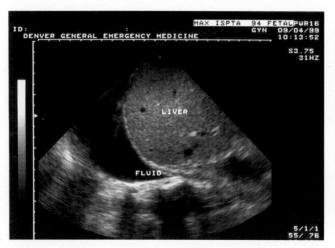

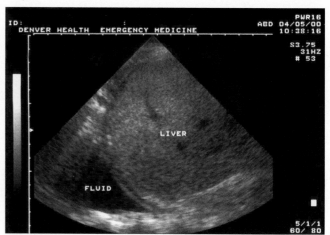

Figure 4.59 a, b. Images of fluid localized to the costophrenic angle.

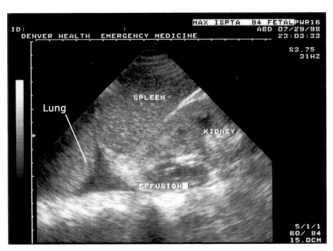 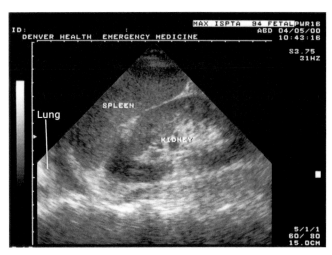

A   B

Figure 4.60 a, b. Ultrasound images demonstrating fluid in the costrophrenic angle and the triangular appearance of lung tissue.

Pneumothorax

The value of the ultrasound for the evaluation of pneumothorax is in its negative predictive value. If the sliding sign, ring down artifact, or the power slide sign are present, the diagnosis of pneumothorax is essentially excluded. Absence of these findings for making the diagnosis of pneumothorax has less diagnostic accuracy and has not been correlated with the size of the pneumothorax.

ARTIFACTS AND PITFALLS

GENERAL ISSUES

A variety of conditions create particular challenges for ultrasound in the trauma patient.

1. Prior surgery with accompanying adhesions can affect how fluid will collect and move within the peritoneal cavity. As a result, fluid may be seen in different areas than those scanned during the standard FAST exam. Particular attention should be paid to the exam performed on patients with evidence of prior abdominal surgery. If the suspicion for injury is high and the ultrasound is negative for fluid, CT scanning is a better method for fully evaluating the peritoneal cavity.
2. Obese patients can be difficult scanning subjects. Increased adipose tissue distances the transducer from the target organ or area. In addition, fat that collects in and around organs can distort normal anatomy.
3. Subcutaneous emphysema is problematic for scanning. Just as air in the lung or bowel distorts the ultrasound signal, air in the subcutaneous tissue prevents penetration of sound waves and limits the usefulness of ultrasound imaging.

Types of Fluid

Ultrasound is extremely sensitive for detecting peritoneal fluid, but it does not discriminate between types of fluid, i.e., blood versus ascites, succus entericus, or urine. The following are types of fluid that may cause false-positive ultrasound exams.

1. Preexisting ascites is the main diagnostic pitfall in the evaluation of trauma patients with free peritoneal fluid (Fig. 4.61). Clues to this condition include physical stigmata of liver disease such as caput medusa, spider angiomas, or jaundice; past medical history for liver

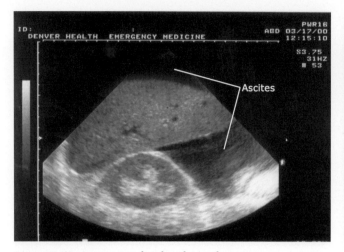

Figure 4.61. Ascites visualized in the perihepatic area.

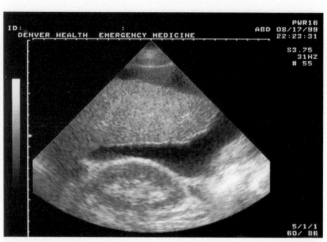

Figure 4.62. Fluid detected in the perihepatic region in a patient with sonographic evidence of liver disease.

disease; or sonographic findings such as a small, contracted, nodular, or echogenic liver (Fig. 4.62).

2. Hollow viscous injuries are another etiology of positive ultrasound exams. Examples include bowel, gallbladder, and intraperitoneal bladder rupture. While these may be considered false-positive exams for hemoperitoneum, in fact, each requires some form of operative intervention and, therefore, in the authors' opinion, should be considered true-positive exams.

Exam quality

While many pathologic findings of the trauma ultrasound exam are straightforward and easy to detect, a poor-quality study can obscure even the most obvious abnormalities. The following are some of the technical factors that can affect the quality of the trauma ultrasound exam.

1. Too much overall gain creates artifact and may obscure the presence of anechoic fluid (Fig. 4.63).
2. "Static imaging," or failing to scan through the full extent of an anatomical area, is a frequent error that limits the exam. At any one moment, ultrasound only provides a two-dimensional image. However, a three-dimensional view can be created by gently

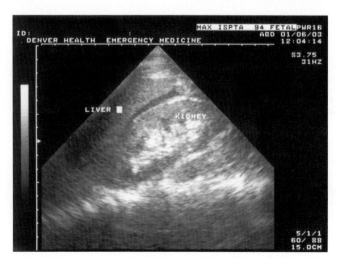

Figure 4.63. Ultrasound image of hemoperitoneum in Morison's pouch. The gain is set too high, making the fluid difficult to discern.

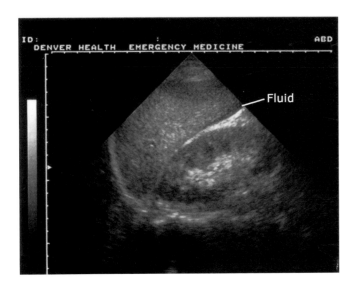

Figure 4.64. Ultrasound image of the perihepatic region that was initially interpreted as negative for free fluid. Further inspection detected a small amount fluid in Morison's pouch.

rocking and maneuvering the transducer to view multiple planes through an anatomical space. Each potential space should be interrogated with biplanar views and frequent angling of the transducer. Static imaging limits the view, minimizes the amount of information gained from the scan, and can miss small fluid collections (Fig. 4.64).

3. Failing to appreciate fluid in "non-classic" areas is another common scanning problem. For example, free fluid may accumulate superior to Morison's pouch, inferior to the left kidney, superior to the dome of the bladder, and inferior to the diaphragm. Dynamic movement of the transducer will allow for visualization of these and other potential spaces that are not considered "classic."

PERIHEPATIC VIEW

1. Perinephric fat may cause a common and sometimes confusing sonographic finding in the right upper quadrant (Fig. 4.65). Fat in the perinephric area creates an echogenic space between the kidney and liver that can be mistaken for organized, clotted peritoneal blood. It can usually be distinguished from hemoperitoneum because it has a more homogeneous echodensity than hematoma and has no anechoic rim. Perinephric fat is adherent and has no motion with respiration, in contrast to hematoma that can move independent of the kidney.

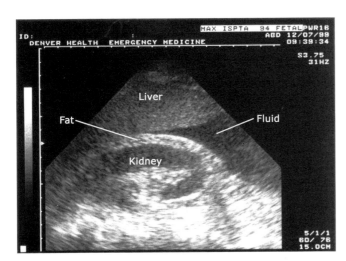

Figure 4.65. The sonographic appearance of perinephric fat in a patient who also has fluid in Morison's pouch.

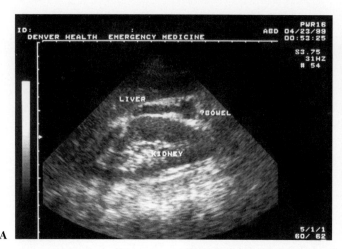 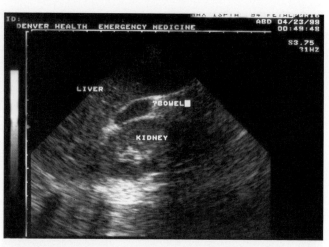

A   B

Figures 4.66 a, b. Ultrasound images demonstrating the appearance of fluid-filled bowel seen in Morison's pouch which can be mistaken for free peritoneal fluid.

2. Either fluid-filled bowel (Fig 4.66) or the gallbladder (Fig. 4.67) can be visualized in the perihepatic area and misinterpreted as free peritoneal fluid. In each case, a careful examination usually demonstrates characteristics of each structure that distinguishes them from peritoneal blood. The gallbladder has echogenic walls, and the rounded fundus is usually visible near the tip of the liver. This is in contrast to fluid in Morison's pouch, which tends to have sharp corners and angles. Fluid-filled bowel is an uncommon finding of the FAST exam (42). It can usually be distinguished by an echogenic wall bounding the lateral aspects of the fluid. As well, there will typically be several discrete, echogenic lines that appear to originate from and run perpendicular to the echogenic wall. These structures represent the valvulae conniventes or haustral sacculations of the bowel (43).

3. Retroperitoneal hemorrhage from a renal parenchyma laceration may initially appear as fluid within Morison's pouch. A more detailed examination will demonstrate that the anechoic fluid collection is deep to the echogenic line of Gerota's fascia (Figure 4.68 **a**). The fluid may also form an anechoic rim surrounding the kidney or the architecture of the kidney may be distorted (4.68 **b**).

4. Clotted blood in Morison's pouch can have a similar echogenic appearance to the liver parenchyma and therefore can be challenging to assess (Fig. 4.45). In most cases there will be a rim of anechoic fluid outlining the clotted blood that helps discern the presence of a pathologic condition (Fig. 4.46).

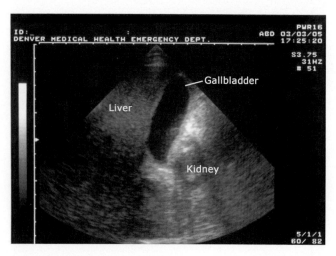

Figure 4.67. The typical appearance of the gallbladder seen during scanning in the perihepatic region.

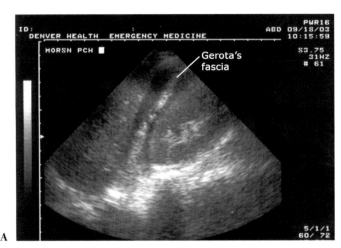

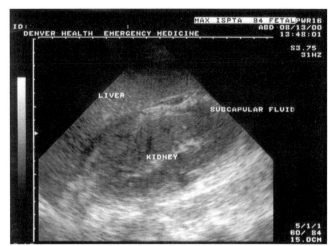

A B

Figure 4.68 (***a***) Ultrasound image of retroperitoneal and intraperitoneal hemorrhage that outlines Gerota's fascia. (***b***) Renal parenchymal injury seen as disruption of the normal renal architecture and subcapsular fluid.

PERISPLENIC VIEW

1. The most challenging aspect of scanning the left upper quadrant is obtaining adequate views. Not only does the spleen offer a much smaller acoustic window than the liver, but it is also more posterior and superior. If an acceptable image of the perisplenic area is not obtained, it is usually because the transducer is not high and posterior enough.

2. Another common error is assuming that fluid in the left upper quadrant collects in a manner similar to the right upper quadrant. The phrenicocolic ligament restricts the amount of fluid that will collect in the splenorenal space, so the focus of the exam should be directed towards the subdiaphragmatic area and the tip of the spleen.

3. The stomach is commonly visualized and may confuse the exam of the perisplenic area. It has a variable sonographic appearance, depending on its contents. If the stomach contains fluid, it may appear anechoic. If it contains mostly food particles, it may appear echogenic (Fig. 4.69). When seen, it almost appears contiguous with the spleen (Fig. 4.70), but angling the transducer slightly posterior will usually remove it from view.

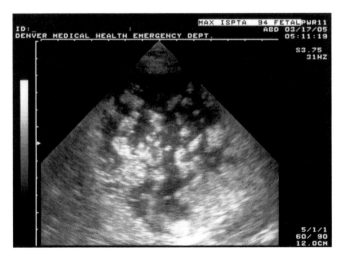

Figure 4.69. Ultrasound image of a fluid and food-filled stomach seen in the left upper quadrant.

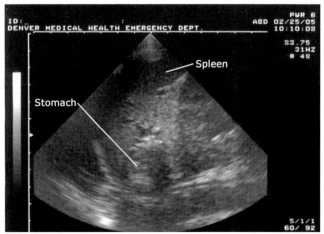

Figure 4.70. A view of the perisplenic region that illustrates the close proximity of the spleen and stomach.

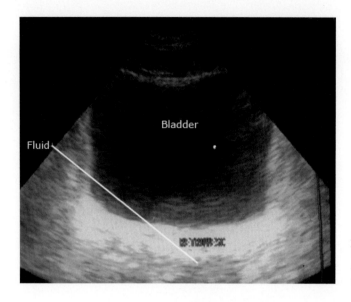

Figure 4.71. Ultrasound image of the male pelvis showing the bladder visualized with too much gain. Note how difficult it is to appreciate the fluid in the retrovesicular space due to the brightness of the image.

PELVIC VIEW

1. Too much gain or acoustic enhancement can dramatically alter images of the retrovesicular area (Fig. 4.71) where fluid typically collects in the pelvis. The retrovesicular area is easiest to image in patients with a filled bladder. However, objects behind fluid-filled structures are enhanced acoustically. While this enhancement allows deeper structures to be visualized, it can also distort them. It may be necessary to minimize the gain to optimize the image behind the bladder and avoid artifact. This can usually be accomplished by decreasing the TGC in the affected area.

2. Ovarian cysts can occasionally be mistaken for peritoneal fluid (Fig. 4.72). A detailed exam that includes different planes of view will demonstrate that these fluid collections have well-demarcated borders and are contained within ovarian tissue.

3. The prostate and seminal vesicles have a hypoechoic appearance posterior to the bladder in male patients (Fig. 4.73). These may be mistaken for free fluid unless a sagittal view of the area is obtained that confirms the inferior, regular appearance of the prostate and the triangular shape of the seminal vesicles. Familiarity with normal ultrasound anatomy in the pelvis will avoid potential misinterpretations.

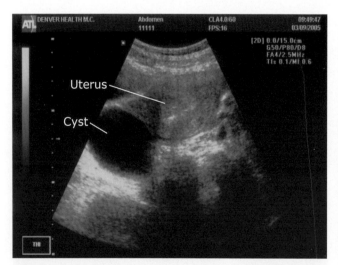

Figure 4.72. Transverse view of the uterus showing a ovarian cyst in the right lower quadrant that could be mistaken for free peritoneal fluid.

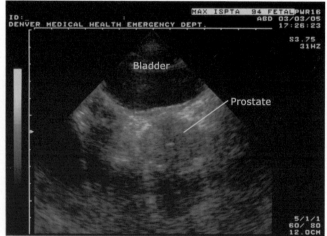

Figure 4.73. The appearance of the prostate posterior to the bladder in the transverse plane.

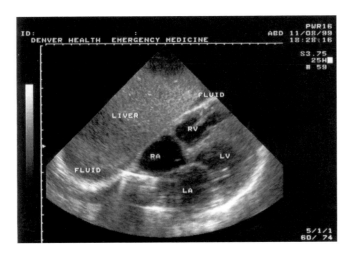

Figure 4.74. Ultrasound image demonstrating the appearance of peritoneal fluid seen from the subxiphoid transducer position.

PERICARDIAL VIEW

1. One of the most common pitfalls in scanning the pericardial area is failing to adjust the depth controls to adequately visualize deep structures. Without optimal depth adjustment, scans may fail to visualize all the cardiac structures and miss posterior pericardial effusions.

2. A pleural effusion, especially on the left side, may mimic a pericardial effusion. The parasternal long-axis view is the best approach to conclusively differentiate pericardial from pleural fluid. Using this transducer position, the descending aorta is viewed in transverse orientation posterior to the heart. Fluid in the pleural space is localized posterior to the descending aorta, whereas pericardial fluid will collect between the posterior wall of the left ventricle and the descending aorta (Fig. 4.54) (44).

3. Occasionally, large amounts of perihepatic fluid can be mistaken for a pericardial effusion when imaged from the subxiphoid transducer position. This can be distinguished from a pericardial effusion by an echogenic band (pericardium) that is between the echo-free space and the free wall of the right ventricle. Additionally, perihepatic fluid collections will conform to Glisson's capsule whereas a pericardial effusion will conform to the rounded aspect of the pericardium adjacent to the apex of the heart (Fig. 4.74).

4. Epicardial fat appears as an echo-free space anterior to the heart that can be as wide as 15 mm (Fig. 4.75). This space will generally narrow toward the apex of the heart, whereas an echo–free space caused by a pericardial effusion tends to be broader near the left ventricular apex than near its base. Additionally, although epicardial fat appears grossly as an echo-free space, there will usually be scattered, soft, isolated reflections adhering to and moving with the myocardium.

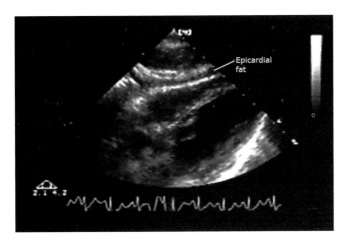

Figure 4.75. Subxiphoid orientation with epicardial fat visualized between the free wall of the right ventricle and the liver.

USE OF THE IMAGE IN MEDICAL DECISION MAKING

The most practical and significant use of ultrasound in all trauma patients is the rapid identification of the source of hypotension and detection of immediate life-threatening injuries, including free intraperitoneal blood and pericardial effusions. In the setting of hypotension and trauma, ultrasound may help identify patients who need immediate surgical intervention, bypassing all other diagnostic procedures. In the setting of mass casualties, ultrasound can help prioritize operative intervention and direct the use of limited resources to those most in need of immediate definitive care. In rural areas and settings remote from trauma centers, ultrasound can help rapidly identify victims who should be moved to higher levels of care. In some cases, ultrasound alone may be sufficient to triage patients to the operating room, while in others, ultrasound will be used in conjunction with CT and DPL. Thus the use of ultrasound in decision making depends upon the stability of the patient, the nature of the trauma, the number of patients undergoing simultaneous evaluation, and the level of care available at the hospital.

BLUNT TRAUMA (FIG. 4.76)

The FAST exam is best known for its role in the detection of free fluid in patients with blunt abdominal trauma. General guidelines for how ultrasound impacts immediate, bedside decisions follow.

Peritoneal free fluid in the unstable patient

The finding of free peritoneal fluid in the unstable traumatized patient suggests the findings of intraperitoneal injury necessitating immediate operative intervention. The decision to operate will depend on the patient's other injuries, the amount and location of free peritoneal fluid, and whether the vital signs stabilize after resuscitation. Large peritoneal fluid collections associated with unstable vital signs usually mandate laparotomy (45,46).

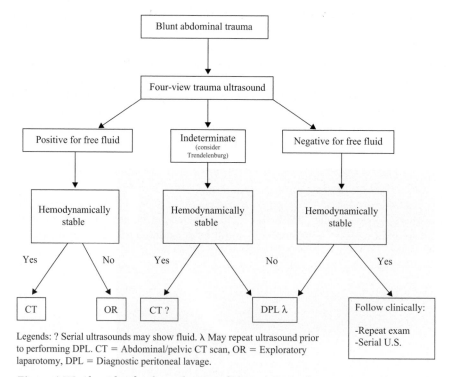

Legends: ? Serial ultrasounds may show fluid. λ May repeat ultrasound prior to performing DPL. CT = Abdominal/pelvic CT scan, OR = Exploratory laparotomy, DPL = Diagnostic peritoneal lavage.

Figure 4.76. Algorithm for the evaluation of blunt abdominal trauma using ultrasound.

Peritoneal free fluid in the stable patient

A patient with stable vital signs, but an ultrasound that demonstrates peritoneal fluid is a candidate for nonoperative management. Therefore, regardless of whether any other ultrasound findings such as specific organ injury are present, a CT of the abdomen and pelvis should be performed. This form of management utilizes the strength of the CT scan for determining the source of hemoperitoneum; thus, it can usually differentiate between lesions that are operable versus those that can be managed nonoperatively.

No free fluid in the unstable patient

Ultrasound is virtually 100% sensitive for hemoperitoneum in the hypotensive patient (47). However, the patient with unstable vital signs and a negative ultrasound remains problematic, since hemoperitoneum remains a lethal, albeit remote, possibility. A few options exist for this diagnostic dilemma. Some have suggested a repeat ultrasound, potentially by a more experienced operator (48). Others opt for an immediate DPL, which is generally more sensitive than ultrasound. However, a negative ultrasound suggests that the source of hypotension is outside the peritoneum. Diagnostic efforts to identify alternative injuries should focus on other common causes, including retroperitoneal injuries and neurogenic shock. In one study of 47 hypotensive trauma patients with a negative ultrasound, none required a laparotomy for acute control of hemorrhage (49). The primary cause of hypotension in these patients was extraperitoneal, such as retroperitoneal hemorrhage caused by pelvic fractures or neurogenic shock.

No free fluid in the stable patient

The finding of no free fluid in a hemodynamically stable patient does not "clear" that patient of injury (50–52). Patients may still have encapsulated solid organ injury, mesenteric or bowel injury, retroperitoneal hemorrhage, or delayed intraperitoneal injury. Patients who are at higher risk include those with lower rib, lumbar spine, or pelvic fractures. Prior to discharge, every patient should have a repeat clinical exam and any new findings of abdominal pain, tenderness, distracting injury, or laboratory abnormalities should prompt further diagnostic evaluation. In this case, management of the patient will be influenced largely by the mechanism of trauma, suspicion of occult injury, and the presence of other injuries.

Indeterminate findings

Certain patients will have indeterminate ultrasound exams. Anatomic defects (pectus excavatum), acquired pathology (open wounds, subcutaneous air), difficult habitus (obesity), and poor acoustic windows (evacuated bladder) are situations that may result in an indeterminate ultrasound exam (53). These patients should receive further clinical, radiographic, or alternative diagnostic evaluation.

Pericardial Effusion (Fig. 4.77)

Transthoracic cardiac ultrasound can detect pericardial effusion associated with blunt cardiac rupture (54–56). Patients with a pericardial effusion should be evaluated for cardiac tamponade, which includes both a targeted physical exam and echocardiographic evaluation. Those with tamponade require an immediate procedure—either pericardiocentesis, pericardiocentesis with pigtail catheter placement, or therapeutic thoracotomy. Those without signs of tamponade might be considered for consultative imaging such as a cardiology echo. Although it is a diagnosis of exclusion, pericardial effusion detected incidentally has been described as a finding of the FAST exam (57).

Solid organ injury

The clinical utility of positive and negative sonographic examinations for specific organ injuries is limited. Some studies have inferred that a negative exam, in certain patients, is sufficient to change medical decision making (58,59). Each of these studies recommended that ultrasound be the initial diagnostic modality for evaluating patients with renal trauma. If a stable, nomotensive patient has a normal renal ultrasound, no hematuria, and no other

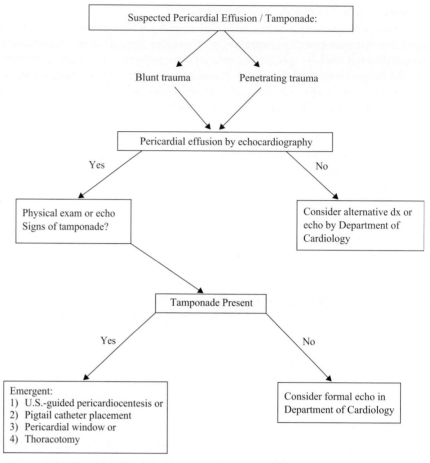

Figure 4.77. Algorithm for the evaluation of pericardial effusion using ultrasound.

significant injuries, then their evaluation was complete. There have been no similar recommendations for the ultrasound evaluation of other organs.

A positive result, on the other hand, may direct certain aspects of the diagnostic evaluation. For instance, in most series, a positive ultrasound exam in a hemodynamically stable patient is an indication for additional diagnostic testing. Commonly this is a CT scan of the abdomen and pelvis, which provides specific information regarding the extent and severity of the organ injuries. Another benefit is that CT scanning can determine whether there are injuries to other organs.

The identification of solid organ injury in the hemodynamically unstable patient provides very little useful information. If a specific etiology for the hypotension is not identified, yet the patient has free intraperitoneal fluid, invariably the patient will undergo laparotomy. Knowing that a specific organ injury exists does not change the approach, technique, or decision making in hemodynamically unstable patients. Another important issue is that ultrasound is poor at identifying injuries to multiple organs, so there is no assurance that an injury identified sonographically is the primary or only etiology of the instability. As a result, there are no widely recognized algorithms that include the presence or absence of specific organ injury identified by ultrasound into clinical decision making.

PENETRATING TRAUMA

Patients with penetrating trauma confront physicians with many of the same diagnostic dilemmas as in blunt trauma: the need to make a diagnosis is imperative, but the diagnostic options are sometimes limited. The utility of ultrasound in this setting should not be underestimated.

Abdomen

Trauma patients with isolated penetrating abdominal wounds who have an obvious indication for laparotomy (eviscerated bowel or peritonitis) do not need an ultrasound, although a positive ultrasound exam is very specific for injury (60,61). Defining the role of ultrasound in the stable patient is problematic as neither a positive or negative exam for peritoneal fluid can be relied upon to absolutely predict or exclude significant injury (61). A patient with a stab wound and a negative ultrasound exam can have significant mesenteric or bowel injury, whereas a positive study may be associated with injuries that can be managed nonoperatively. However, in patients with multiple penetrating wounds, the sonographic evaluation of the peritoneum and pericardium can direct the operative approach to the chest, abdomen, or both. As well, the presence or absence of hemopericardium from gapping or even innocuous–appearing wounds to the chest or epigastrium can be definitively assessed with sonographic evaluation of the pericardial space. As in blunt abdominal trauma, ultrasound can also quantitate the amount of free fluid and potential for sudden deterioration.

Chest (Fig. 4.77)

The ultrasound finding of pericardial fluid can rapidly identify patients who need immediate treatment to avoid hemodynamic deterioration secondary to cardiac tamponade. In the setting of penetrating trauma to the torso, the presence of pericardial fluid suggests penetration of the pericardium and possible injury to a cardiac chamber (62,63). Sonographic signs of impending cardiovascular collapse include right atrial systolic collapse, right ventricular diastolic collapse, a dilated inferior vena cava without respiratory variation, and intraventricular septal flattening.

The patient with penetrating trauma to the torso and no pericardial fluid should have a period of observation prior to ruling out the possibility of cardiac injury (64,65). Delayed presentations of pericardial effusions have occurred, especially with injuries to the right atrium and ventricle, which are low pressure chambers that may not leak until increased intravascular volume causes clot breakdown. Another concern is the presence of a left-sided pleural effusion. It should alert the resuscitating physician that penetration of both anterior and posterior surfaces of the pericardium may have occurred, thus allowing spontaneous evacuation of the pericardial effusion into the pleural space (66,67).

EXPANDED APPLICATIONS: THORACIC TRAUMA

In addition to the primary clinical applications for the FAST exam, other uses for ultrasound in trauma patients have recently been suggested. These include the sonographic assessment of the pleural spaces for blood or air.

Pleural fluid

The detection of hemothorax in a supine trauma patient can be problematic as the supine portable chest radiograph can be insensitive for small fluid collections. Ultrasound, on the other hand, has been estimated to detect as little as 20 mL of pleural fluid (68). Ultrasound may be useful for the detection of hemothorax in both blunt and penetrating thoracic trauma, however this is an evolving standard that has not yet been widely accepted (69–71). Pleural fluid detected during trauma ultrasound should be interpreted in the clinical context of the effusion. Patients with decreased breath sounds, evidence of chest trauma, hypoxemia, chest radiography with pleural effusion, hypotension, or other findings suggestive of tension hemothorax, may be aided by the sonographic findings of fluid in the pleural space. Decompression and evacuation procedures can then proceed. However, an ultrasound exam that does not demonstrate pleural fluid should not be interpreted as eliminating traumatic pleural effusion from the differential, especially in the patient with blunt chest trauma (71).

Pneumothorax

The use of ultrasound to evaluate for pneumothorax is a relatively new concept, and its role in trauma decision making is evolving. At this time, it is an adjunctive technique that may identify pneumothorax earlier than chest radiography, especially in the supine patient or those with small pneumothoraces. Several studies provide support for the use of ultrasound to detect or exclude pneumothorax in the trauma patient (72,73). In one study, a single ultrasound exam of the anterior thorax was 95% sensitive and 100% specific for pneumothoraces that were detected by chest radiography (72). A second study found similar results (73), adding weight to this conclusion. Standard radiographs for the detection of pneumothorax may be limited by patient position. Air that collects anteriorly or inferiorly, rather than in the apices, may be difficult to appreciate on a supine chest radiograph. Ultrasound findings that suggest pneumothorax include the absence of a sliding sign or comet tail artifact. These findings should be followed by clinical correlation of breath sounds and chest radiography. Ultrasound is probably most useful in its negative predictive value. In other words, if the ultrasound exam performed by an experienced sonographer is interpreted as negative for pneumothorax, the diagnosis can be excluded or considered less likely.

SPECIAL CONSIDERATIONS

Obstetric patients

The use of ultrasound for the diagnostic evaluation of the pregnant blunt trauma patient has the benefits of not exposing the mother and fetus to ionizing radiation and invasive procedures, while also being able to assess for peritoneal fluid and fetal viability (74–76). The primary application of trauma ultrasound in the pregnant patient is no different than that in the nonpregnant patient, which is the noninvasive evaluation of the peritoneal and thoracic cavities for blood. While the peritoneal anatomy will change in pregnancy, especially in the late second and third trimesters, the FAST exam technique is the same and fluid is still readily identifiable in the standard potential spaces.

Another equally useful application of ultrasound in the pregnant trauma patient is the assessment of fetal gestational age and fetal cardiac activity. In later pregnancy, the easiest estimation of gestational age is obtained by measuring the biparietal diameter. Although there is some institutional variation, fetuses greater than 24 weeks gestational age are considered viable. Fetal cardiac activity should be assessed for presence and rate as bradycardia is a marker of fetal distress caused by poor perfusion or hypoxia. Blood may be shunted away from the fetus before the mother exhibits obvious signs of hypotension.

Pediatric patients

One of the primary roles of emergency sonography of pediatric patients is the evaluation of blunt abdominal trauma. While the finding of peritoneal fluid is a similar primary goal for adult and pediatric patients, results have been somewhat discouraging for the latter (77–82). This is surprising, because one of the limitations of sonography, obesity, is encountered much less commonly in pediatric patients. Although the sensitivity is reported to be lower in pediatric patients, the specificity is still excellent.

Even more discouraging have been the pediatric studies citing the accuracy of ultrasound in the evaluation of solid organ injury. Little useful information can be gleaned from an ultrasound to evaluate the solid organs; CT is far superior in this regard.

Ultimately, the role of ultrasound in pediatric blunt abdominal trauma is limited by the increasingly conservative management of solid organ injuries in children. While ultrasound may detect free peritoneal fluid, this information has little impact on management since CT and clinical observation will determine the course of action in pediatric patients with splenic and liver injuries.

Pelvic Fracture

There are a number of confounding factors to be considered when interpreting an ultrasound exam in the patient with a pelvic fracture. The first is that a significant amount of bleeding from a pelvic fracture may be isolated to the retroperitoneum, which is an area where ultrasound is unreliable (52). Another concern is the association of intraperitoneal bladder rupture with pelvic fractures, especially in the patient with hemodynamic instability (83). In this case, free fluid detected by ultrasound may represent urine, not blood.

As a result, it has been suggested that the patient with a positive ultrasound and severe pelvic fractures undergo a DPL as their next diagnostic test (83).

Triage of multiple patients or disaster situations
Ultrasound has qualities, such as being quick, noninvasive, portable, and sensitive, that make it an ideal imaging modality for the evaluation of large numbers of traumatically injured patients. In trauma centers it is not unusual to experience the simultaneous presentation of multiple, potentially critically injured patients. Decisions regarding patient priority for the operating room, CT scan, or procedural intervention are magnified when resources are stretched to their limits. One study demonstrated that the results of a FAST exam could be used to determine patient priority for operative intervention (84). Others have incorporated an ultrasound exam into the evaluation of patients sustaining injuries on the battlefield and during a natural disaster (85,86).

COMPARISON WITH OTHER DIAGNOSTIC MODALITIES

The diagnostic approach to the traumatically injured patient typically involves a variety of diagnostic tests, including plain radiographs, DPL, ultrasound, CT, and clinical observation with serial exams. Each test has advantages and disadvantages and the integration of each in the management of trauma is influenced by many factors, including the nature of the trauma and the stability of the patient (Table 4.1).

Patients with blunt abdominal trauma present a distinct challenge to physicians. The workup for blunt abdominal trauma primarily focuses on the detection of free intraperitoneal fluid. The physical exam for significant injuries is notoriously unreliable with error rates reported to be as high as 45% (87) and accuracy rates at best being 65% (88). DPL has a long history in the evaluation of patients with blunt abdominal trauma, but it is invasive, time-consuming, not specific for organ injury, and sometimes overly sensitive, resulting in nontherapeutic laparotomies. CT comprises the majority of diagnostic imaging in blunt abdominal trauma, however it is expensive, time-consuming, and requires that the patient be stable in order to be transported out of the ED. Ultrasound offers many advantages compared with DPL and CT. It is sensitive for hemoperitoneum, noninvasive, can be performed quickly and simultaneously with other resuscitative measures, and provides immediate information at the patient's bedside. Ultrasound has not completely replaced CT or DPL, but has assumed a primary role in the early bedside assessment of blunt trauma.

Table 4.1: Comparison of Common Diagnostic Modalities for the Trauma Patient

Comparison Category	US	DPL	CT
Speed	2.5 min	20 min	20–60 min
Cost	Low	Low	High
Bedside Test	+++	+++	−
Repeatable	+++	−	++
Blunt Trauma	+++	+++	+++
Penetrating Trauma	++	++	+++
Unstable Patient	+++	++	−
Identifies Bleeding Site	+/−	−	++
Nonoperative Management	++	−	+++
Retroperitoneal / Renal	++	−	+++
Pancreas	+/−	+	+++
Pelvic Fracture	+/−	−	+++
Accuracy	94–97%	97.6%	92–98%

While detecting intraperitoneal fluid is of some importance, the more critical issue is whether a laparotomy is indicated. In the past, this question was often answered by the results of a DPL. A positive DPL by either initial aspiration or subsequent cell counts was an indication for an exploratory laparotomy. While looking for a noninvasive, less time-consuming alternative to DPL, a number of studies have assessed the ability of ultrasound as an adjunct in making this decision (4–8,89). All of these studies report favorable results when comparing sensitivity and specificity of ultrasound to DPL. Many trauma centers, therefore, have abandoned the use of DPL in favor of ultrasonography.

There are a few exceptions to the generalization that ultrasound can entirely replace DPL. The unstable hypotensive patient with blunt trauma and a negative ultrasound and the patient with penetrating abdominal trauma are important exceptions. While it has been suggested that a negative ultrasound for peritoneal fluid in the hemodynamically unstable patient is reliable enough to prompt a search for an extraperitoneal source of instability (49), in some EDs, DPL will still be the study of last resort after a thorough consideration for other sources of shock. As well, the results of an ultrasound exam in a patient with an abdominal stab wound can be deceiving; many centers will opt to proceed with wound exploration, DPL, laparoscopy, or laparotomy.

Detecting hemoperitoneum or predicting the need for laparotomy are significant diagnostic endpoints for the emergency physician, but it is also important to determine the extent of specific organ injury. Recently this has become even more relevant as many surgeons are managing splenic and liver injury nonoperatively. In most centers indications for laparotomy are currently based, to some extent, on CT grading of organ injury. Enthusiasm for a similar role for ultrasound has been present for some time (90). Despite the early interest, investigators have failed to establish a definitive role for ultrasound in specific organ injury detection. Not only is ultrasound not accurate for evaluating retroperitoneal hemorrhage or bowel injuries, but it also cannot be relied upon to grade the severity of organ injury, detect active bleeding, or isolate injury to a single organ. These limitations of ultrasound are in competition with the fact that access, speed, and accuracy of CT scanning has increased significantly in recent years. Therefore, in trauma centers, where timely access to high-speed CT scanners is not limited, there is little sound evidence for ultrasound supplanting CT scan in the diagnostic evaluation of the stable blunt abdominal trauma patient.

Unfortunately, unlimited access to abdominal CT scanning is not always available. Trauma centers may be presented with multiple stable patients requiring CT scanning and ultrasound may be used to triage which, and in what order, patients should be scanned. As well, patients can present with blunt abdominal trauma to hospitals where there is limited or no access to a CT scanner. A positive ultrasound exam in this setting can be used to mobilize a CT technologist from home, alert a trauma surgeon on call, or initiate immediate transport to a trauma center.

It is important to recognize the limitation of physical exams for detecting traumatic intraperitoneal injuries (87,88). Many physicians rely on the physical exam to detect occult injuries from relatively minor trauma from mechanisms such as falls or low-speed motor vehicle accidents. This is potentially a dangerous practice. One case series reported on six alert, non-intoxicated patients with seemingly minor trauma who had no complaints of abdominal pain or tenderness, yet were found to have significant hemoperitoneum detected incidentally by ultrasound (91). While the true incidence of this scenario is unknown, the presentation of these cases is still alarming and suggests that even patients with minor blunt trauma should have an ultrasound exam, rather than relying on a physical exam alone to exclude significant intraperitoneal injury.

INCIDENTAL FINDINGS

As clinicians apply bedside ultrasound, they will inevitably encounter a variety of incidental conditions, both normal and pathological. The responsible clinician should be prepared to recognize common variants and appreciate abnormalities that require follow-up.

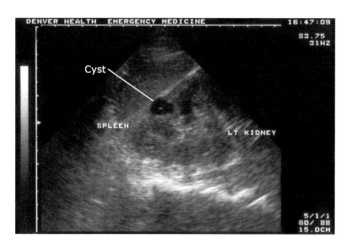

Figure 4.78. The appearance of a renal cyst that was detected during a FAST exam.

Cysts

Cysts may be found in the liver, spleen, kidneys, or ovaries. Sonographically, benign cysts appear as unilocular round structures that exhibit good sound transmission, lack internal projections, and have thin walls and an anechoic center (Fig. 4.78). All cysts, whether or not they appear benign, should have follow-up arranged after their ED visit or inpatient hospitalization.

Masses

Masses may take different forms with variable patterns of echogenicity (Fig. 4.79). Concerning findings include heterogeneity of solid organs, abnormal patterns of normal layers, and abnormal organ size. All masses should have confirmatory diagnostic testing and follow-up.

Abnormal Organ Size or Chambers

The FAST exam may also detect organs that appear smaller or larger than normal. Examples include cardiomegaly, abdominal aortic aneurysm, small or absent kidneys, or large uteri or ovaries. The severity of the abnormality and clinical circumstances will dictate the immediacy, type, and location of the follow-up.

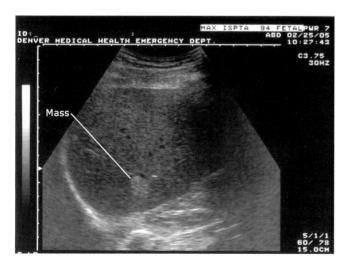

Figure 4.79. Ultrasound image of a lesion in the liver that was detected during a FAST exam. It was determined by CT to be a hemangioma.

CLINICAL CASES

CASE ONE

A 31-year-old male was brought in by paramedics after being involved in a head-on motor vehicle accident. His initial blood pressure was 110/40 mm Hg with a pulse rate of 130 beats per minute. The patient is intubated and unresponsive to all stimuli. He has been given 750 cc of crystalloid via two intravenous lines. On arrival to the ED, his primary survey is significant for decreased breath sounds bilaterally with associated vital signs of a pulse of 140 beats per minute and a blood pressure of 70 mm Hg systolic. Blood products are given and an ultrasound is performed simultaneously with radiographs of the chest and pelvis. The chest and pelvis x-rays were interpreted as normal. The FAST exam findings are shown in Figures 4.80–4.81.

The resuscitating physician's impression of the trauma ultrasound was that free peritoneal fluid was present in Morison's pouch, the pelvis, and the right pleural cavity. The left flank and the subxiphoid view were interpreted as negative for fluid. Based on the patient's ultrasound findings and hemodynamic status, the decision was made to insert a right tube thoracostomy and then proceed directly to the operating room. The exploratory laparotomy was significant for a grade-4 spleen laceration with 1500 cc of associated hemoperitoneum. The patient had a splenectomy with control in peritoneal bleeding and made an uneventful post-operative recovery.

CASE TWO

A 45-year-old male was brought to the ED by ambulance with a single stab wound to the left anterior chest. The injury occurred approximately 20 minutes prior to ED arrival by an unknown assailant with an unknown object. Prehospital vital signs were a systolic blood pressure of 110 mm Hg, pulse of 100 beats per minute, and respirations of 24 per minute. Upon arrival to the ED, the patient's vital signs were a systolic blood pressure of 70 mm Hg, pulse rate of 110 beats per minute, and a respiratory rate of 30 breaths per minute. His physical exam was remarkable for a 2-centimeter wound to the left anterior chest with no other wounds visualized after full exposure. The patient was awake, alert, diaphoretic, and in moderate distress. The physical exam was otherwise unremarkable. An ultrasound exam of his heart was performed immediately on arrival which was significant for a moderate-

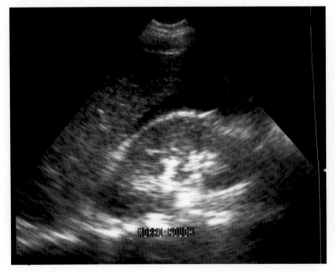

Figure 4.80. Case One. FAST exam, image 1.

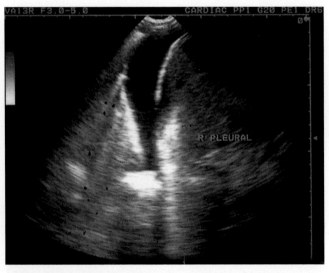

Figure 4.81. Case One. FAST exam, image 2.

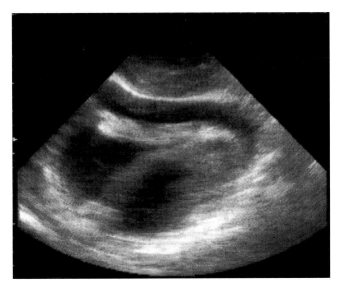

Figure 4.82. Case Two. An ultrasound exam of the heart significant for a moderate sized pericardial effusion.

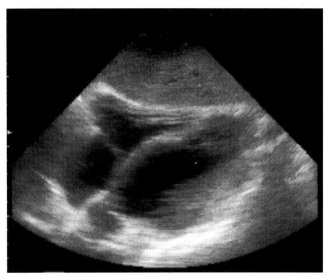

Figure 4.83. Case Two. A repeat ultrasound done 4 minutes after the first was interpreted as being free of pericardial fluid.

sized pericardial effusion (Fig 4.82). The patient was then intubated and a successful pericardiocentesis was performed. A repeat ultrasound done 4 minutes after the first was interpreted as being free of pericardial fluid (Fig 4.83). The patient was taken emergently to the operating room where a 1-centimeter laceration in his right ventricle was repaired. He was discharged from the hospital two days later after an uneventful hospital course.

REFERENCES

1. Goldberg BB, Goodman GA, Clearfield HR. Evaluation of ascites by ultrasound. Radiology 1970; 96:15–22.
2. Goldberg BB, Clearfield HR, Goodman GA, et al. Ultrasonic determination of ascites. Arch Intern Med 1973; 131:217–220.
3. Goldberg BB. Ultrasonic evaluation of intraperitoneal fluid. JAMA 1976; 235:2427–2430.
4. Gruessner R, Mentges B, Duber C, et al. Sonography versus peritoneal lavage in blunt abdominal trauma. J Trauma 1989; 29:242–244.
5. Bode PJ, Niezen RA, van Vugt AB, et al. Abdominal ultrasound as a reliable indicator for conclusive laparotomy in blunt abdominal trauma. J Trauma 1993; 34:27–31.
6. Glaser K, Tschmelitsch J, Klingler P, et al. Ultrasonography in the management of blunt abdominal and thoracic trauma. Arch Surg 1994; 129:743–747.
7. McKenney M, Lentz K, Nunez D, et al. Can ultrasound replace diagnostic peritoneal lavage in the assessment of blunt trauma? J Trauma 1994; 37:439–441.
8. Lentz KA, McKenney MG, Nunez DB Jr, et al. Evaluating blunt abdominal trauma: role for ultrasonography. J Ultrasound Med 1996; 15:447–451.
9. Tso P, Rodriguez A, Cooper C, et al. Sonography in blunt abdominal trauma: a preliminary progress report. J Trauma 1992; 33:39–43; discussion 43–44.
10. Rozycki GS, Shackford SR. Ultrasound, what every trauma surgeon should know. J Trauma 1996; 40:1–4.
11. Scalea TM, Rodriguez A, Chiu WC, et al. Focused Assessment with Sonography for Trauma (FAST): results from an international consensus conference. J Trauma 1999; 46:466–472.
12. Stengel D, Bauwens K, Sehouli J, et al. Discriminatory power of 3.5 MHz convex and 7.5 MHz linear ultrasound probes for the imaging of traumatic splenic lesions: a feasibility study. J Trauma 2001; 51:37–43.
13. Biffl WL, Moore EE, Kendall J. Postinjury torso ultrasound: FAST should be SLOH. J Trauma 2000; 48:781–782.

14. Henderson SO, Sung J, Mandavia D. Serial abdominal ultrasound in the setting of trauma. J Emerg Med 2000; 18:79–81.

15. Blaivas M, DeBehnke D, Phelan MB. Potential errors in the diagnosis of pericardial effusion on trauma ultrasound for penetrating injuries. Acad Emerg Med 2000; 7:1261–1266.

16. Ma OJ, Kefer MP, Mateer JR, et al. Evaluation of hemoperitoneum using a single- vs multiple-view ultrasonographic examination. Acad Emerg Med 1995; 2:581–586.

17. Rozycki GS, Ochsner MG, Feliciano DV, et al. Early detection of hemoperitoneum by ultrasound examination of the right upper quadrant: a multicenter study. J Trauma 1998; 45:878–883.

18. Jehle D, Guarino J, Karamanoukian H. Emergency department ultrasound in the evaluation of blunt abdominal trauma. Am J Emerg Med 1993; 11:342–346.

19. Islam NB, Levy PD. Emergency bedside ultrasound to detect pneumothorax. Acad Emerg Med 2003; 10:819–820; author reply 820–821.

20. Forsby J, Henriksson L. Detectability of intraperitoneal fluid by ultrasonography. An experimental investigation. Acta Radiol Diagn (Stockh) 1984; 25:375–378.

21. Branney SW, Wolfe RE, Moore EE, et al. Quantitative sensitivity of ultrasound in detecting free intraperitoneal fluid. J Trauma 1995; 39:375–380.

22. Branney SW, Wolfe RE, Albert NP. The reliability of estimating intraperitoneal fluid volume with ultrasound. Acad Emerg Med (abstract) 1995; 2:345.

23. Jehle D, Adams B, Sukumvanich P, et al. Ultrasound for the detection of intraperitoneal fluid: the role of Trendelenburg positioning. Acad Emerg Med (abstract) 1995; 2:407.

24. Von Kuenssberg Jehle D, Stiller G, Wagner D. Sensitivity in detecting free intraperitoneal fluid with the pelvic views of the FAST exam. Am J Emerg Med 2003; 21:476–478.

25. Abrams BJ, Sukumvanich P, Seibel R, et al. Ultrasound for the detection of intraperitoneal fluid: the role of Trendelenburg positioning. Am J Emerg Med 1999; 17:117–120.

26. Tiling T, Bouillon B, Schmid A, et al. Ultrasound in blunt abdominothoracic trauma. In: Border J, Algoewer M, Reudi T, eds. *Blunt multiple trauma*. New York: Marcel Dekker Inc, 1990.

27. Goletti O, Ghiselli G, Lippolis PV, et al. The role of ultrasonography in blunt abdominal trauma: results in 250 consecutive cases. J Trauma 1994; 36:178–181.

28. Meyers MA. The spread and localization of acute intraperitoneal effusions. Radiology 1970; 95:547–554.

29. Hahn DD, Offerman SR, Holmes JF. Clinical importance of intraperitoneal fluid in patients with blunt intra-abdominal injury. Am J Emerg Med 2002; 20:595–600.

30. van Sonnenberg E, Simeone JF, Mueller PR, et al. Sonographic appearance of hematoma in liver, spleen, and kidney: a clinical, pathologic, and animal study. Radiology 1983; 147: 507–510.

31. Yoshii H, Sato M, Yamamoto S, et al. Usefulness and limitations of ultrasonography in the initial evaluation of blunt abdominal trauma. J Trauma 1998; 45:45–50; discussion 50–51.

32. Lam AH, Shulman L. Ultrasonography in the management of liver trauma in children. J Ultrasound Med 1984; 3:199–203.

33. Froelich JW, Simeone JF, McKusick KA, et al. Radionuclide imaging and ultrasound in liver/spleen trauma: a prospective comparison. Radiology 1982; 145:457–461.

34. Richards JR, McGahan JP, Pali MJ, et al. Sonographic detection of blunt hepatic trauma: hemoperitoneum and parenchymal patterns of injury. J Trauma 1999; 47:1092–1097.

35. Weill F, Bihr E, Rohmer P, et al. Ultrasonic study of hepatic and splenic traumatic lesions. Eur J Radiol 1981; 1:245–249.

36. Richards JR, McGahan JP, Jones CD, et al. Ultrasound detection of blunt splenic injury. Injury 2001; 32:95–103.

37. Richards JR, McGahan PJ, Jewell MG, et al. Sonographic patterns of intraperitoneal hemorrhage associated with blunt splenic injury. J Ultrasound Med 2004; 23:387–394, quiz 395–396.

38. Singh S, Wann LS, Schuchard GH, et al. Right ventricular and right atrial collapse in patients with cardiac tamponade—a combined echocardiographic and hemodynamic study. Circulation 1984; 70:966–971.

39. Reddy PS, Curtiss EI, Uretsky BF. Spectrum of hemodynamic changes in cardiac tamponade. Am J Cardiol 1990; 66:1487–1491.

40. Moreno FL, Hagan AD, Holmen JR, et al. Evaluation of size and dynamics of the inferior vena cava as an index of right-sided cardiac function. Am J Cardiol 1984; 53:579–585.

41. Kircher BJ, Himelman RB, Schiller NB. Noninvasive estimation of right atrial pressure from the inspiratory collapse of the inferior vena cava. Am J Cardiol 1990; 66:493–496.

42. Kendall JL, Ramos JP. Fluid-filled bowel mimicking hemoperitoneum: a false-positive finding during sonographic evaluation for trauma. J Emerg Med 2003; 25:79–82.

43. Fleischer AC, Dowling AD, Weinstein ML, et al. Sonographic patterns of distended, fluid-filled bowel. Radiology 1979; 133:681–685.

44. Lewandowski BJ, Jaffer NM, Winsberg F. Relationship between the pericardial and pleural spaces in cross-sectional imaging. J Clin Ultrasound 1981; 9:271–274.

45. Ma OJ, Kefer MP, Stevison KF, et al. Operative versus nonoperative management of blunt abdominal trauma: Role of ultrasound-measured intraperitoneal fluid levels. Am J Emerg Med 2001; 19:284–286.

46. McKenney KL, McKenney MG, Cohn SM, et al. Hemoperitoneum score helps determine need for therapeutic laparotomy. J Trauma 2001; 50:650–654; discussion 654–656.

47. Rozycki GS, Ballard RB, Feliciano DV, et al. Surgeon-performed ultrasound for the assessment of truncal injuries: lessons learned from 1540 patients. Ann Surg 1998; 228:557–567.

48. Forster R, Pillasch J, Zielke A, et al. Ultrasonography in blunt abdominal trauma: influence of the investigators' experience. J Trauma 1993; 34:264–269.

49. Wherrett LJ, Boulanger BR, McLellan BA, et al. Hypotension after blunt abdominal trauma: the role of emergent abdominal sonography in surgical triage. J Trauma 1996; 41:815–820.

50. Chiu WC, Cushing BM, Rodriguez A, et al. Abdominal injuries without hemoperitoneum: a potential limitation of focused abdominal sonography for trauma (FAST). J Trauma 1997; 42:617–623; discussion 623–625.

51. Sirlin CB, Brown MA, Deutsch R, et al. Screening US for blunt abdominal trauma: objective predictors of false-negative findings and missed injuries. Radiology 2003; 229:766–774.

52. Sirlin CB, Brown MA, Andrade–Barreto OA, et al. Blunt abdominal trauma: clinical value of negative screening US scans. Radiology 2004; 230:661–668.

53. Boulanger BR, Brenneman FD, Kirkpatrick AW, et al. The indeterminate abdominal sonogram in multisystem blunt trauma. J Trauma 1998; 45:52–56.

54. Pretre R, Chilcott M. Blunt trauma to the heart and great vessels. N Engl J Med 1997; 336:626–632.

55. Schiavone WA, Ghumrawi BK, Catalano DR, et al. The use of echocardiography in the emergency management of nonpenetrating traumatic cardiac rupture. Ann Emerg Med 1991; 20:1248–1250.

56. Brevetti GR, Zetterlund P, Spowart G. Delayed cardiac tamponade complicating airbag deployment. J Trauma 2002; 53:104–105.

57. Lukan JK, Franklin GA, Spain DA, et al. "Incidental" pericardial effusion during surgeon-performed ultrasonography in patients with blunt torso trauma. J Trauma 2001; 50:743–745.

58. Furtschegger A, Egender G, Jakse G. The value of sonography in the diagnosis and follow-up of patients with blunt renal trauma. Br J Urol 1988; 62:110–116.

59. Rosales A, Arango O, Coronado J, et al. The use of ultrasonography as the initial diagnostic exploration in blunt renal trauma. Urol Int 1992; 48:134–137.

60. Udobi KF, Rodriguez A, Chiu WC, et al. Role of ultrasonography in penetrating abdominal trauma: a prospective clinical study. J Trauma 2001; 50:475–479.

61. Soffer D, McKenney MG, Cohn S, et al. A prospective evaluation of ultrasonography for the diagnosis of penetrating torso injury. J Trauma 2004; 56:953–957; discussion 957–959.

62. Plummer D, Brunette D, Asinger R, et al. Emergency department echocardiography improves outcome in penetrating cardiac injury. Ann Emerg Med 1992; 21:709–712.

63. Tayal VS, Beatty MA, Marx JA, et al. FAST (focused assessment with sonography in trauma) accurate for cardiac and intraperitoneal injury in penetrating anterior chest trauma. J Ultrasound Med 2004; 23:467–472.

64. Harris DG, Janson JT, Van Wyk J, et al. Delayed pericardial effusion following stab wounds to the chest. Eur J Cardiothorac Surg 2003; 23:473–476.

65. Nagy KK, Lohmann C, Kim DO, et al. Role of echocardiography in the diagnosis of occult penetrating cardiac injury. J Trauma 1995; 38:859–862.

66. Meyer DM, Jessen ME, Grayburn PA. Use of echocardiography to detect occult cardiac injury after penetrating thoracic trauma: a prospective study. J Trauma 1995; 39:902–907; discussion 907–909.

67. Chan D. Echocardiography in thoracic trauma. Emerg Med Clin North Am 1998; 16:191–207.

68. Rothlin MA, Naf R, Amgwerd M, et al. Ultrasound in blunt abdominal and thoracic trauma. J Trauma 1993; 34:488–495.

69. Sisley AC, Rozycki GS, Ballard RB, et al. Rapid detection of traumatic effusion using surgeon-performed ultrasonography. J Trauma 1998; 44:291–296; discussion 296–297.

70. Ma OJ, Mateer JR. Trauma ultrasound examination versus chest radiography in the detection of hemothorax. Ann Emerg Med 1997; 29:312–315; discussion 315–316.

71. Abboud PA, Kendall J. Emergency department ultrasound for hemothorax after blunt traumatic injury. J Emerg Med 2003; 25:181–184.

72. Dulchavsky SA, Schwarz KL, Kirkpatrick AW, et al. Prospective evaluation of thoracic ultrasound in the detection of pneumothorax. J Trauma 2001; 50:201–205.

73. Knudtson JL, Dort JM, Helmer SD, et al. Surgeon-performed ultrasound for pneumothorax in the trauma suite. J Trauma 2004; 56:527–530.

74. Ma OJ, Mateer JR, DeBehnke DJ. Use of ultrasonography for the evaluation of pregnant trauma patients. J Trauma 1996; 40:665–668.

75. Goodwin H, Holmes JF, Wisner DH. Abdominal ultrasound examination in pregnant blunt trauma patients. J Trauma 2001; 50:689–693; discussion 694.

76. Bochicchio GV, Haan J, Scalea TM. Surgeon-performed focused assessment with sonography for trauma as an early screening tool for pregnancy after trauma. J Trauma 2002; 52:1125–1128.

77. Thourani VH, Pettitt BJ, Schmidt JA, et al. Validation of surgeon-performed emergency abdominal ultrasonography in pediatric trauma patients. J Pediatr Surg 1998; 33:322–328.

78. Partrick DA, Bensard DD, Moore EE, et al. Ultrasound is an effective triage tool to evaluate blunt abdominal trauma in the pediatric population. J Trauma 1998; 45:57–63.

79. Coley BD, Mutabagani KH, Martin LC, et al. Focused abdominal sonography for trauma (FAST) in children with blunt abdominal trauma. J Trauma 2000; 48:902–906.

80. Emery KH, McAneney CM, Racadio JM, et al. Absent peritoneal fluid on screening trauma ultrasonography in children: a prospective comparison with computed tomography. J Pediatr Surg 2001; 36:565–569.

81. Holmes JF, Brant WE, Bond WF, et al. Emergency department ultrasonography in the evaluation of hypotensive and normotensive children with blunt abdominal trauma. J Pediatr Surg 2001; 36:968–973.

82. Ong AW, McKenney MG, McKenney KA, et al. Predicting the need for laparotomy in pediatric trauma patients on the basis of the ultrasound score. J Trauma 2003; 54:503–508.

83. Jones AE, Mason PE, Tayal VS, et al. Sonographic intraperitoneal fluid in patients with pelvic fracture: two cases of traumatic intraperitoneal bladder rupture. J Emerg Med 2003; 25:373–377.

84. Blaivas M. Triage in the trauma bay with the focused abdominal sonography for trauma (FAST) examination. J Emerg Med 2001; 21:41–44.

85. Miletic D, Fuckar Z, Mraovic B, et al. Ultrasonography in the evaluation of hemoperitoneum in war casualties. Mil Med 1999; 164:600–602.

86. Sarkisian AE, Khondkarian RA, Amirbekian NM, et al. Sonographic screening of mass casualties for abdominal and renal injuries following the 1988 Armenian earthquake. J Trauma 1991; 31:247–250.

87. Olsen WR, Hildreth DH. Abdominal paracentesis and peritoneal lavage in blunt abdominal trauma. J Trauma 1971; 11:824–829.

88. Powell DC, Bivins BA, Bell RM. Diagnostic peritoneal lavage. Surg Gynecol Obstet 1982; 155:257–264.

89. Porter RS, Nester BA, Dalsey WC, et al. Use of ultrasound to determine need for laparotomy in trauma patients. Ann Emerg Med 1997; 29:323–330.

90. Asher WM, Parvin S, Virgillo RW, et al. Echographic evaluation of splenic injury after blunt trauma. Radiology 1976; 118:411–415.

91. Blaivas M, Sierzenski P, Theodoro D. Significant hemoperitoneum in blunt trauma victims with normal vital signs and clinical examination. Am J Emerg Med 2002; 20:218–221.

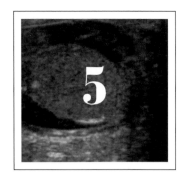

ECHOCARDIOGRAPHY

Christopher L. Moore
Henry Lin

INTRODUCTION

Emergency echocardiography (echo) is one of the most challenging ultrasound examinations for the emergency physician to become comfortable with, but is potentially among the most rewarding. Images and landmarks can be difficult to obtain consistently, orientation is sometimes confusing, and there is a wide range of pathology, some of which is beyond the scope of the emergency physician to diagnose with confidence. However, the ability to diagnose and exclude pericardial effusion and evaluate gross cardiac motion is well within the scope of all emergency physicians and can provide immediate, valuable diagnostic information.

Emergency echo also differs from other emergency ultrasound applications in that echocardiograms performed by another specialist (typically a cardiologist) can be much more difficult to obtain than other forms of ultrasound, especially in off hours. While the amount of training required to perform echocardiography may be controversial, with goal-directed training it is not difficult to determine the presence of a large pericardial effusion or evaluate gross cardiac motion (1–5). Emergency echocardiography offers great diagnostic potential for patients with a variety of presentations, from arrest situations to unexplained shock, dyspnea, or chest pain. The challenge is to discern what information emergency physicians can reliably obtain and use with focused emergency echo.

CLINICAL APPLICATIONS

Emergency echocardiography has been shown to provide diagnostic and prognostic information in an emergency department (ED) population with a variety of suspected cardiac-related symptoms (6–10). Emergency echocardiography is most likely to be effective when it is used in populations with a relatively high likelihood of pathology that is discernible by focused emergency echo: pericardial effusion, left ventricular systolic dysfunction, or severe right ventricular strain. The great benefit of emergency echo is that it lowers the threshold for testing, and may aid in making diagnoses that might otherwise be missed if obtaining an echocardiogram is time-consuming, difficult, or even impossible in the ED setting. While much research still needs to be done regarding the training and utility of echo by emergency physicians, the most high-yield presentations that may benefit from emergency echocardiography, especially when the diagnosis is in doubt, are: circulatory shock, shortness of breath, and chest pain. The use of emergency echo may provide valuable information in the detection and diagnosis of hypovolemia, congestive heart failure, pulmonary embolus, cardiogenic shock, pulseless electrical activity (PEA), and pericardial effusion with tamponade. It can also assist in bedside procedures such as pericardiocentesis and pacemaker placement as well as aid in the identification of mechanical pacer capture (either external or internal) (11–16) (See Chapter 13).

IMAGE ACQUISITION

There are three basic sonographic windows to the heart: subxiphoid, parasternal long axis (PSLA), and apical four-chamber views (Fig. 5.1–5.5). Many emergency physicians are most familiar with the subxiphoid (or subcostal) view as it is commonly taught as part of the trauma exam, although in our experience the parasternal window may be easier to obtain and often provides superior visualization of many cardiac structures. It is a rare patient who can be visualized well from all approaches, but comfort with different views should allow some visualization in even the most difficult patients.

Begin with patients supine and completely flat if they are able to tolerate the position. Some windows may also be improved by having the patient assume a left lateral decubitus position, which pulls the heart away from behind the sternum and toward the ribs of the left chest. Because the heart is on the left side of the body, some sonographers choose to position the machine on this side of the patient, although scanning from the right side of the patient is typically not too difficult and may be more comfortable if other examinations are done from this side. The transducer choice is typically a small footprint (i.e., small size to the face) transducer with a frequency range of 2–5 MHz, allowing visualization between the ribs. A phased array transducer is ideal if available, although a larger footprint transducer may be fine for a subxiphoid window. Many machines have a cardiac setting or application for the transducer that typically has higher contrast than abdominal settings, allowing improved differentiation between myocardium and blood. If available, tissue harmonic imaging may enhance visualization as well.

In contrast to many other areas of the body in which there are well-defined and separate external anatomic landmarks, the landmarks for sonographic images of the heart

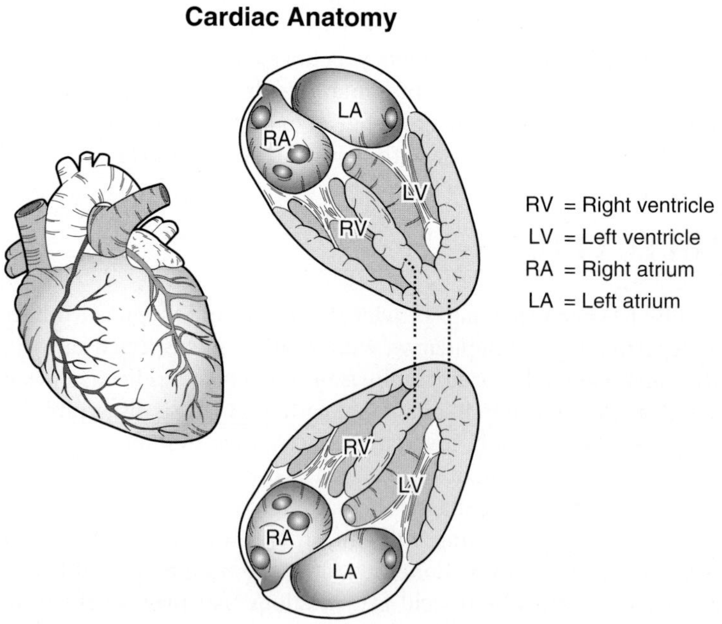

Cardiac Anatomy

RV = Right ventricle
LV = Left ventricle
RA = Right atrium
LA = Left atrium

Figure 5.1. Cardiac Anatomy. The heart is cut from the apex to the base (long axis) and folded down to expose the internal anatomy. The lower cut shows the structures in the orientation obtained from a subxiphoid window.

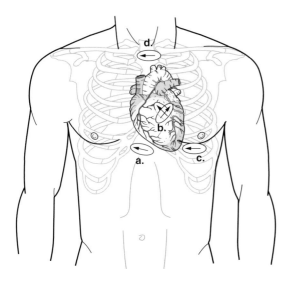

Figure 5.2. Transducer Placement. This diagram shows transducer placement and direction for the three primary windows (subxiphoid, parasternal long axis, and apical four-chamber) as well as two secondary windows (parasternal short axis and suprasternal). The arrow indicates direction of the indicator, generally to the patient's right or patient's head. (**a.** subxiphoid; **b.** long and short axis parasternal; **c.** apical; **d.** suprasternal)

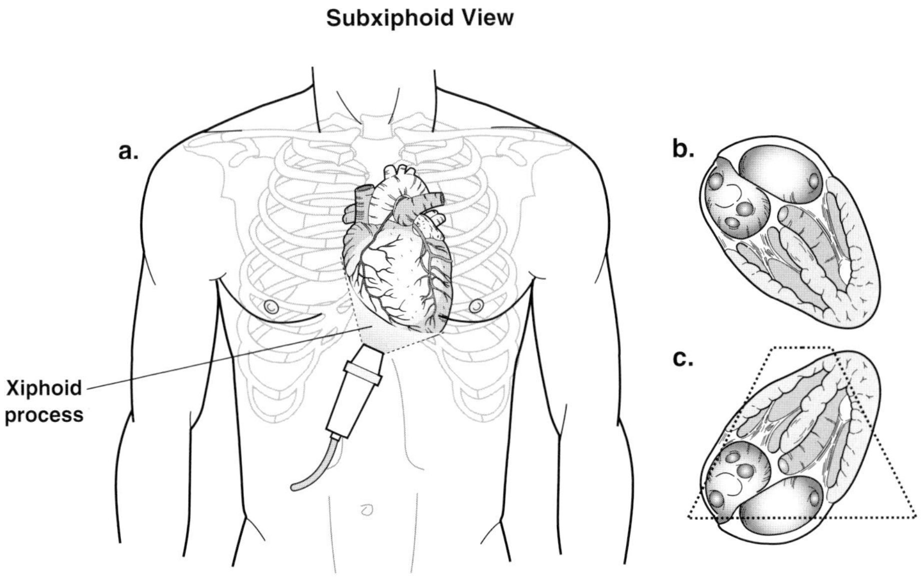

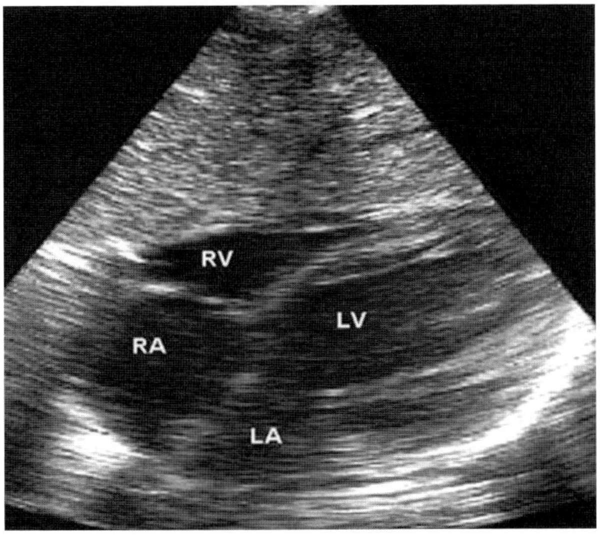

Subxiphoid View

Figure 5.3. Transducer placement, orientation, and anatomy for the subxiphoid (subcostal) cardiac view. Transducer placement is below the xiphoid process with the indicator to the patient's right and the beam angled up into the chest (**a**). The heart is seen as if it were cut in the plane of the ultrasound beam and folded down (**b**), with the lower image showing the anatomy as it appears on the ultrasound screen (**c**). Ultrasound image of the heart seen from the subxiphoid transducer position (**d**).

Parasternal Long Axis View

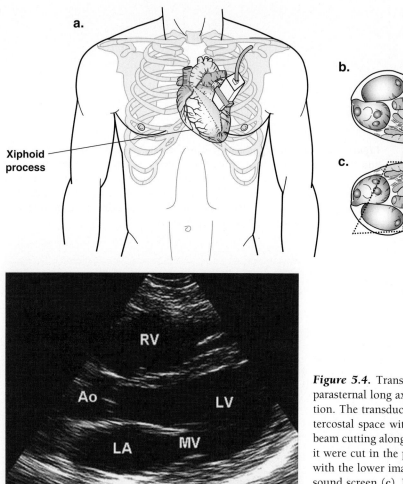

d.

Figure 5.4. Transducer placement, orientation, and anatomy for the parasternal long axis cardiac view in the emergency medicine orientation. The transducer is placed to the left of the sternum at the 4th intercostal space with indicator to the patient's right shoulder and the beam cutting along the long axis of the heart (**a**). The heart is seen as if it were cut in the plane of the ultrasound beam and folded down (**b**), with the lower image showing the anatomy as it appears on the ultrasound screen (**c**). Ultrasound image of the heart seen in the long axis parasternal transducer position (**d**). Note how the emergency medicine long axis orientation has left-sided structures, such as the apex of the heart, on the right side of the screen, which is the opposite of traditional cardiology orientation.

are internal structures within the heart itself. The position of the heart may vary remarkably from patient to patient. Obese patients tend to have a heart that is high up in the chest with a more transverse axis while patients with chronic obstructive lung disease often have a heart in a nearly longitudinal axis and dropped down almost to the costal margin.

Scanning technique and transducer orientation may be a source of confusion in echocardiography. Cardiologists typically perform echocardiography from the left side of the patient, with the transducer indicator corresponding to the right side of the screen. This is in contrast to other emergency ultrasound examinations that are typically performed from the right side of the patient with the indicator corresponding to the left side of the screen. The net result is that in emergency echo, two of the three primary cardiac windows (subxiphoid and apical four-chamber) are consistent with a cardiology orientation. However, the PSLA view traditionally described by cardiologists is flipped so that the apex of the heart appears on the left side of the screen. This leaves the emergency physician with two choices in obtaining the PSLA view: Either reverse the indicator in order to get an image that differs from typical emergency ultrasound orientation, or obtain a PSLA view that is consistent with abdominal applications, but reversed from a typical cardiology scan. In this text we have chosen to use an orientation consistent with the rest of emergency ultrasound, in which all windows (including the PSLA) are obtained by keeping the transducer to the patient's right, with right-sided cardiac structures appearing on the left side of the screen as they are viewed. Regarding the primary cardiac views, the only image that will appear significantly different from illustrations in cardiology texts is the PSLA. With practice using a consistent orientation (indicator in the arc from the patient's right to patient's head), each of the three views will meld into a coherent picture of the heart, with the PSLA being slightly higher than the subxiphoid and rotated clockwise from the apical view, but with structures remaining consistently oriented on the same side of the screen throughout (Fig. 5.6).

Apical Four Chamber View

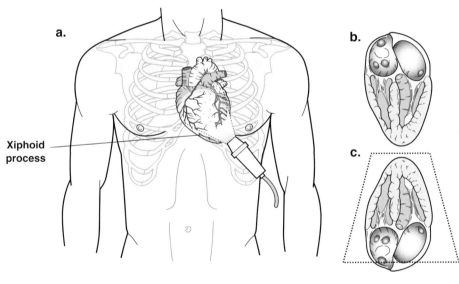

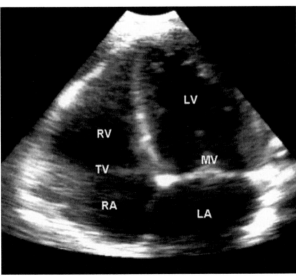

Figure 5.5. Transducer placement, orientation, and anatomy for the apical four-chamber cardiac view. The transducer is placed lateral to the nipple line with the indicator directed to the patient's right (may be toward the ceiling on the lateral chest wall of a supine patient) (**a**). The heart is seen as if it were cut in the plane of the ultrasound beam (**b**) and folded down, with the lower image showing the anatomy as it appears on the ultrasound screen (**c**). Ultrasound image of the heart seen in the apical transducer position (**d**).

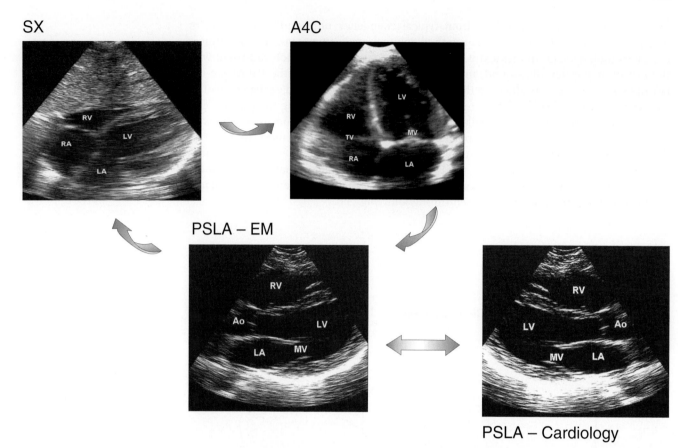

Figure 5.6. Primary emergency medicine cardiac windows. The subxiphoid (SX), apical four chamber (A4C), and parasternal long axis (PSLA) views are shown. Note how the subxiphoid is similar to the apical four-chamber, only the apical four-chamber image is rotated slightly counterclockwise. The parasternal long axis is very similar to the subxiphoid, only the parasternal long axis is at a higher level (includes aortic root). The image typically seen in a cardiology parasternal long axis is shown for reference; it is flipped 180 degrees. If desired, this image may be obtained by rotating the probe 180 degrees or flipping the screen orientation.

NORMAL ULTRASOUND ANATOMY AND PRIMARY CARDIAC WINDOWS

The heart is a three-dimensional structure that sits obliquely in the chest. The base of the heart, which includes the atria and major valves, is to the right and slightly posterior, while the apex of the heart points to the left, anteriorly and inferiorly (Fig. 5.1). Blood flowing from the right-sided inferior vena cava (IVC) joins the right atrium (RA), then proceeds through the tricuspid valve to the right ventricle (RV). Typically, hepatic veins in the liver can be followed sonographically into the IVC and then through the RA to the RV from a subxiphoid approach, which is often a useful maneuver for ultrasound orientation. The RV is anterior and to the right, with the free wall frequently seen adjacent to the liver. The left atrium (LA) is posterior and drains across the mitral valve to the muscular left ventricle (LV). The left ventricular outflow tract (aortic valve and aortic root) is in the center of the base of the heart and is typically best seen on the PSLA view.

In this text we will discuss three primary sonographic windows to the heart: the subxiphoid, the PSLA, and the apical four-chamber window. Additional windows that may be of particular use to the emergency physician are the parasternal short axis and the suprasternal notch view (Fig. 5.2). In general, the "long axis" of the heart may be thought of as a line that runs from the center of the base of the heart to the apex, corresponding to a line from the patient's right shoulder to left lower flank. A long axis view is one in which the ultrasound plane is parallel to this line, while a short axis is perpendicular to this axis and typically cuts across the left ventricle providing a "donut" type of image.

SUBXIPHOID WINDOW (FIG. 5.3)

The subxiphoid view is obtained by placing the transducer below the sternum at the costal margin with the transducer indicator to the patient's right (Fig. 5.3). The plane of the ultrasound transducer should be angled up towards the left chest, with the transducer pressed nearly flat on the abdomen and a firm amount of pressure applied in order to get the plane of the ultrasound beam below the rib cage. A helpful technique is to ask patients to bend their knees slightly to allow the physician to press the transducer flat and into the abdomen more deeply below the costal margin. Although it may be somewhat counterintuitive (as the heart is a left-sided structure) it is also sometimes helpful to move the transducer slightly to the right to use the liver as a sonographic window into the left chest. Remember that the subxiphoid window is obtained from the abdomen and the heart is in the chest and requires the ultrasound beam to be directed cephalad. One of the most frequent causes of novice sonographers being unable to obtain a subxiphoid image is that they are placing the transducer on the abdominal wall and imaging straight down (i.e., toward the back), instead of flattening the transducer against the abdomen and applying adequate pressure to image the chest cavity. Placing the scanning hand over the top of the transducer with the thumb on the indicator and pressing into the abdomen with the transducer nearly flat on the abdomen will help to avoid this tendency.

When correctly obtained the subxiphoid view is a four-chamber image that includes the RA, RV, LA, and LV (Figs. 5.3, 5.7). The RA, tricuspid valve, and RV are somewhat anterior and to the right. The LA, mitral valve, and LV are more posterior. The apex of the LV should be anterior and to the right side of the screen (patient's left). It may be helpful to sonographically trace the hepatic veins draining from the liver into the IVC and up into the RA. The subxiphoid view is an excellent view for pericardial effusion; which is typically seen as a significant anechoic space between the right ventricular free wall and the liver, corresponding to an inferior location of the fluid around the heart but seen anteriorly on the screen (near the transducer). Be aware that the subxiphoid window may overemphasize the relative size of the RV if it cuts across it in an oblique plane. The subxiphoid view is typically excellent in patients with chronic obstructive lung disease, as chest hyperexpansion moves the heart closer to the abdomen, but may be limited in patients who are obese or have other causes of abdominal distension. If the patient

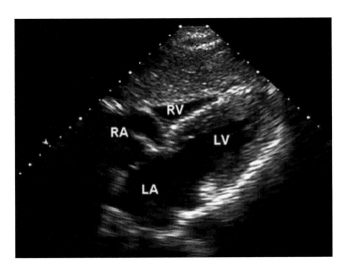

Figure 5.7. Subxiphoid view. The RV is seen as a small wedge against the liver.

is cooperative, the subxiphoid view may often be enhanced by having the patient take and hold a deep breath.

Parasternal Long Axis (PSLA) View (Fig. 5.4)

The PSLA view is an excellent window to the heart and is often complementary to the subxiphoid view. Patients with a heart that is high up in the chest or with abdominal distension often have a poor subxiphoid window but an excellent PSLA window. Conversely, patients with hyperexpanded lungs (chronic lung disease or on a ventilator) typically have a good subxiphoid view but lack the PSLA view.

The PSLA view is obtained in an emergency medicine orientation with the transducer lateral to the sternum at the fourth or fifth intercostal space and the indicator directed towards the patient's right shoulder, keeping the ultrasound plane along the long axis of the heart (Fig. 5.4). If a cardiology orientation for the PSLA view is desired, the indicator can be reversed (either on the machine or by directing the transducer indicator towards the patient's left hip). Keep in mind that if a cardiology orientation is used for the PSLA view the apex of the heart (physically on the patient's left) will be seen on the left of the screen as it is viewed, in contrast to other cardiac and emergency ultrasound views.

The PSLA view typically includes the RV anteriorly, with LA, mitral valve, LV, and left ventricular outflow tract more posteriorly (Figs. 5.4, 5.8). The anterior and posterior leaflets of the mitral valve are often clearly seen, along with the accompanying chordae tendinae and papillary muscles. The aortic valve can usually be seen to open in systole. Occasionally the descending aorta can be seen passing down the chest posterior to the left ventricle (Fig. 5.8).

Small pericardial effusions are often located posteriorly on the PSLA view (Fig. 5.9). As they enlarge they may also be seen anteriorly between the RV free wall and the pericardium as well as circumferentially, and it may be helpful to tilt the transducer in order to include the apex of the heart (Figs. 5.10, 5.11). Again, be careful to visualize the posterior (deep) pericardium as well, which may harbor an isolated effusion (Fig. 5.12). If feasible, the PSLA window may be enhanced by having the patient lie in a left lateral decubitus position, allowing gravity to pull the heart from behind the sternum into a better window.

Apical Four-Chamber View (Fig. 5.5)

The apical four-chamber view is typically the most difficult of the three primary windows to obtain, but also holds the most potential information (Fig. 5.5). The ability to obtain an apical view may be greatly enhanced by having the patient assume a left lateral decubitus position, allowing the apex of the heart to be pressed against the left chest. Because of the difficult nature in scanning between the ribs for the apical view, a phased array transducer will help significantly in obtaining good windows.

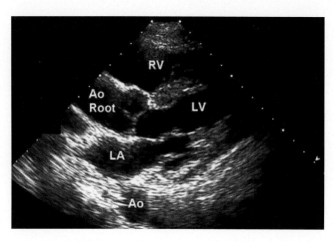

Figure 5.8. Parasternal long axis view. The aortic valve and aortic root are clearly seen. Note the descending aorta (Ao).

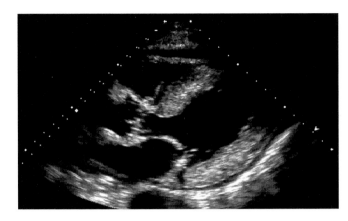

Figure 5.9. Parasternal long axis view. Small pericardial fluid is seen both posteriorly and anteriorly.

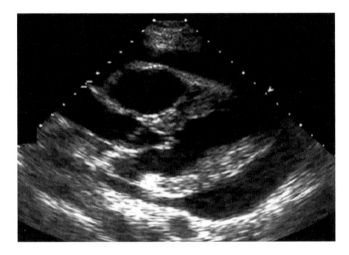

Figure 5.10. Parasternal long axis view with large pericardial effusion, both posterior and anterior.

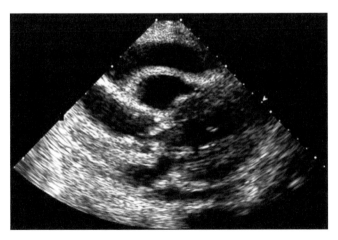

Figure 5.11. Parasternal long axis view, fluid seen posteriorly as well as anteriorly.

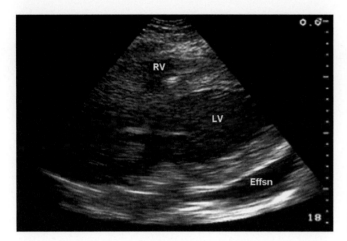

Figure 5.12. Parasternal long axis view. Isolated posterior pericardial effusion (Effsn). This is a moderate sized effusion, but no fluid is seen anteriorly.

The apical view is obtained laterally at about the level of the nipple in males. In females, the transducer will frequently need to be placed lateral to and somewhat beneath the breast tissue. As in all emergency ultrasounds, the transducer indicator should be directed to the patient's right, although this may be more toward the ceiling in a supine patient when obtaining a very lateral apical view. (Think of the direction of the indicator as wrapping around the torso.) To obtain a window, a rib interspace should be found. The transducer may need to be rotated somewhat to obtain an unobstructed view between the ribs.

In a properly obtained apical view, the apex of the heart is close to and near the center of the transducer face. The ventricles will be toward the face of the transducer, and the atria will be deeper. The interventricular septum should run nearly vertically down the screen, with the right-sided structures (RV and RA) on the left of the screen as they are viewed and the left-sided structures (LV and LA) on the right side of the screen as they are viewed. The tricuspid valve should be seen between the RV and RA and the mitral valve between the LV and LA (Fig. 5.13). A common pitfall with this approach is not being sufficiently lateral on the patient when obtaining the image, resulting in an image that appears more like a subxiphoid view, with the septum running diagonally towards the apex on the right side of the screen. When properly obtained this view is excellent for effusion, often providing a circumferential view (Fig. 5.14). Left ventricular function as well as RV size

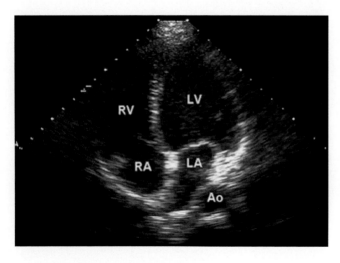

Figure 5.13. Apical four-chamber view. The closed mitral valve is clearly seen between LA and LV. Note the descending aorta (Ao).

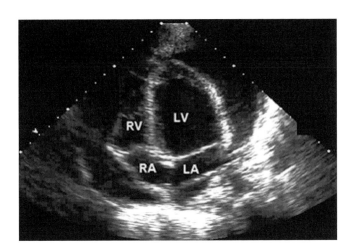

Figure 5.14. Apical four-chamber view showing a large circumferential pericardial effusion.

relative to LV are well-assessed with this view (Fig. 5.15). Although typically beyond the scope of the emergency physician, this view is the ideal one for obtaining Doppler flow across the tricuspid and mitral valves.

ALTERNATE VIEWS

Of the numerous other cardiac windows, two are of particular interest to the emergency physician: the parasternal short axis and suprasternal notch views. The parasternal short axis view is obtained by obtaining a PSLA view and rotating the transducer 90 degrees clockwise. This view cuts across the ventricle in sort of a "donut" configuration, and may allow for excellent assessment of overall circumferential LV contraction. There are several levels for the short axis (Fig. 5.16). Typically the papillary muscle level is most useful, with higher levels showing the mitral and aortic valves. The parasternal short axis may also show effusion, often posterior if small (Fig. 5.17).

The suprasternal notch view is obtained by placing the transducer just above the sternum. This view is difficult because of the small size of this notch as well as the many vascular structures that cross the superior mediastinum, but when properly obtained will show the aortic arch (Fig. 5.18).

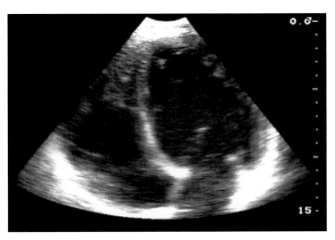
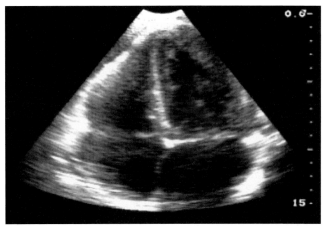

A   B

Figure 5.15. Apical four-chamber view, diastole (**A**) and systole (**B**).

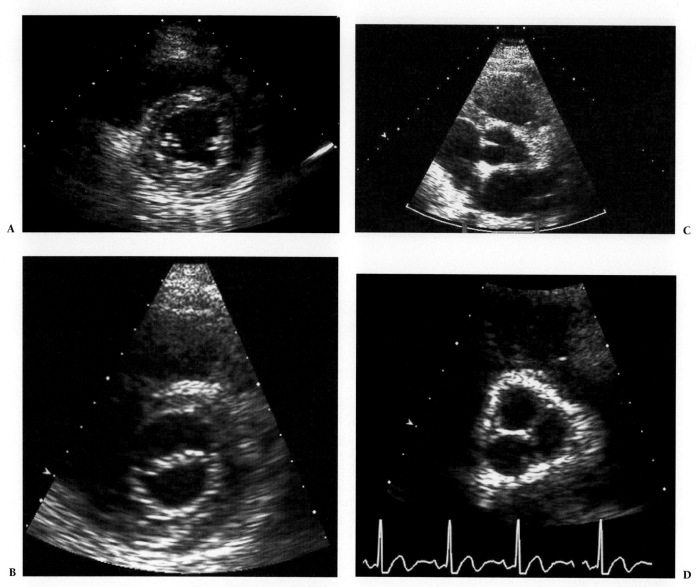

A

B

C

D

Figure 5.16. Parasternal short axis view showing the typical donut view of the LV. Papillary muscle level (**A**), mitral valve level (**B**), aortic valve level (**C**). Figure **D** is a zoomed view of the trileaflet aortic valve in short axis showing the "Mercedes Benz" sign.

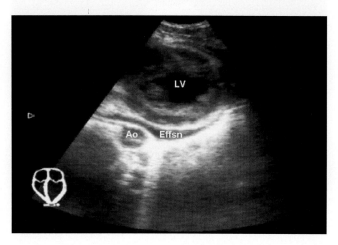

Figure 5.17. Parasternal short axis view, small pericardial effusion. The effusion is seen only posteriorly. Note the descending aorta (Ao).

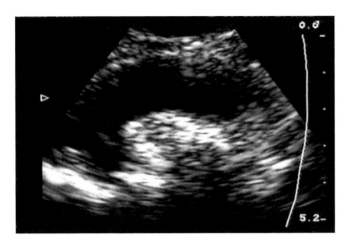

Figure 5.18. Aortic arch, seen via the suprasternal notch. The aortic root is to the left of the screen.

PATHOLOGY

PERICARDIAL EFFUSION, TAMPONADE

The space between the epicardium and pericardium typically has a small amount of epi-cardial fat and may contain up to 10 ml of serous physiologic fluid. A variety of traumatic and medical conditions may cause this area to be filled by fluid, pus, or blood. Ultimately fluid collecting in this space impedes the ability of the right side of the heart to fill, causing tamponade. Ultrasound is an excellent modality for assessing the presence of pericardial effusion. Ultrasound may also provide evidence of tamponade physiology, although true tamponade requiring immediate intervention is a clinical diagnosis: circulatory collapse secondary to pericardial effusion.

The amount of fluid necessary to cause tamponade typically depends on how rapidly it has accumulated. An acute traumatic tamponade may result from as little as 50 ml in the pericardial space, especially in the presence of other sources of blood loss, while the grad-ual accumulation of pericardial fluid in a cancer patient may be relatively well tolerated over 200 ml. Because small effusions tend to collect inferiorly and posteriorly, the subxiphoid approach is typically the best window, providing a view of the inferior pericardium between the liver and RV (Figs. 5.19–5.21). Particular care should be taken to look posteriorly if only

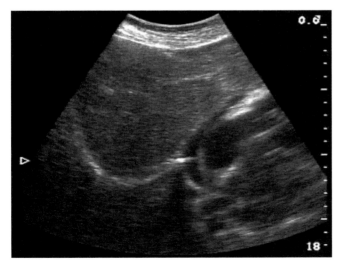

Figure 5.19. Small pericardial effusion, seen only between the RV free wall and liver in this subxiphoid view. This effusion was not seen on the parasternal view.

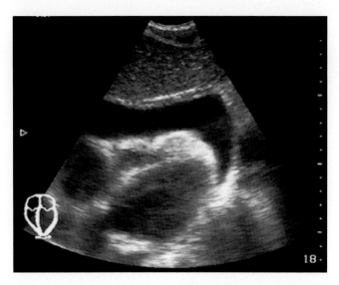

Figure 5.20. Subxiphoid view, moderate to large pericardial effusion.

a parasternal view is obtained (Figs. 5.12, 5.17). As effusions increase in volume they may be seen anteriorly and circumferentially (Figs. 5.9–5.11, 5.14). Pericardial effusions are typically characterized as small, moderate, or large. This is often somewhat subjective and grading systems differ, but typically an effusion is considered small if the posterior echo-free space is measured <10 mm, moderate if 10–15 mm, and large if over 15 mm (17). Other authors have suggested adding the anterior and posterior spaces, with large effusions being those that measure more than 20 mm together (18,19).

Echocardiographic evidence of tamponade is present when there is diastolic collapse of the right side of the heart (RA or RV) (Figs. 5.22–5.24) (20). This is indicative of pericardial fluid preventing diastolic filling and may be visualized with two-dimensional ultrasound when the RV or RA collapse or do not fill after tricuspid valve opening. Be careful not to confuse atrial contraction, which occurs with atrial systole, with diastolic collapse. In addition to right-sided diastolic collapse, a plethoric IVC with lack of inspiratory collapse is also frequently noted with tamponade, because the blood is prevented from flowing into the heart and backs up into the IVC. Doppler examination showing marked inspiratory increase in flow across the mitral or tricuspid valves also indicates tamponade physiology (the ultrasound version of pulsus paradoxus), although this may be outside of the scope of the emergency physician to assess (21).

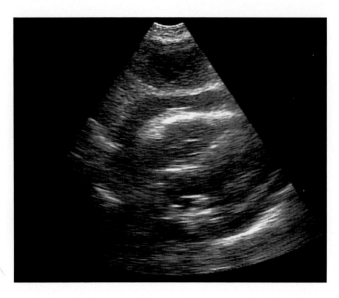

Figure 5.21. Subxiphoid view, small circumferential pericardial effusion.

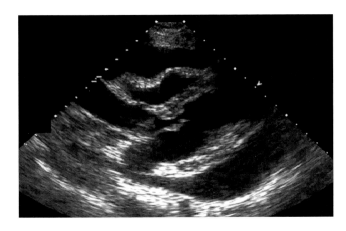

Figure 5.22. Parasternal long axis view, large effusion with evidence of RV collapse, seen anteriorly.

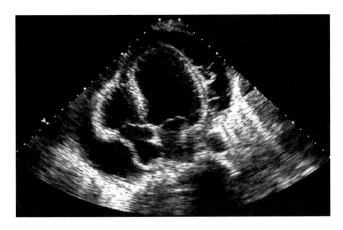

Figure 5.23. Apical four-chamber view with large circumferential effusion and evidence of right atrial collapse. Note the fibrinous material adjacent to the left ventricle.

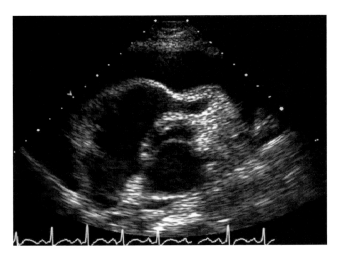

Figure 5.24. Short axis view showing an anterior effusion with RV collapse.

LEFT VENTRICULAR SYSTOLIC FUNCTION

Left ventricular systolic function is typically quantified as an ejection fraction, representing the percentage of blood ejected from the ventricle during systole. While there are quantitative methods for estimating the ejection fraction, it is frequently determined by visual estimation using echo (22). It has been shown that with goal-directed training, emergency physicians can learn to estimate left ventricular systolic function and are accurate when compared to cardiologists (5,23). A normal ejection fraction is typically 55% or above, and may be qualitatively graded as normal (>50%), moderately depressed (30–50%), or severely depressed (<30%). The most severe degree of left ventricular systolic dysfunction is the absence of detectable cardiac activity. Occasionally there may be valvular motion with no detectable cardiac motion, but this typically signifies only agonal cardiac activity.

When attempting to estimate left ventricular systolic function it is important to watch the border of the endocardium, which usually appears slightly echogenic and represents the innermost layer of the heart. The myocardium should thicken uniformly as the endocardium moves in a healthy heart. When possible, the left ventricular cavity should be imaged in two planes, ideally orthogonal to each other (for example PSLA and parasternal short axis). Harmonic imaging may be helpful if available. A uniformly and circumferentially contracting endocardium that moves significantly from diastole to systole is indicative of good function. While better seen with dynamic images, Figure 5.25 shows a heart with good function in diastole and systole contrasted with a dilated LV that is minimally contractile (Fig. 5.26). Poor LV function is often coupled with a dilated or plethoric IVC, indicating fluid overload and congestive heart failure (Fig. 5.27).

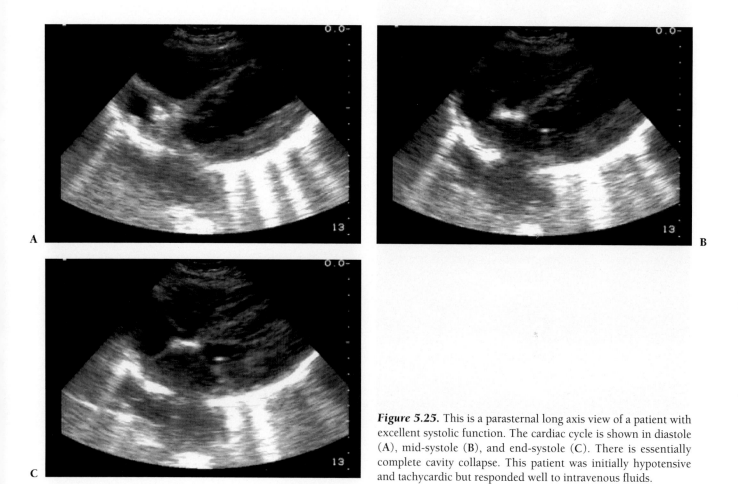

Figure 5.25. This is a parasternal long axis view of a patient with excellent systolic function. The cardiac cycle is shown in diastole (**A**), mid-systole (**B**), and end-systole (**C**). There is essentially complete cavity collapse. This patient was initially hypotensive and tachycardic but responded well to intravenous fluids.

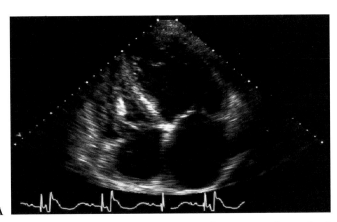 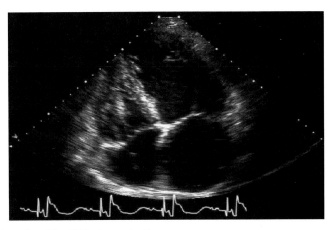

A
B

Figure 5.26. Apical four-chamber view of a patient with systolic dysfunction. The LV is shown in diastole (A) and end-systole (B). It appears dilated with little change in volume. Formal echocardiography estimated the ejection fraction to be 20%.

It is tempting to look for focal wall motion abnormalities, as these may be indicative of cardiac ischemia. While occasionally these may be grossly obvious, the interobserver variability is high even among cardiologists and this is generally beyond the scope of emergency echo.

RIGHT VENTRICULAR STRAIN

In the absence of a shunt, the change in volume from diastole to systole is the same per cardiac cycle in both the RV and the LV. However, the thin-walled and lower-pressure RV is anatomically wrapped around the muscular LV and thus appears to be less wide on most ultrasound windows, particularly the PSLA and apical views. In a process where there is outflow obstruction the RV will bow into the LV septum making it appear to enlarge relative to the LV. This finding may be appreciated by echo. Other echo signs of RV strain include RV hypokinesis and paradoxical septal motion, where the interventricular septum actually appears to bow out somewhat towards the LV during systole. While many processes may cause RV strain, the acute process causing increased RV outflow obstruction and RV dilatation that is of most interest to the emergency physician is massive pulmonary embolus, which may be dramatic, life-threatening, and potentially aided by rapid diagnosis and treatment with anticoagulants, including thrombolytics in some cases.

A normal RV:LV ratio is less than 0.6:1 when measured across the tips of the valves on a PSLA or apical view. Specificity increases with a higher cutoff, and if the RV:LV ratio is 1:1 or greater (i.e., RV appears to be larger than the LV) it is safe to say there is significant RV

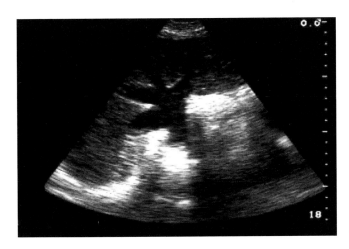

Figure 5.27. IVC in a patient with congestive heart failure. The IVC is grossly dilated and does not collapse with inspiration.

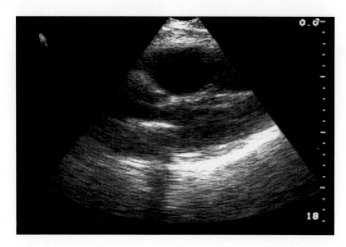

Figure 5.28. Parasternal long axis view, showing RV dilatation relative to LV. The ratio of RV to LV is greater than 1:1.

strain (Figs. 5.28, 5.29) (24). Although acute RV strain is poorly sensitive for pulmonary embolus, it may be reasonably specific (25). RV strain provides prognostic information in patients with proven pulmonary emboli, and mortality of patients with pulmonary emboli and RV strain is ten times the mortality without RV strain (26,27). While some authors have suggested that RV strain in the presence of proven pulmonary embolism may be an indication for thrombolytic therapy, a definite mortality benefit has not been demonstrated (28,29).

It is important to keep in mind that there are many chronic conditions that cause RV strain, including chronic lung disease, pulmonary hypertension, pulmonary stenosis, and others. Typically these are accompanied by RV hypertrophy, and an RV free wall in excess of 5 mm likely indicates a more chronic condition (Figs. 5.30, 5.31).

The identification of RV strain should be made with caution by the emergency physician and followed by consultative echocardiography if the situation allows. RV strain is not sensitive for pulmonary embolus, as many pulmonary emboli do not have any identifiable increase in RV pressure, even by consultative echo. However, identification of RV strain by emergency echo may at times be fairly obvious and dramatic, and may help to guide the diagnostic and therapeutic course in patients with suspected pulmonary emboli.

INCIDENTAL FINDINGS

Goal-directed echo should focus primarily on finding and ruling out the pathologic findings described above. Inevitably, as more echocardiograms are performed, other findings

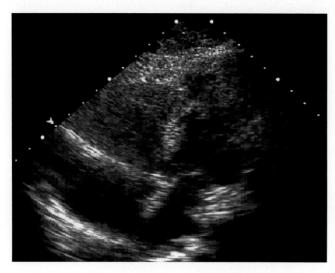

Figure 5.29. Apical four-chamber view showing a dilated RV. This patient was found to have a saddle embolus. The view is slightly medial, as the apex of the heart is off the screen with the septum not quite vertical.

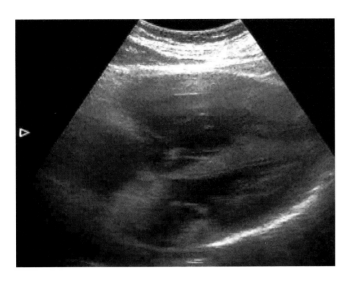

Figure 5.30. RV dilatation with RV hypertrophy. This patient had a history of pulmonic stenosis.

will be discovered. Some of these are simple and may be obvious from the patient's history and electrocardiogram (EKG), i.e., presence of a pacer wire (Fig. 5.32) or left ventricular hypertrophy (Fig. 5.33). Others may be infrequent but require attention, i.e., thoracic aortic dilatation (Fig. 5.34), intracardiac mass (Fig. 5.35), or ventricular aneurysm (Fig. 5.36). When unusual findings that may require change in management are discovered we recommend liberal use of consultative echo or other imaging modalities as available.

USE OF THE IMAGE IN CLINICAL DECISION MAKING

CIRCULATORY SHOCK—CODE SITUATION TO UNEXPLAINED HYPOTENSION

Perhaps the most dramatic use of emergency echo is in assessing the patient in circulatory shock, whether from a medical or traumatic cause. Circulatory shock may be considered as a spectrum from true PEA, to hypotension/tachycardia, or even occult shock (shock with a normal blood pressure and/or pulse). A visual picture of the heart and IVC may quickly establish whether poor perfusion is due to a "pump problem" or a "volume problem."

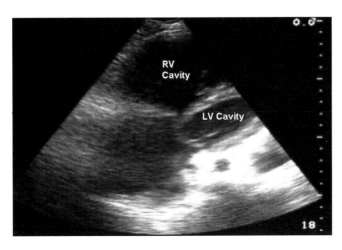

Figure 5.31. Massive RV dilatation. This was secondary to chronic pulmonary hypertension.

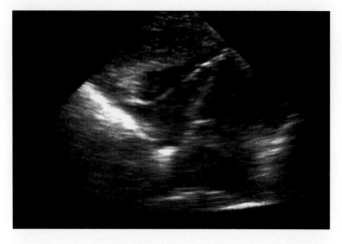

Figure 5.32. Pacer wire, subxiphoid view. The wire can be seen traveling from the right atrium through the RV to the RV apex.

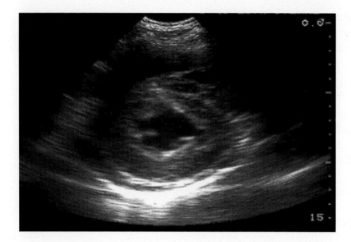

Figure 5.33. Parasternal short axis view, left ventricular hypertrophy. The short axis is a particularly good view for seeing the concentric myocardium.

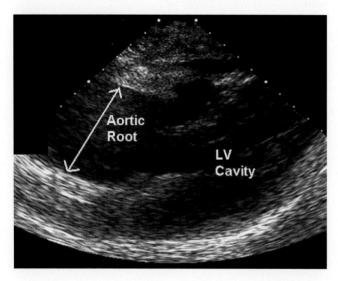

Figure 5.34. Thoracic aortic dilatation. Normal is usually considered below 4 cm. (Also see figure 5.39).

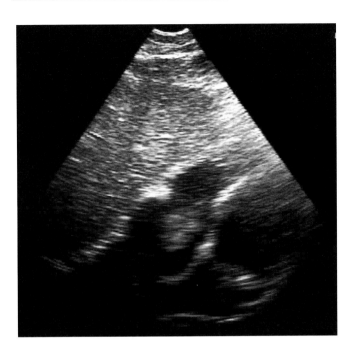

Figure 5.35. Intracardiac mass, subxiphoid view. The mass can be seen prolapsing across the tricuspid valve between the RA and RV. The differential diagnosis includes myxoma, thrombus, or endocardial vegetation. This turned out to be a clot in a patient with metastatic renal carcinoma.

In true arrest situations emergency echo may be valuable in assessing the need for further interventions (30). In a series of 169 patients in a code situation absence of cardiac activity by ultrasound was found to be 100% predictive of death in the ED (31). In patients without organized electrical activity, either asystole or ventricular fibrillation, it is not expected that there would be any degree of left ventricular contraction. However, ultrasound may be useful in distinguishing between the two and some authors have suggested that fine ventricular fibrillation may at times be misinterpreted as asystole (32). The ultrasound appearance of fibrillation is that of a "shivering" myocardium.

PEA was formerly known as electromechanical dissociation, however emergency echo showed that in many cases there was some cardiac activity, thus this description is a misnomer (33). For patients who are in PEA, ultrasound may be able to quickly diagnose or exclude several treatable causes, most notably tamponade and hypovolemia (34). The typical appearance of hypovolemia is a well contracting endocardium and a flat IVC (Figs. 5.25, 5.37), as contrasted with a poorly contractile LV and a dilated IVC indicating cardiogenic shock (Figs. 5.26, 5.27, 5.38).

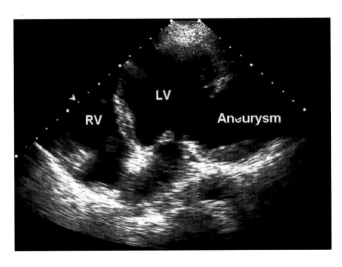

Figure 5.36. Apical four-chamber view, left ventricular aneurysm.

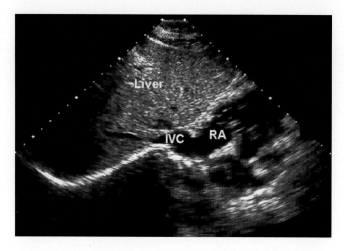

Figure 5.37. Subxiphoid view of IVC during inspiration. The IVC nearly collapses, indicating a low preload.

In patients with penetrating chest trauma, especially those with shock, emergency echo may be truly lifesaving in its ability to rapidly identify traumatic tamponade. In a retrospective review of patients with penetrating cardiac injury, immediate emergency echo decreased time to operative intervention and increased survival (35).

Emergency echo has shown great potential for patients with nontraumatic unexplained hypotension. Emergency echo may be incorporated as a portion of a focused sonographic examination that quickly screens for important and treatable causes of hypotension or PEA. An ultrasound protocol for the undifferentiated hypotensive patient has been suggested, utilizing views of the heart for effusion as well as imaging the abdominal aorta and peritoneal spaces for free fluid (36). A trial of over 200 patients presenting with nontraumatic hypotension randomized patients to immediate or delayed ultrasound evaluation that included seven sonographic windows, both cardiac and abdominal. They found a significant improvement in speed and diagnostic accuracy for patients who underwent initial versus delayed ultrasound (18,37).

When approaching the patient with unexplained hypotension an echocardiogram should first rule out effusion, then assess overall LV function with attention to volume status. Transthoracic echo by emergency physicians has been shown to be accurate in determining left ventricular function in patients with unexplained hypotension (23). A collapsed IVC with a well contracting LV indicates the need for initial fluid resuscitation while adequate volume status with LV dysfunction may indicate the need for additional

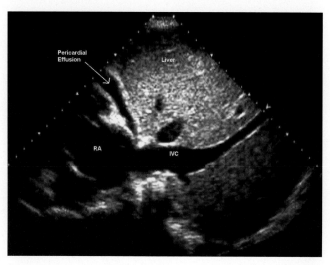

Figure 5.38. Sagittal view of the IVC showing a dilated IVC. This subxiphoid view is obtained with the transducer indicator directed toward the patient's head. It is a particularly useful view for watching the IVC during inspiration, as diaphragmatic movement will not move the IVC out of view (as in a transverse view). Note the small inferior pericardial effusion.

pressor agents. The presence of severe RV strain may indicate the possibility of a large pulmonary embolus or other pulmonary process resulting in cor pulmonale and hypotension.

SHORTNESS OF BREATH

When patients present with shortness of breath emergency physicians typically look first for a pulmonary cause. When the physical exam and initial studies fail to determine the cause of dyspnea, echo offers a useful adjunct to detect etiologies such as pericardial effusion, congestive heart failure, myocardial infarction, and pulmonary embolism. One study of ED patients who presented with dyspnea of unclear etiology following standard evaluation found that the incidence of pericardial effusion found by emergency echo was nearly 14%, with a significant number of large pericardial effusions (17).

Emergency echo may also be able to demonstrate evidence of congestive heart failure that may be difficult to determine from physical examination alone (38). In addition to the assessment of left ventricular systolic function, evidence of increased central venous pressure may be assessed by examining the IVC during inspiration. Dilatation of the IVC with absence of inspiratory collapse indicates fluid overload, while a collapsed IVC is unlikely in congestive heart failure (Figs. 5.27, 5.37, 5.38). Recent work has also indicated that the measurement of the meniscus in the internal jugular vein may be even more accurate for fluid overload than IVC measurement, although this meniscus is visible in the minority of patients (39). Ultrasound is one of the most sensitive indicators of pleural effusion, often present with heart failure (40). A screening examination that includes an examination of the heart, IVC or internal jugular vein, and pleural spaces (for both effusion and pneumothorax) may quickly add to the evaluation of the patient with unexplained shortness of breath.

It is important to note that several cardiac causes of shortness of breath, particularly valvular dysfunction and diastolic dysfunction, require more sophisticated echo techniques using Doppler and M-mode. Attempting to diagnose causes for murmurs, stenotic lesions, or valvular regurgitation, for example, can be difficult and misleading for patient care and should only be performed by a physician who is well trained in advanced echocardiography.

CHEST PAIN

In a study of 124 patients with "suspected cardiac disease," including chest pain, dyspnea, palpitations, and syncope, a screening ultrasound performed by an emergency physician was helpful in diagnosing significant abnormalities not found by initial evaluation as well as providing prognostic value for length of stay of admitted patients (41). While a consultative echocardiogram may be sensitive for ischemia if chest pain is ongoing, it is not recommended that emergency physicians attempt to determine if focal wall motion abnormalities are present in ruling out myocardial infarction (42). However, the presence of significant left ventricular systolic dysfunction may indicate more serious disease.

Because the differential diagnosis for chest pain is broad, emergency echocardiography can help limit the possible causes and etiologies. In patients presenting with chest pain concerning for pericarditis, emergency echo can determine if there is any significant pericardial effusion. Although not a primary indication for emergency echo, demonstration of a dilated aortic root, aortic flap, or pericardial effusion may be present in patients with thoracic aortic aneurysm or dissection (Figs. 5.34, 5.39) (43,44). Transesophageal echocardiography is a superior modality for the diagnosis of aortic pathology (Fig. 5.40).

As with many ultrasound applications, findings on echocardiography tend to be more specific than sensitive. When findings are present in the patient with chest pain they may be helpful in diagnosis. However, the absence of findings by emergency echo should not generally be used to exclude many of the life-threatening causes of chest pain.

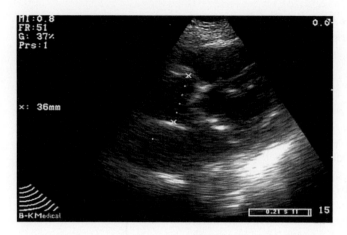

Figure 5.39. Measurement of the aortic root on parasternal long axis view. This is borderline dilated, but less than the cutoff of 4 cm.

ARTIFACTS AND PITFALLS

ARTIFACTS

The most common sonographic artifacts encountered in echo are mirror image and side lobe artifact.

1. Mirror image artifact occurs when sound encounters a strong reflector, and the more proximal structure appears to be duplicated on the other side of the reflector. Occasionally there may appear to be another structure contracting on the other side of the pericardium due to mirror image.
2. Side lobe artifact occurs when sound is deflected from the sides of a fluid-filled object. While more typically encountered in the urinary bladder or gallbladder, side lobe may occasionally make it appear as if there is a mass inside the atrial or ventricular cavity. If artifact is suspected, imaging the structure in a different window usually will identify it. Confirmatory or follow-up consultative echoes should occur if there still appears to be an abnormality.

PITFALLS

1. Perhaps the greatest potential pitfall of emergency echo is the temptation to call or rule out diagnoses that are beyond the scope of the typical emergency physician, especially

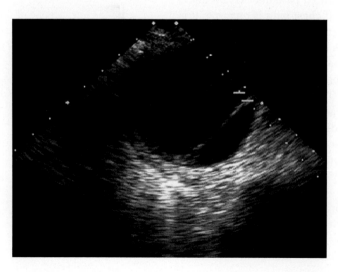

Figure 5.40. Transesophageal echocardiogram showing the descending aorta with an intimal flap (dissection). This is the preferred echocardiographic approach for diagnosis of dissection, if available.

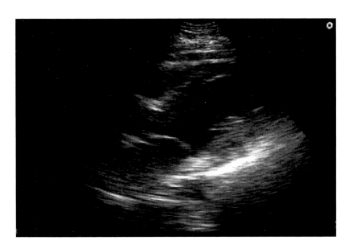

Figure 5.41. Anterior fat pad, seen on parasternal long axis view. The echo-free space may be mistaken for pericardial effusion, but is small and not seen in the posterior pericardium. With dynamic images the space diminishes in diastole.

in the absence of accurate Doppler evaluation. These include, but are not limited to, valvular stenosis or regurgitation, diastolic dysfunction, focal wall motion abnormalities, and endocarditis.

2. It takes some experience to distinguish between epicardial fat and normal or physiologic fluid in the pericardial space from small effusions (Figs. 5.41, 5.42) (45). A key to this is appreciating the mottled echogenicity of fat in contrast to the typically anechoic effusion. Take care that the gain is neither too low nor too high, and watch to see if an anechoic space continues to be present throughout the cardiac cycle. A space that appears and disappears is less likely to be a significant effusion. If effusion is suspected on any view, it is helpful to try to confirm using another view. If obtainable, the subxiphoid is typically most helpful and sensitive. While large effusions may track anteriorly they typically do not exist there in isolation. In particular, the anterior pericardium in the PSLA view often appears to have a small echo-free space that should not be taken to be effusion if there is no fluid seen posteriorly or on the subxiphoid view.

3. Fluid in other spaces, particularly the pleural spaces, may be mistaken for pericardial fluid. On the right side, the IVC should be followed and may show a border between the vessel and the effusion (Figs. 5.43, 5.44). A left pleural effusion may be particularly difficult to distinguish as it may appear to be directly against the ventricular free wall of the apex of the heart (Fig. 5.45). When differentiating fluid on the left side of the heart as pleural or pericardial effusion, if possible it is helpful to visualize the descending

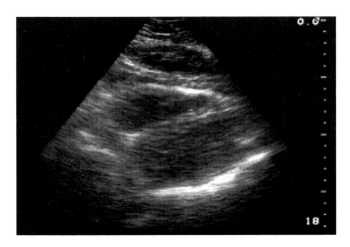

Figure 5.42. Subxiphoid view, showing a fat pad anterior to the RV. There appear to be some echoes in the space, indicating fat and not fluid.

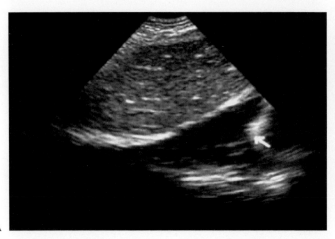

A

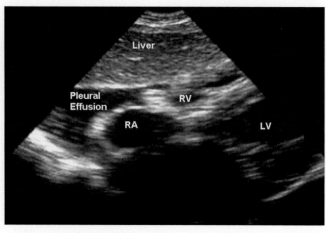

B

Figure 5.43. Right pleural effusion, from subxiphoid approach. In (**A**) the arrow shows the edge of the RA. In (**B**) the RA can be seen as separate from the pleural effusion.

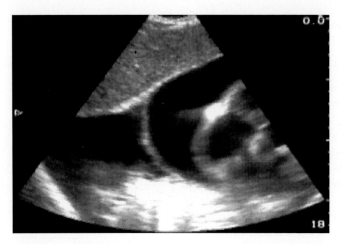

Figure 5.44. Pleural and pericardial fluid, subxiphoid view. The pericardium is seen between the large right pleural effusion and the pericardial effusion.

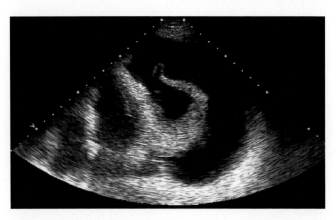

Figure 5.45. Apical view, large left pleural effusion. The serpiginous structure is tissue within the pleural effusion.

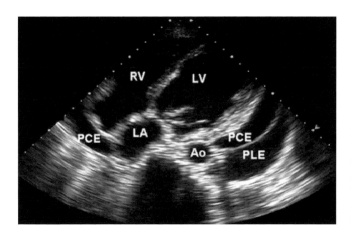

Figure 5.46. Pleural and pericardial effusion, low parasternal view. The circular structure is the descending aorta (Ao), sitting on the thoracic spine. The line on the right side of the screen is the pericardium, separating pericardial (PCE) from pleural fluid (PLE). Note how the pericardial fluid is beginning to interpose itself between the heart and descending aorta, while the pleural effusion is lateral to the aorta.

aorta. Pericardial fluid will tend to interpose itself between the posterior heart and aorta, while pleural fluid will not (Fig. 5.46).

In either case, if pleural effusion is suspected a quick coronal view in the right and left flanks (as in a trauma scan) should be able to establish whether there is fluid in the pleural space. If pleural fluid is present, use caution in calling a pericardial effusion in addition to the pleural effusion unless fluid can be seen on both sides of the pericardium (Figs. 5.44, 5.46).

4. When attempting to determine overall left ventricular systolic function two orthogonal views should be obtained (i.e., PSLA and parasternal short axis), allowing for the possibility of significant focal wall motion abnormalities.

5. Right ventricular dilatation is best visualized from a PSLA or apical view, as the subxiphoid view may cut obliquely across the RV, overemphasizing the size.

CASE

A 65-year-old male presents with a chief complaint of shortness of breath which he states has been progressive for the last three days. He has some sharp chest discomfort that is worse with movement. He is otherwise healthy and takes no medications, but does note that last week he had a brief febrile illness with a slightly persistent cough. Further review of systems is unremarkable. His blood pressure is 105/85, pulse is 106 beats per minute, temperature is 99.6 °F, and oxygen saturation is 99% on room air. He does not appear markedly uncomfortable. On physical examination his lungs are clear and there is no evident jugular venous distension. His heart is tachycardic without audible gallop, murmur, or rub. An electrocardiogram shows sinus tachycardia with nonspecific T-wave abnormalities and no ST-segment changes. Laboratory studies are pending. A chest radiograph is obtained, shown in Figure 5.47. It is interpreted as mild cardiomegaly without pulmonary infiltrate.

Consultative echocardiography is not available and the emergency physician performs a bedside echocardiography that demonstrates a large pericardial effusion with evidence of right ventricular collapse (Fig. 5.48). Cardiology is consulted and the patient is given intravenous fluids. The patient is admitted and an urgent pericardial window is placed. Serous fluid (350 cc) is drained, which later shows malignant cells on pathology. The patient is found to have metastatic colon cancer.

While certainly few would argue that the above patient requires admission, the most likely diagnostic concern with the above patient following initial workup is heart failure, although certainly not severe. The treatment for heart failure is typically diuretics, opposite of the treatment for pericardial effusions, which require fluids to keep preload high. An alternate echo finding that would be equally plausible in this patient is shown in Figure 5.49, which shows a dilated LV (with significant systolic dysfunction on real-time echo).

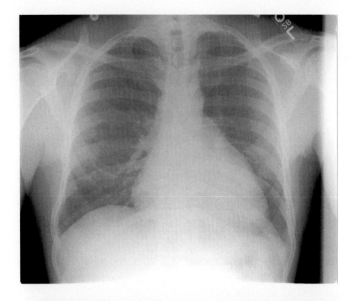

Figure 5.47. Chest x-ray. Interpreted as mild cardiomegaly.

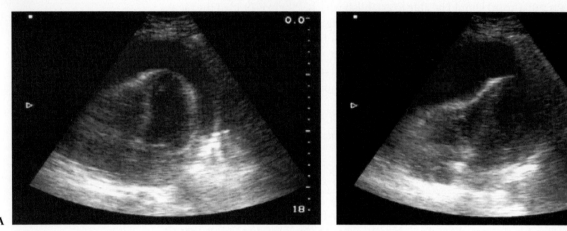

A   B

Figure 5.48. Apical four-chamber view showing a large pericardial effusion (**A**). Evidence of diastolic RV collapse is seen (**B**).

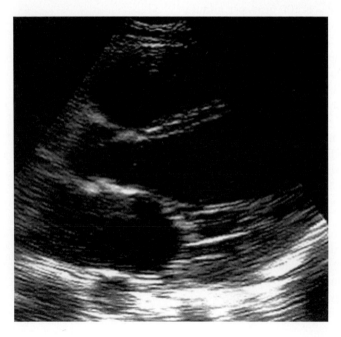

Figure 5.49. Parasternal long axis view. While better seen with dynamic images, the LV is clearly dilated and was seen to be hypocontractile with an estimated ejection fraction of 15%.

If these were the findings intravenous diuretics would be appropriate. In this case the ability of the emergency physician to perform echocardiography provides definitive diagnosis and markedly alters patient treatment and course.

REFERENCES

1. Stewart WJ, Douglas PS, Sagar K, et al. Echocardiography in Emergency Medicine: A Policy Statement by the American Society of Echocardiography and the American College of Cardiology. The Task Force on Echocardiography in Emergency Medicine of the American Society of Echocardiography and the Echocardiography TPEC Committees of the American College of Cardiology. *J Am Soc Echocardiogr.* 1999;12:82–84.
2. Mateer J, Plummer D, Heller M, et al. Model curriculum for physician training in emergency ultrasonography. *Ann Emerg Med.* 1994;23:95–102.
3. Krause RS. Re: Echocardiography in emergency medicine: A policy statement by the American Society of Echocardiography and the American College of Cardiology. *J Am Soc Echocardiogr.* 1999;12:607–608.
4. Stahmer SA. The ASE Position Statement on Echocardiography in the Emergency Department. *Acad Emerg Med.* 2000;7:306–308.
5. Jones AE, Tayal VS, Kline JA. Focused training of emergency medicine residents in goal-directed echocardiography: a prospective study. *Acad Emerg Med.* 2003;10:1054–1058.
6. Mayron R, Gaudio FE, Plummer D, et al. Echocardiography performed by emergency physicians: impact on diagnosis and therapy. *Ann Emerg Med.* 1988;17:150–154.
7. Hauser AM. The emerging role of echocardiography in the emergency department. *Ann Emerg Med.* 1989;18:1298–1303.
8. Oh JK, Meloy TD, Seward JB. Echocardiography in the emergency room: Is it feasible, beneficial, and cost-effective? *Echocardiography.* 1995;12:163–170.
9. Sanfilippo AJW, Arthur E. The role of echocardiography in managing critically ill patients. *J Crit Illn.* 1988;3:27–44.
10. Sabia P, Abbott RD, Afrookteh A, et al. Importance of two-dimensional echocardiographic assessment of left ventricular systolic function in patients presenting to the emergency room with cardiac-related symptoms. *Circulation.* 1991;84:1615–1624.
11. Callahan JA, Seward JB, Nishimura RA, et al. Two-dimensional echocardiographically guided pericardiocentesis: experience in 117 consecutive patients. *Am J Cardiol.* 1985;55:476–479.
12. Mazurek B, Jehle D, Martin M. Emergency department echocardiography in the diagnosis and therapy of cardiac tamponade. *J Emerg Med.* 1991;9:27–31.
13. Ettin D, Cook T. Using ultrasound to determine external pacer capture. *J Emerg Med.* 1999;17:1007–1009.
14. Macedo W Jr, Sturmann K, Kim JM, et al. Ultrasonographic guidance of transvenous pacemaker insertion in the emergency department: a report of three cases. *J Emerg Med.* 1999;17:491–496.
15. Aguilera PA, Durham BA, Riley DA. Emergency transvenous cardiac pacing placement using ultrasound guidance. *Ann Emerg Med.* 2000;36:224–227.
16. Harper RJC, Michael L. Pericardiocentesis and Intracardiac Injections. In: Roberts JRH, Jerris R, ed. *Clinical Procedures in Emergency Medicine.* Philadelphia: WB Saunders, 1998: 231–253.
17. Blaivas M. Incidence of pericardial effusion in patients presenting to the emergency department with unexplained dyspnea. *Acad Emerg Med.* 2001;8:1143–1146.
18. Shabetai R. Pericardial effusion: haemodynamic spectrum. *Heart.* 2004;90:255–256.
19. Soler-Soler J, Sagrista-Sauleda J, Permanyer-Miralda G. Management of pericardial effusion. *Heart.* 2001;86:235–240.
20. Sanfilippo AJW, Arthur E. Pericardial Disease. In: Weyman AA, ed. *Principles and Practice of Echocardiography.* Philadelphia: Lippincott Williams & Wilkins; 1994: 1102–1134.
21. Choong CY. Left Ventricle V: Diastolic Function—Its Principles and Evaluation. In: Weyman AA, ed. *Principles and Practice of Echocardiography.* Philadelphia: Lippincott Williams & Wilkins; 1994: 771–772.
22. Rumberger JA, Behrenbeck T, Bell MR, et al. Determination of ventricular ejection fraction: a comparison of available imaging methods. The Cardiovascular Imaging Working Group. *Mayo Clin Proc.* 1997;72:860–870.
23. Moore CL, Rose GA, Tayal VS, et al. Determination of left ventricular function by emergency physician echocardiography of hypotensive patients. *Acad Emerg Med.* 2002;9:186–193.
24. Nazeyrollas P, Metz D, Jolly D, et al. Use of transthoracic Doppler echocardiography combined with clinical and electrocardiographic data to predict acute pulmonary embolism. *Eur Heart J.* 1996;17:779–786.

25. Grifoni S, Olivotto I, Cecchini P, et al. Utility of an integrated clinical, echocardiographic, and venous ultrasonographic approach for triage of patients with suspected pulmonary embolism. *Am J Cardiol*. 1998;82:1230–1235.

26. Kasper W, Konstantinides S, Geibel A, et al. Prognostic significance of right ventricular afterload stress detected by echocardiography in patients with clinically suspected pulmonary embolism. *Heart*. 1997;77:346–349.

27. Ribeiro A, Lindmarker P, Juhlin-Dannfelt A, et al. Echocardiography Doppler in pulmonary embolism: right ventricular dysfunction as a predictor of mortality rate. *Am Heart J*. 1997;134:479–487.

28. Come PC, Kim D, Parker JA, et al. Early reversal of right ventricular dysfunction in patients with acute pulmonary embolism after treatment with intravenous tissue plasminogen activator. *J Am Coll Cardiol*. 1987;10:971–978.

29. Goldhaber SZ, Haire WD, Feldstein ML, et al. Alteplase versus heparin in acute pulmonary embolism: randomised trial assessing right-ventricular function and pulmonary perfusion. *Lancet*. 1993;341:507–511.

30. Cardenas E. Limited bedside ultrasound imaging by emergency medicine physicians. *West J Med*. 1998;168:188–189.

31. Blaivas M, Fox JC. Outcome in cardiac arrest patients found to have cardiac standstill on the bedside emergency department echocardiogram.[comment]. *Acad Emerg Med*. 2001;8:616–621.

32. Amaya SC, Langsam A. Ultrasound detection of ventricular fibrillation disguised as asystole. *Ann Emerg Med*. 1999;33:344–346.

33. Bocka JJ, Overton DT, Hauser A. Electromechanical dissociation in human beings: an echocardiographic evaluation. *Ann Emerg Med*. 1988;17:450–452.

34. Tayal VS, Kline JA. Emergency echocardiography to detect pericardial effusion in patients in PEA and near-PEA states. *Resuscitation*. 2003;59:315–8.

35. Plummer D, Brunette D, Asinger R, et al. Emergency department echocardiography improves outcome in penetrating cardiac injury. *Ann Emerg Med*. 1992;21:709–712.

36. Rose JS, Bair AE, Mandavia D, et al. The UHP ultrasound protocol: a novel ultrasound approach to the empiric evaluation of the undifferentiated hypotensive patient.[comment]. *Am J Emerg Med*. 2001;19:299–302.

37. Jones AE, Tayal VS, Sullivan DM, et al. Randomized, controlled trial of immediate versus delayed goal-directed ultrasound to identify the cause of nontraumatic hypotension in emergency department patients. *Crit Care Med*. 2004;32:1703–1708.

38. Chizner MA. The diagnosis of heart disease by clinical assessment alone. *Curr Probl Cardiol*. 2001;26:285–379.

39. Jang T, Aubin C, Naunheim R, et al. Ultrasonography of the internal jugular vein in patients with dyspnea without jugular venous distension on physical examination. *Ann Emerg Med*. 2004;44:160–168.

40. Ma OJ, Mateer JR. Trauma ultrasound examination versus chest radiography in the detection of hemothorax. *Ann Emerg Med*. 1997;29:312–315; discussion 315–316.

41. Kimura BJ, Bocchicchio M, Willis CL, et al. Screening cardiac ultrasonographic examination in patients with suspected cardiac disease in the emergency department. *Am Heart J*. 2001;142:324–330.

42. Peels CH, Visser CA, Kupper AJ, et al. Usefulness of two-dimensional echocardiography for immediate detection of myocardial ischemia in the emergency room. *Am J Cardiol*. 1990;65:687–691.

43. Erbel R, Engberding R, Daniel W, et al. Echocardiography in diagnosis of aortic dissection. *Lancet*. 1989;1:457–460.

44. Roudaut RP, Billes MA, Gosse P, et al. Accuracy of M-mode and two-dimensional echocardiography in the diagnosis of aortic dissection: an experience with 128 Cases. *Clin Cardiol*. 1988;11:553–562.

45. Blaivas M, DeBehnke D, Phelan MB. Potential errors in the diagnosis of pericardial effusion on trauma ultrasound for penetrating injuries. *Acad Emerg Med*. 2000;7:1261–1266.

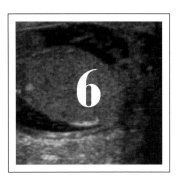

FIRST TRIMESTER PREGNANCY

Kristen Nordenholz
Jean Abbott
John Bailitz

INTRODUCTION

Emergency Department (ED) pelvic ultrasound is an accurate and efficient tool that can facilitate the triage, diagnosis, and management of patients who present to the ED with symptoms or signs related to pregnancy in the first trimester. The primary role of ED ultrasound is to detect ectopic pregnancy in a timely fashion by identifying intrauterine pregnancy (IUP) and thereby excluding ectopic pregnancy in a majority of patients. In addition, emergency physicians can use ultrasound to determine gestational age and establish fetal viability. In the unstable patient, the addition of the Focused Assessment with Sonography for Trauma (FAST) examination for free fluid in the abdomen to the pelvic ED ultrasound can rapidly identify patients requiring emergent surgical intervention for a presumed ectopic pregnancy or other hemorrhagic complication of the first trimester.

The diagnosis of pregnancy can be made at a very early gestational age with remarkable accuracy. The early diagnosis of pregnancy results in an increased ability to recognize complications before they are overtly symptomatic: ectopic pregnancy prior to rupture, an embryonic pregnancy or intrauterine fetal demise before clinical passage of tissue occurs, as well as molar pregnancy and other less common complications of early pregnancy.

CLINICAL APPLICATIONS

The primary responsibility of emergency physicians in symptomatic early pregnancy is to recognize ectopic pregnancy before significant morbidity or mortality occurs. History and physical examination are inadequate to this task. Only half of patients with symptomatic ectopic pregnancy have identifiable risk factors, such as a previous ectopic pregnancy, use of an intrauterine device, history of pelvic inflammatory disease, tubal ligation, in vitro fertilization, or infertility (1). The history in early ectopic pregnancy is neither sensitive nor specific. Patients with ectopic pregnancy can initially be pain-free or have midline crampy abdominal pain. They may have passed "tissue"; some even present without a missed menses. Physical examination findings of tenderness, masses, or peritoneal irritation increase the risk of an ectopic pregnancy, but are likewise inadequate to discriminate patients who can be excluded from consideration of an ectopic pregnancy (2). Furthermore even patients with hemoperitoneum from a ruptured ectopic pregnancy may demonstrate a relative bradycardia, and correlation of vital signs with volume of hemoperitoneum is poor (3). Other ancillary studies are also inaccurate: serum β-hCG levels and progesterone can be helpful over time, or in differentiating a healthy pregnancy from an unhealthy one, but not in locating the pregnancy. Early pregnancy hormonal levels are also frequently in the nondiagnostic range. Ultrasound is the most efficient means of identifying an early IUP and virtually excludes an ectopic pregnancy in the majority of cases (4–6). Pelvic ultrasound markedly decreases the number of patients left with an indeterminate location and viability of pregnancy who must receive close follow-up to make a definitive diagnosis. In a series of 481 consecutive symptomatic ED patients in the first trimester, Kaplan et al showed that transvaginal ultrasound was diagnostic (IUP or ectopic) in 75% of women (4). In other ED studies, 70% of symptomatic first trimester patients were diagnosed with an IUP by pelvic sonography performed by trained ED physicians (7,8).

Secondary roles for early pregnancy pelvic ED ultrasound are diagnosing pregnancy and determining the gestational age and viability of an IUP. A rapid screen during trauma evaluation may detect a new pregnancy and protect against avoidable teratogenic interventions. Early recognition of IUP loss is often not medically necessary. It is still important for patient care to advise a woman of an accurate gestational age when possible, to reassure her of the health of the pregnancy at the time of evaluation, or to prepare her for the high likelihood that the pregnancy is not normal. In addition, urgency and other aspects of follow-up care are clearer when a viable or a nonviable IUP can be suspected based on bedside ultrasound results.

ED ultrasound is well-established as easily repeatable, safe, and nonirradiating for both the mother and the embryo, and it can be accomplished at the bedside rapidly. The emergency physician both performs and interprets the exam, guided by the clinical question, "Is there an IUP present?" Transabdominal ultrasound (Fig. 6.1) successfully identifies IUPs in a majority of women with gestations over 7 to 8 weeks. Transvaginal ultrasound allows definitive diagnosis of a significantly greater number of women, especially in the 5-to-6–week gestational age time period when the risk of ectopic pregnancy is particularly great.

IMAGE ACQUISITION

TRANSABDOMINAL IMAGE OF THE NORMAL PREGNANT UTERUS (FIGS. 6.1–6.3)

The transabdominal view of the uterus is seen best when the bladder is full and can act as an acoustic window. The full bladder also displaces loops of bowel that scatter ultrasound waves. The uterus should be visualized in the both the sagittal and transverse views.

For the sagittal view of the uterus, a standard curvilinear 3–5 MHz transducer is placed in the midline of the abdomen just above the symphysis pubis (Fig. 6.2). The transducer is held such that the most cephalad point of the transducer (often designated by a marker) is oriented to the left side of the ultrasound screen. This is standard sagittal orientation, which places the most cephalad portion of the image at the left side of the screen. It is important to sweep the transducer cephalad and caudad, as well as from left to right such that the entire uterus and retro-uterine space (the cul-de-sac) is seen. If the uterus is anteverted, the uterus will be seen just left of the anechoic, urine-filled bladder. The bowel contents are seen on the far field (bottom) of the screen.

To visualize the uterus in the transverse plane, the transducer is rotated 90 degrees in the counterclockwise position, which orients the right side of the patient to the left of the screen in the standard convention (Fig. 6.3). As in the longitudinal view, the sonographer should sweep the transducer to both sides to ensure that the entire uterus is visualized.

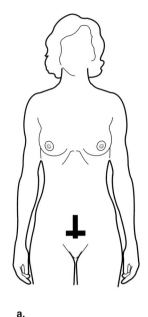

a.

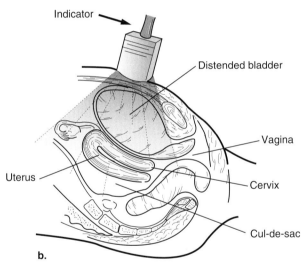

b.

Figure 6.1. Transabdominal Scan.
- Place the transducer in the midline just above the pubis (**A**).
- Place the transducer indicator to project the patient's head to the left of the screen to obtain a sagittal view.
- Rotate the transducer 90° counterclockwise to obtain a transverse view.
- In each view, gently rock the transducer to obtain a 3-dimensional view of the uterus and adnexa.
- When possible, scan with a distended bladder to optimize the acoustic window to the pelvis (**B**).
- The internal landmarks of the transabdominal scan are visualized in **B**.

(**B** is redrawn from Simon and Snoey, eds. *Ultrasound in Emergency and Ambulatory Medicine.* St. Louis, MO: Mosby–Year Book, 1997.)

TRANSVAGINAL IMAGE OF THE NORMAL PREGNANT UTERUS (FIGS. 6.4–6.6)

The transvaginal ultrasound approach to the uterus capitalizes on the shortened distance from the uterus to the transducer, and therefore allows a higher frequency transducer to produce images of improved resolution. However because of the proximity, it is also common to overshoot the target of interest and miss the uterus altogether, imaging only bowel. It is best to ask the patient to empty her bladder, since a large bladder will occupy most of the scan field and make it difficult to visualize the uterus. A small amount of urine in the bladder helps to orient the sonographer.

The examiner should explain this procedure to the patient, obtain the patient's verbal consent, and discuss that this procedure is similar to the gynecologic pelvic examination. In order to prepare the endovaginal transducer, ultrasound gel is applied directly to the transducer and a cover is placed over the transducer to serve as a barrier to infectious dis-

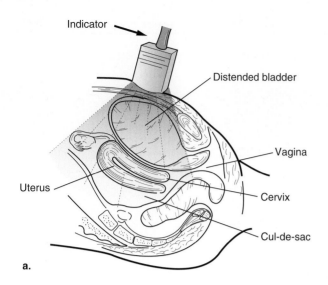

a.

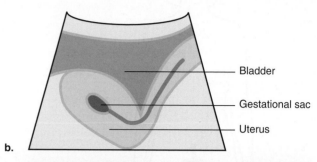

b.

Bladder
Gestational sac
Uterus

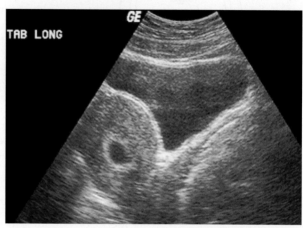

TAB LONG

c.

Figure 6.2. Transabdominal ultrasound of an early IUP, sagittal orientation. (**A**) The transducer is placed in the midline, just above the pubis, using the bladder as an acoustic window. The arrow notes the indicator positioned toward the patient's head to obtain a sagittal orientation (**A**). (**B**) A schemata of the anatomy of an early IUP is shown. (**C**) Ultrasound of a normal early IUP. (**A** is redrawn from Simon and Snoey, eds. *Ultrasound in Emergency and Ambulatory Medicine*. St. Louis, MO: Mosby–Year Book, 1997.)

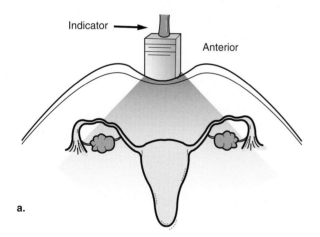

a.

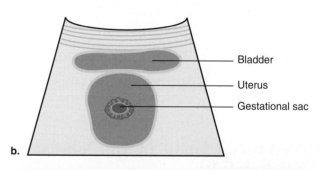

b.

Bladder
Uterus
Gestational sac

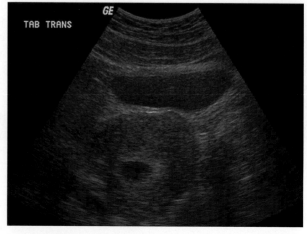

TAB TRANS

c.

Figure 6.3. Transabdominal ultrasound of an early IUP, transverse orientation. The transducer is placed in the midline, just above the pubis, in a transverse orientation. The indicator points to the patient's right (arrow) (**A**). A schemata of a normal early pregnancy is seen in transverse orientation (**B**). Ultrasound of a normal early pregnancy in transverse orientation (**C**). (**A** is redrawn from Simon and Snoey, eds. *Ultrasound in Emergency and Ambulatory Medicine*. St. Louis, MO: Mosby–Year Book, 1997.)

ease, taking care not to trap air bubbles. A specifically manufactured sheath or condom can be used as an appropriate barrier. Then a water-based lubricant should be applied on top of the cover because the conducting gel can be a vaginal irritant. It is important to understand the pelvic anatomy and the orientation of the endovaginal transducer before placing it in the vagina. For the sagittal view, the superior aspect of the endovaginal transducer corresponds to the most anterior portion of the vaginal vault and projects the bladder on the left side of the screen. If the uterus is anteverted, it will appear as an elongated structure with the fundus most anterior or, by convention, pointing toward the left side of the screen (Fig. 6.5). If the uterus is retroverted, the fundus is directed posteriorly or, by convention, points toward the right side of the screen (Fig. 6.7). The sonographer may need to rotate or move the transducer slightly until the midline of the uterus, noted by the endometrial stripe, is easily visualized. The sonographer then sweeps the transducer laterally to both sides to visualize the uterus in its entirety, because it is often deviated to one side. The cul-de-sac is seen inferior to the uterus in the far field, and it should be assessed for the presence of free peritoneal fluid.

Once the uterus is seen in its long axis, the transducer is rotated 90 degrees to the left (counterclockwise), in order to obtain the coronal view, or short-axis (Fig. 6.6). Although this rotation produces a coronal view through the patient, the image appears as a transverse section through the uterus because the uterus is perpendicular to the transducer. It is not possible to obtain a true transverse image of the uterus because the transducer cannot be placed beside the uterus.

Once the sagittal and coronal planes are identified the transducer is swept laterally, as well as anteriorly and posteriorly, such that the entire uterus and surrounding areas are visualized in all planes, to ensure that the boundaries of the uterus are identified. The cul-de-sac is seen inferior to the uterus, or in the far field, in all images. It is important to determine if there is free fluid present in the cul-de-sac, taking care not to confuse fluid in the rectal lumen with free peritoneal fluid. The endometrial stripe should be identified and visualized in its entirety. At least 5 mm of myometrial mantle should surround a gestational sac in all planes to ensure that it is fully within the uterus.

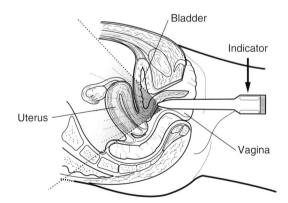

Figure 6.4. The Transvaginal Scan.
- Begin in the sagittal plane with the transducer indicator pointed up (see arrow).
- Advance only as far as necessary to visualize the uterus.
- Find the endometrial stripe to identify the midline of the uterus.
- Rotate the transducer 90° counterclockwise (indicator pointing toward the patient's right side) to obtain a coronal view.
- In each orientation, gently rock the transducer in all planes to obtain a 3-dimensional view of the uterus and adnexa.

(Redrawn from Simon and Snoey, eds. *Ultrasound in Emergency and Ambulatory Medicine*. St. Louis, MO: Mosby–Year Book, 1997.)

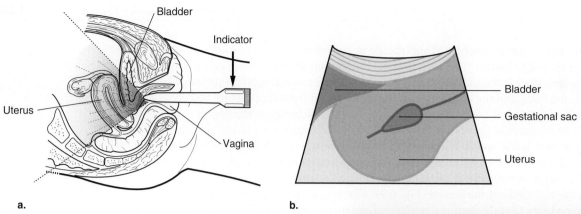

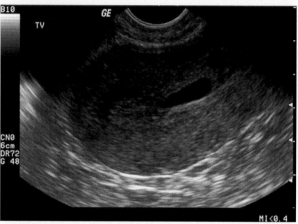

Figure 6.5. Transvaginal ultrasound of an early IUP, sagittal orientation. The transducer is placed in the vaginal vault and advanced until the uterus is seen (**A**). The indicator is positioned up to obtain a sagittal orientation (**A**). The normal anatomy of an early IUP (**B**). An ultrasound of a normal anteverted uterus with an early IUP is seen in sagittal orientation (**C**). (**A** is redrawn from Simon and Snoey, eds. *Ultrasound in Emergency and Ambulatory Medicine.* St. Louis, MO: Mosby–Year Book, 1997.)

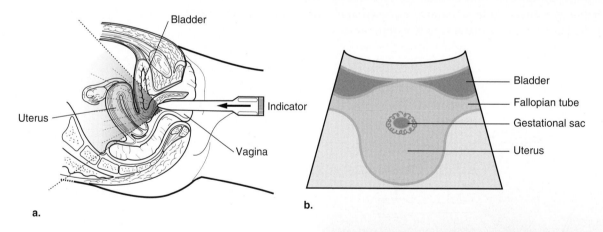

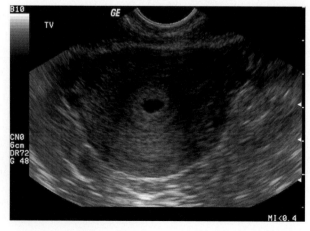

Figure 6.6. Transvaginal ultrasound of an early IUP, coronal orientation. (**A**) The transducer is placed in the vaginal vault and advanced until the uterus is seen. The indicator is positioned toward the patient's right to obtain a coronal orientation. (**B**) A schemata of a normal early pregnancy is seen. (**C**) Ultrasound of a normal early pregnancy as seen in coronal orientation.

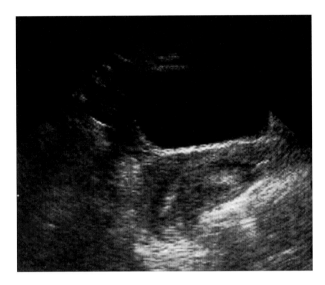

Figure 6.7. Retroverted Uterus. Image courtesy of Mark Deutchman, MD.

VISUALIZATION OF OVARIES

The ovaries are not the primary focus of emergency ultrasound. However, with experience most sonographers will become competent in visualizing the ovaries and benefit from the information they provide. The ovaries are ovoid structures that have the gray echotexture characteristic of soft tissue punctuated by smooth-walled anechoic cystic structures along their periphery (follicles). The ovaries are lateral to the uterus and usually lie anterior to the internal iliac veins and medial to external iliac vessels (Figs. 6.8, 6.9). If the uterus is retroverted the ovaries may lie more anteriorly.

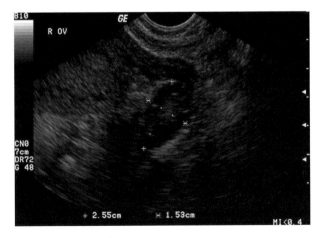

Figure 6.8. Normal Ovary.

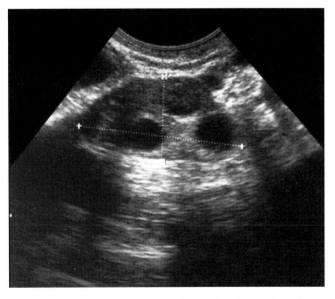

Figure 6.9. Normal Ovary. Reprinted from Kendall JL, Deutchman M. *Ultrasound in Emergency Medicine and Trauma.* Nashville: Healthstream Inc. 2001, with permission.

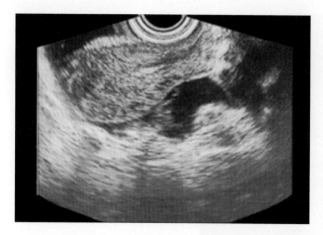

Figure 6.10. Free fluid along the posterior wall of the uterus. Reprinted from Kendall JL, Deutchman M. *Ultrasound in Emergency Medicine and Trauma.* Nashville: Healthstream Inc. 2001, with permission.

FLUID IN THE CUL-DE-SAC (FIGS. 6.10, 6.11)

A small amount of anechoic (black) or hypoechoic free fluid may be present normally in the pelvis and is more likely to be detected by transvaginal scans than transabdominal. There is no consistent, standardized method for grading the amount of fluid in the cul-de-sac; however, there are generally accepted guidelines. According to conventions established by Dart et al., the amount of fluid is considered "small" if it tracks less than a third of the way up the posterior wall of the uterus. Free fluid is considered "moderate" if it tracks two-thirds up the posterior wall of the uterus but is not free-flowing in the peritoneum. The amount of fluid is considered "large" if it tracks beyond two-thirds of the posterior uterine wall, or if it is free-flowing in the peritoneum or seen in Morison's pouch or the splenic recess (9). In one study, 43 of 68 patients diagnosed with ectopic pregnancy had free intraperitoneal fluid seen by ultrasound in amounts ranging from small (23 patients) or moderate (16 patients) to large (4 patients). However, 30% of nonectopics also had visible free fluid, making this neither a sensitive nor specific sign. Most (88%) ectopic pregnancies with cul-de-sac fluid had echoes within the fluid typical of blood and clot; this additional finding should raise the suspicion of ectopic pregnancy (10). Fluid collections are also likely to vary with patient positioning.

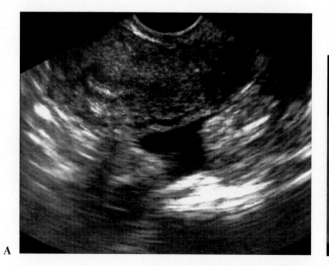
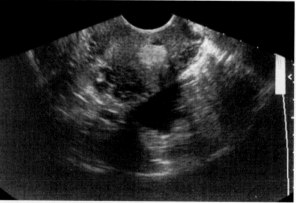

A   B

Figure 6.11. Free fluid tracking along the posterior wall of the uterus (A). Fluid seen in the posterior cul-de-sac in a transverse view of the uterus (B). Reprinted from Kendall JL, Deutchman M. *Ultrasound in Emergency Medicine and Trauma.* Nashville: Healthstream Inc. 2001, with permission.

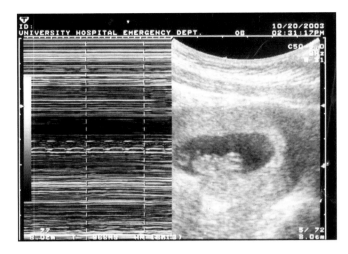

Figure 6.12. M-Mode demonstrates fetal heart activity.

RECOGNITION OF EMBRYONIC HEART RATE USING M-MODE

If an IUP is visualized, cardiac activity can be documented by using M (motion)-mode imaging (Fig. 6.12). It is necessary to become familiar with the specifics of each ultrasound manufacturer's M-mode function. However, the basic principle is that an M-mode beam is placed through the moving heart, and documents the motion waveform over time. A software calculation will then determine the heart rate and record this on the image. Color Doppler or pulse-wave Doppler techniques of measuring cardiac activity should not be used, because potential adverse effects on the fetus have not been ruled out (11).

SONOGRAPHIC FINDINGS IN NORMAL FIRST TRIMESTER PREGNANCY

Both recognition of the possibility of an ectopic pregnancy and assessment of intrauterine gestational age and viability require an understanding of the ultrasound anatomy and landmarks of normal early pregnancy. A timeline of pertinent landmarks of early pregnancy is depicted in Figure 6.13 (Timeline) and Table 6.1.

Table 6.1: Sonographic Landmarks of Normal Pregnancy

	TVS (TAS)		
GA (in weeks)	*US Finding*	*MSD (mm)*	*Embryo/CRL (mm)*
5 (5)	Gestational Sac	5 (5)	—
5.5 (7)	Yolk Sac	8 (20)	—
6 (8)	Cardiac Activity/Embryo	16 (25)	5* (9)

TVS = transvaginal sonography
TAS = transabdominal sonography
MSD = mean sac diameter
CRL = crown rump length
GA = gestational age
Adapted from: Laing FC, Frates MC. "Ultrasound Evaluation During the First Trimester." In: Callen PW, ed. *Ultrasonography in Obstetrics and Gynecology*, 4th ed. Philadelphia: WB Saunders Co, 2000:124.

gestational age	Range of BhCG

4½ weeks   75 – 2,600

5 weeks   2,600

Figure 6.13. Timeline of Normal Pregnancy. Sonographic findings and corresponding range of β-hCG levels are shown.

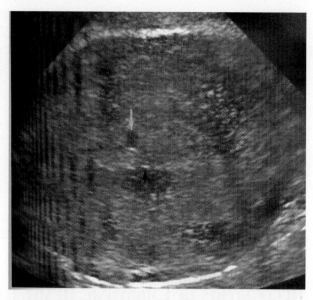

a. Intradecidual Sign. Reprinted from Brant WE. Ultrasound. The Core Curriculum. Philadelphia: Lippincott Williams & Wilkins 2001:231, with permission.

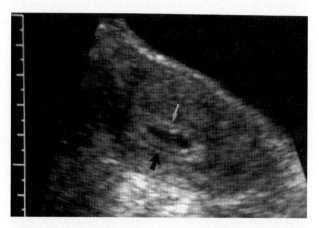

b. Double Decidual Sign. Reprinted from Brant WE. Ultrasound. The Core Curriculum. Philadelphia: Lippincott Williams & Wilkins 2001:235, with permission

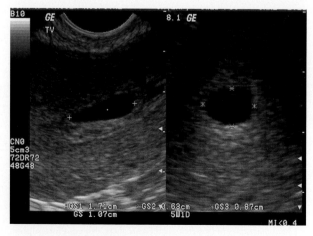

c. Early gestational sac, 5 weeks gestational age, transvaginal scan, sagittal and coronal views.

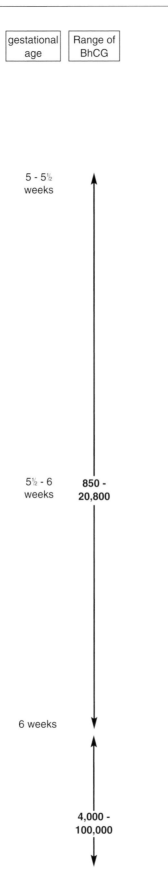

gestational age	Range of BhCG
5 - 5½ weeks	
5½ - 6 weeks	850 - 20,800
6 weeks	
	4,000 - 100,000

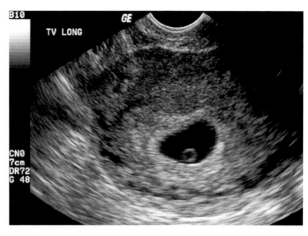

d. 5½ week gestation with yolk sac.

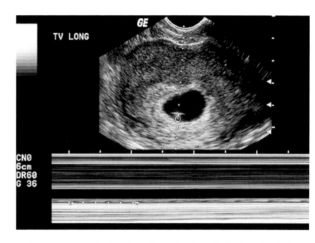

e. 5½ week gestation with embryonic plate. Fetal heart activity is seen in M-mode.

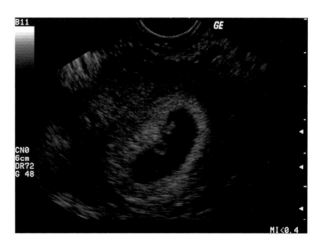

f. 5.5 - 6 week gestation with yolk sac and fetal pole.

Figure 6.13. *(continued)* Timeline of Normal Pregnancy, 5–6 weeks.

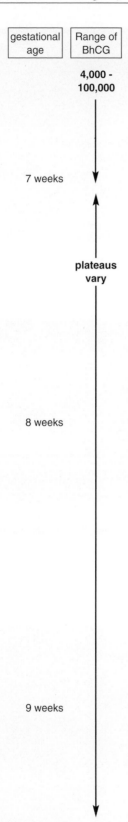

gestational age	Range of BhCG
	4,000 - 100,000

7 weeks

plateaus vary

8 weeks

9 weeks

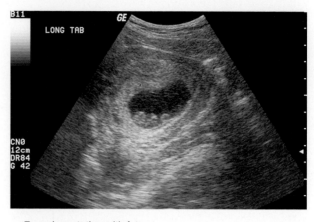

g. 7 week gestation with fetus.

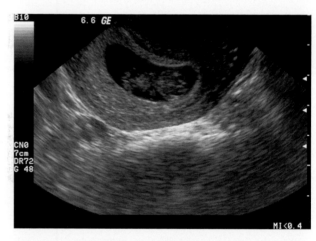

h. 8 week gestation with fully formed fetus and early limb buds.

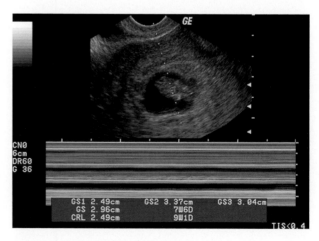

i. 9 week gestation with growing fetus.

Figure 6.13. *(continued)* Timeline of Normal Pregnancy, 7–9 weeks.

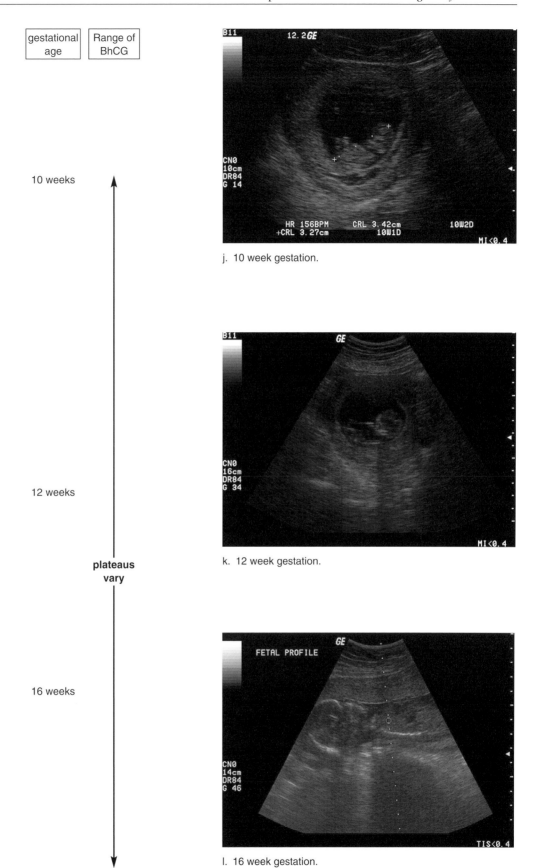

gestational age	Range of BhCG

10 weeks

j. 10 week gestation.

12 weeks

k. 12 week gestation.

plateaus vary

16 weeks

l. 16 week gestation.

Figure 6.13. *(continued)* Timeline of Normal Pregnancy, 10–16 weeks.

ULTRASOUND FINDINGS SUGGESTIVE OF AN EARLY IUP

A number of findings are suggestive of, but not definitive for, intrauterine pregnancy. The earliest sonographic sign of an intrauterine pregnancy is the "intradecidual sign," which is an embryo completely embedded within the endometrial decidua, but that does not displace the endometrial stripe (Fig. 6.13A) (12). Because this is technically difficult to recognize, clinicians must depend on finding more definitive evidence of an IUP and the value of this finding is limited clinically.

It is somewhat easier to see the "double decidual sac sign" by transvaginal ultrasound between 5 and 6 weeks gestational age, before the yolk sac can be seen (Fig. 6.13B). The double decidual sac sign refers to two rings: the decidua capsularis (the inner ring) and the decidua vera (the outer ring), separated by a thin hypoechoic layer, all of which surround the gestational sac. Misinterpretation of the double decidual sac sign is common, however, and this should also not be used as a definitive sign of an IUP. When the double decidual sac sign is suspected, transvaginal ultrasound should be performed, because transvaginal imaging offers a more diagnostic image by the fifth week gestation (12,13).

At 5 weeks a gestational sac, also known as the chorionic sac, can be visualized by transvaginal ultrasound. This occurs when the mean sac diameter is 5 mm (Fig. 6.13C, Table 6.1) (13). The gestational sac is a fluid-filled structure that appears "empty." At this stage of development, it is difficult to distinguish between a true gestational sac and a pseudogestational sac, a collection of fluid within the uterus that occurs in ectopic pregnancies due to hormonal stimulation of the endometrium. Thus, detecting a fluid collection should not be interpreted as a gestational sac or as evidence that a pregnancy is intrauterine.

DEFINITIVE FINDINGS OF IUP

As the pregnancy progresses, ultrasound findings become more definitive. Between 5 and 6 weeks the yolk sac becomes visible within the gestational sac by transvaginal ultrasound; this is considered to be the first reliable sign of an IUP and may be difficult to see on transabdominal scans (Figs. 6.13D, 6.14) (12,13). The yolk sac is a highly echogenic round structure. However, depending on the lateral resolution of the ultrasound transducer, it may initially appear as a set of parallel lines (Fig. 6.13E). These may be very faint and challenging to demonstrate, and the sonographer must be confident of the finding to definitively diagnose IUP at this stage.

Between 5 and 6 weeks an embryo ("fetal pole") appears by transvaginal ultrasound at the border of the yolk sac (Fig. 6.13F). Initially this is only 2 to 3 mm and can be difficult

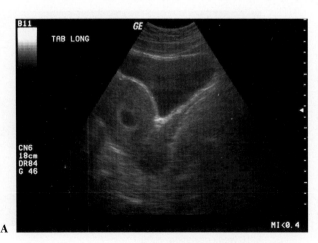

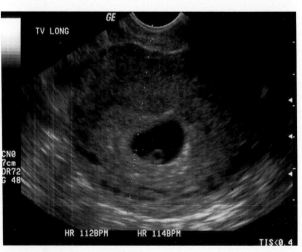

Figure 6.14. Transabdominal view of the uterus of a pregnant patient shows an empty gestational sac that is insufficient to establish an IUP (and exclude ectopic) (**A**). In the same patient, a transvaginal scan demonstrates a gestational sac with a yolk sac, establishing an IUP (**B**).

to visualize. At 6 weeks the embryo is a definite structure that can be measured. In addition, cardiac activity can be seen on transvaginal scans. Normal embryonic heart rate may be as low as 70 to 100 beats per minute range during early gestation, but soon rises to the fetal normal range of 120 to 160 beats per minute by 9 to 10 weeks gestational age (14).

At 7 weeks gestation the head of the embryo is seen on transvaginal scanning (Fig. 6.13G). This is also the time when the yolk sac and the first fetal heart tones can be seen by transabdominal ultrasound. Cardiac activity should be seen by the time the embryo is 5 mm in length (11). After 8 weeks the head of the embryo has a ventricle visible by transvaginal scans, seen as an anechoic structure. At the same time, the amniotic sac can begin to be visualized as a thin echogenic line surrounding the embryo. This fuses with the chorion after 14 weeks gestation. At 10 weeks the embryo is now termed a fetus, since organogenesis is complete.

DETERMINING GESTATIONAL AGE

The gestational age in early pregnancy can be accurately determined from a number of different measurements, based on sonographic findings at different stages of pregnancy. Standard measurements of gestational age are referenced from the onset of the last normal menstrual period, about 2 weeks before the actual time of conception. The following measurements define gestational age.

1. Mean Sac Diameter (MSD), or Gestational Sac Size (GSS). In early pregnancy the gestational age can be determined from the size of the gestational sac using the MSD. The earliest that the gestational sac can be visualized by transvaginal ultrasound is at a diameter of 2 to 3 mm, which correlates with a gestational age between 4 and 5 weeks. MSD can be calculated by obtaining measurements of the diameter of the gestational sac in three planes and dividing by 3. The gestational age (GA) is calculated from the formula: MSD *(mm)* + 30 = GA +/− 4 days. MSD is normally 5 mm at 5 weeks gestational age. Charts are available correlating the MSD with gestational age (12, 13). An embryo should be visible within a gestational sac with a MSD of 16 mm by transvaginal scans, or 25 mm by transabdominal scans (Fig. 6.15, Table 6.1).
2. Crown Rump Length (CRL). When an embryo is present, the CRL can be measured with calipers defining the length of embryo (excluding the legs and yolk sac) (Fig. 6.16). The gestational age can be measured using the formula: CRL *(in cms)* + 42 = GA (days) between 6 and 9.5 weeks (12). The CRL increases by about 1 mm per day, as does the MSD.
3. Once the fetus has reached 13 weeks gestational age, other methods of determining gestational age are used, such as head circumference (HC), biparietal diameter (BPD), abdominal circumference (AC) and femur length (FL) (Fig. 6.17) (12).

While these guidelines are useful, most ultrasound machines are equipped with software to provide estimates of gestational age based on these measurements.

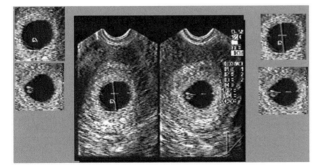

Figure 6.15. The Mean Sac Diameter (MSD), also known as Gestational Sac Size (GSS). Obtained by taking three measurements of the diameter of the gestational sac in three dimensions, as shown here. Reprinted from Kendall JL, Deutchman M. *Ultrasound in Emergency Medicine and Trauma.* Nashville: Healthstream Inc. 2001, with permission.

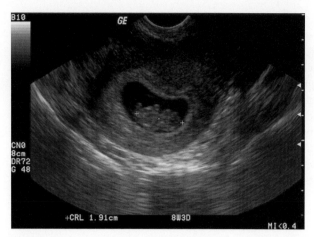

Figure 6.16. A crown rump length measurement of an 8-week–3-day-old fetus.

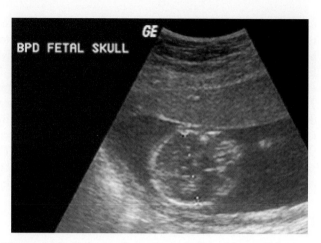

Figure 6.17. Gestational age determined by biparietal diameter (BPD).

PATHOLOGY

ABNORMAL PREGNANCY

If pregnancy does not proceed according to the guidelines in Table 6.1, the pregnancy is probably abnormal. In several series of patients presenting to EDs in the first trimester with vaginal bleeding or pain, only about half of women have normal pregnancies, and 7 to 13% have ectopic pregnancies (4,15,16). Definitive diagnosis of early pregnancy failure usually requires serial examinations or a follow-up consultative ultrasound. Normal pregnancy parameters are shown in Table 6.1, and criteria suggestive for early pregnancy failure are listed in Table 6.2. It is important to remember that either an intra- or extrauterine pregnancy problem may exist if ultrasound findings do not correlate with β-hCG levels described in the timeline of Figure 6.13 and Table 6.1. In addition, women with multiple gestations have elevated β-hCG levels for a given gestational age, and therefore the embryos may not be visible by singleton β-hCG landmarks. Likewise infertility patients with multiple gestations may have an ectopic pregnancy in addition to an IUP (heterotopic pregnancy) and can present a special diagnostic challenge.

SPONTANEOUS ABORTION

Spontaneous abortion occurs in about 20 to 25% of chemically diagnosed pregnancies. About 80% of early fetal loss occurs in the first trimester. Intrauterine fetal loss occurs at several stages. Anembryonic gestation, (blighted ovum or unsuccessful development), in which the embryo never develops within the gestational sac, is defined as the absence of an embryo when the mean gestational sac diameter is 25 mm or more (Fig. 6.18, Table 6.2) (17,18). Abnormal embryonic growth (embryonic demise or failed pregnancy) is in-

Table 6.2: Sonographic Suspicion for Abnormal Pregnancy
No gestational sac at a β-hCG of 3000 mIU/ml or ≥ 38 days since onset last menses Absent embryo with gestational sac of 25 mm mean diameter (by TAS) Embryo of 5 mm crown rump length with no heartbeat No fetal heart tones after 10 to 12 weeks gestational age
Adapted from Dart RG. Role of pelvic ultrasound in evaluation of symptomatic first trimester pregnancy. *Ann Emerg Med.* 1999;33:310.

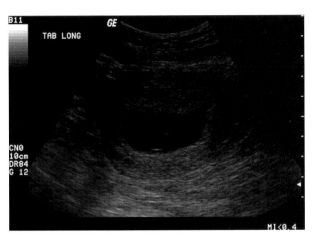

Figure 6.18. Transabdominal scan of a gestational sac without a well-defined fetus, consistent with a blighted ovum.

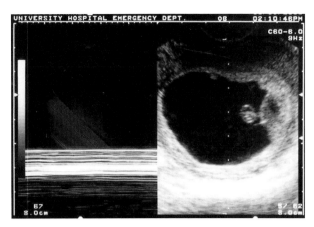

Figure 6.19. Failure of pregnancy to progress and absent fetal heart activity confirm an intrauterine fetal demise.

dicated by the absence of fetal heart activity by transvaginal ultrasound at the normal gestational age of 8 weeks (Fig. 6.19) (7,12). Some intrauterine fetal demise occurs after fetal heart activity develops, secondary to subchorionic hemorrhage, faulty implantation or genetic flaws. Intrauterine fetal demise is often suggested by an abnormal gestational sac (Fig. 6.20). Therefore not only is the gestational sac size not appropriate for dates, but

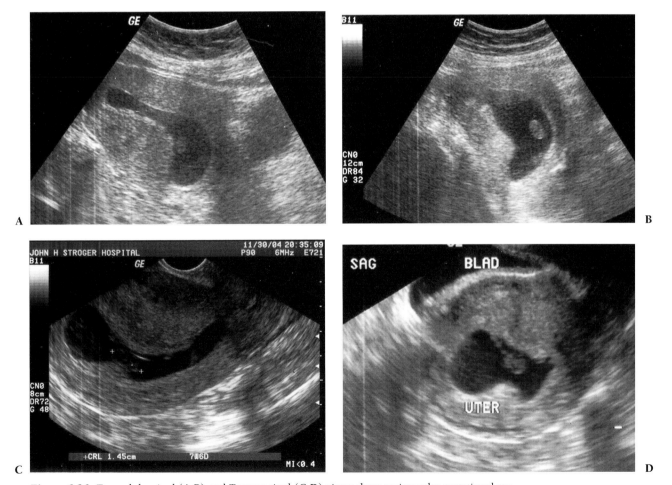

Figure 6.20. Transabdominal (**A,B**) and Transvaginal (**C,D**) views show an irregular gestational sac with poorly defined content consistent with an intrauterine fetal demise.

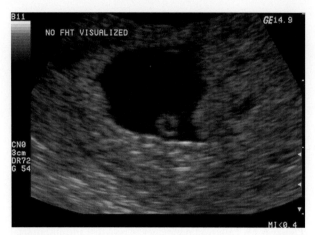

Figure 6.21. Scalloping of the gestational sac in an abnormal pregnancy.

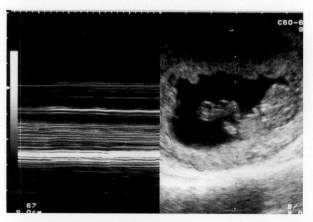

Figure 6.22. Scalloped gestational sac.

the edges are irregular and may be scalloped in appearance (Figs. 6.21, 6.22). Further, a gestational sac positioned near the cervix or low in the uterus is suggestive of demise. Loss of identifiable fetal parts and a thickened, irregular endometrium may reflect debris of a fetal loss (Fig. 6.23). The likelihood of spontaneous loss without symptoms of bleeding or pain has been reported to be only about 5 to 10% after fetal cardiac activity is detected by transabdominal ultrasound (which is almost the same rate as in patients with symptoms). With transvaginal ultrasound the likelihood of pregnancy loss is higher after fetal heart tones are seen, due to the earlier gestational age at which the heartbeat can be detected. While spontaneous abortion rates in younger women (< 36 years) after a heartbeat is identified by transvaginal ultrasound is still in the 5% range, rates of loss after documented fetal heart tones have been reported as high as 30% in patients over 40 years of age (11).

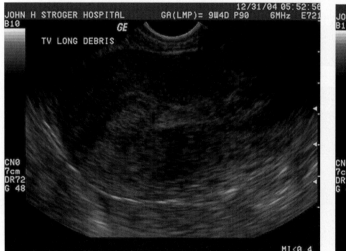

A

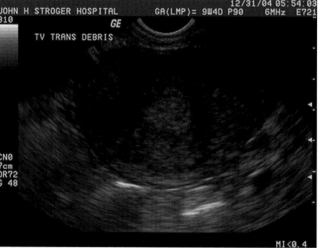

B

Figure 6.23. Failed pregnancy with debris. Transvaginal scan, longitudinal orientation (**A**). Transvaginal scan, coronal orientation (**B**).

ECTOPIC PREGNANCY (FIGS. 6.24–6.39)

Ectopic pregnancy occurs in about 2% of pregnancies. Ectopic locations for pregnancy implantation vary. Most commonly an ectopic pregnancy is within the fallopian tubes, but interstitial locations (at the edge of the uterus adjacent to the tubes), cornual (in one horn of a bicornuate uterus), cervical, ovarian, and abdominal implantations may occur (Figs. 6.24, 6.25). Interstitial pregnancies are particularly problematic, since the location on the myometrium at the edge of the uterus allows the pregnancy to develop further before rupture occurs (often at 10 to12 weeks gestation), thus accounting for the disproportionate mortality of interstitial ectopics (19,20).

Occasionally an ectopic gestation is directly visualized by ultrasound (Figs. 6.24–6.32). In one series of 45 ectopic pregnancies reported by radiologists, an extrauterine fetal pole (with or without cardiac activity) could be visualized by transvaginal scans in up to one-third of cases; a few were seen by transabdominal scans (21). However, most ectopic pregnancies are not visualized directly by pelvic ultrasound. The emergency sonographer should recognize that even when an ectopic gestation is not seen, the ultrasound may detect other abnormalities that would increase suspicion for an ectopic pregnancy. Indirect evidence suspicious for ectopic pregnancy includes adnexal masses, contained extrauterine fluid collections, or significant free fluid in the cul-de-sac in the setting of failure to detect an intrauterine embryo at any β-hCG level (Figs. 6.33–6.39).

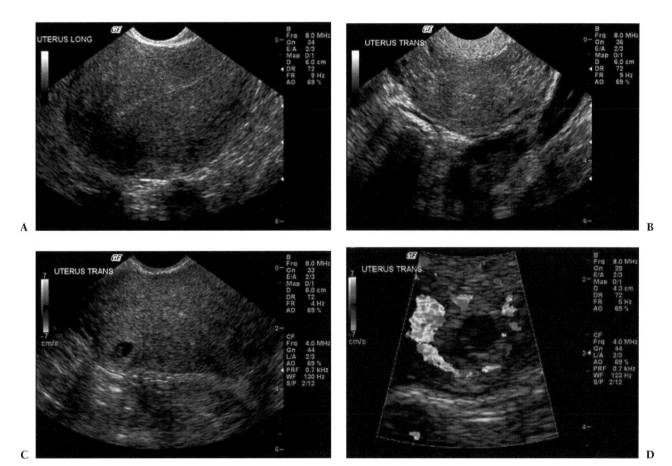

Figure 6.24. Interstitial pregnancy in a pregnant patient with vaginal bleeding. No IUP is seen by transvaginal ultrasound in longitudinal (**A**) and transverse (**B**) views through the midline of the uterus. Further survey of the pelvis reveals an interstitial pregnancy with active fetal heart activity (**C**). A ring of fire is seen by Doppler indicating hypervascularity around the gestational sac (**D**). (See color insert for color image of Part D.) Images courtesy of Cory Cunningham, PA-C, and Karen Cosby, MD.

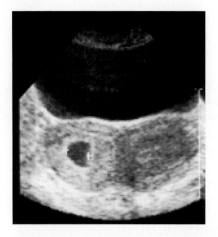

Figure 6.25. IUP in a Bicornate Uterus. Image courtesy of Kendall JL, Deutchman M. *Ultrasound in Emergency Medicine and Trauma*. Nashville:Healthstream 2001.

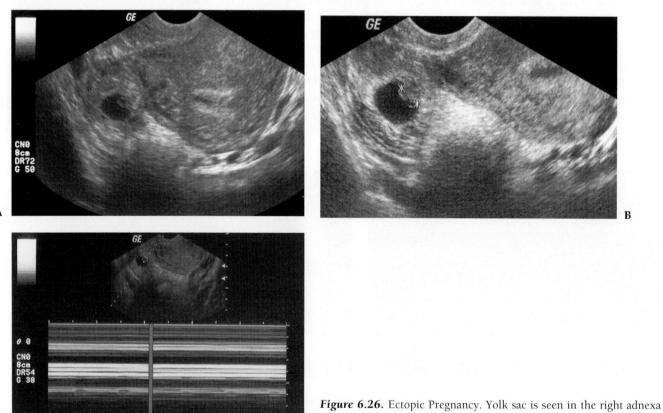

A

B

C

Figure 6.26. Ectopic Pregnancy. Yolk sac is seen in the right adnexa (A). Fetal pole (B) with fetal heart activity is visualized (C). Image courtesy of Karen Cosby, MD.

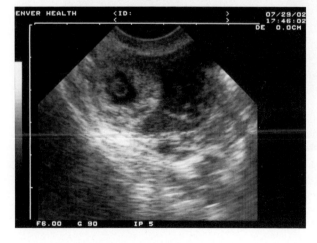

Figure 6.27. An ectopic pregnancy is seen outside the uterus. Image courtesy of John Kendall, MD.

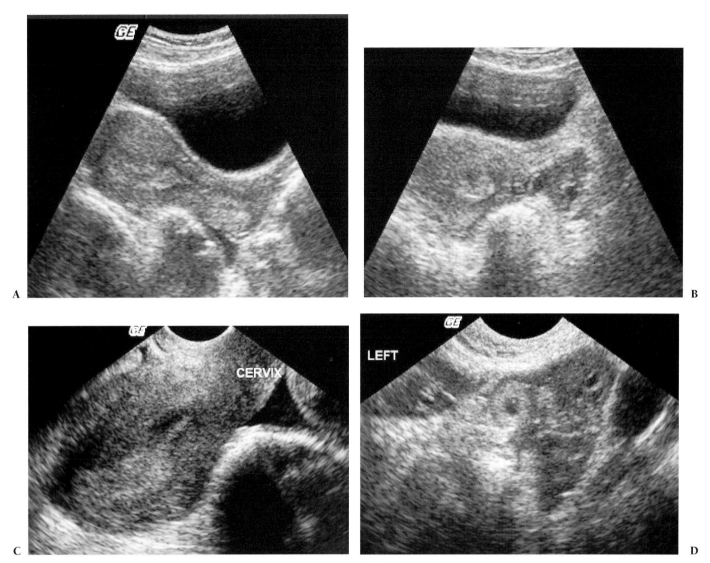

Figure 6.28. Ectopic Pregnancy. A transabdominal scan shows a small amount of free fluid in the cul-de-sac (**A**) and a suspicious left adnexal mass (**B**). The transvaginal scan confirms fluid in the cul-de-sac (**C**) and visualizes the ectopic on the left (**D**). Image courtesy of Karen Cosby, MD.

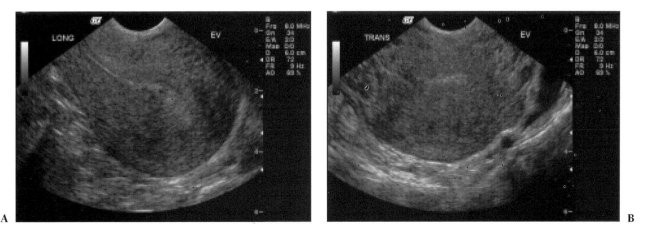

Figure 6.29. Ectopic Pregnancy. A transvaginal scan through the midline of the uterus fails to find an IUP in this pregnant patient with a β-hCG of 2,477 (**A** and **B**).

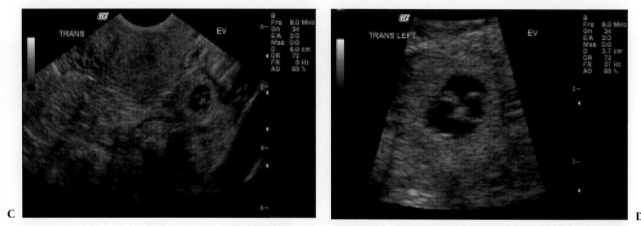

C   D

Figure 6.29. *(continued)* On closer inspection an ectopic pregnancy is seen in the adnexa (**C** and **D**). Image courtesy of Karen Cosby, MD.

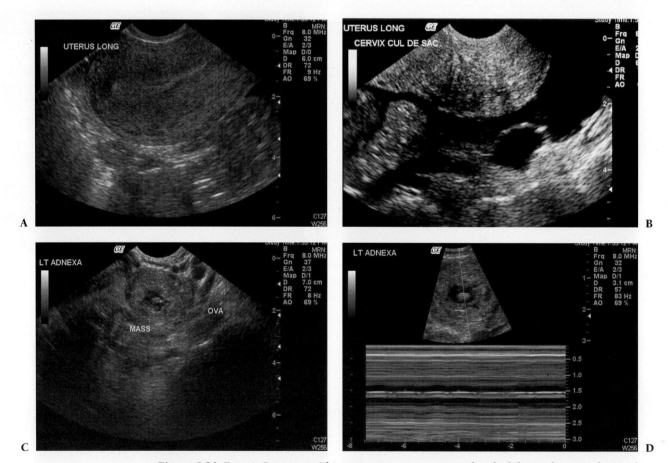

A   B

C   D

Figure 6.30. Ectopic Pregnancy. This pregnant patient presented with abdominal pain and vaginal bleeding. Her β-hCG was 8,664. A transvaginal scan failed to find an IUP (**A**), but did find a large amount of free fluid in the pelvis (**B**). Closer inspection visualized a complex mass in the left adnexa (**C**) and a fetal pole with active cardiac activity (**D**). Image courtesy of Karen Cosby, MD.

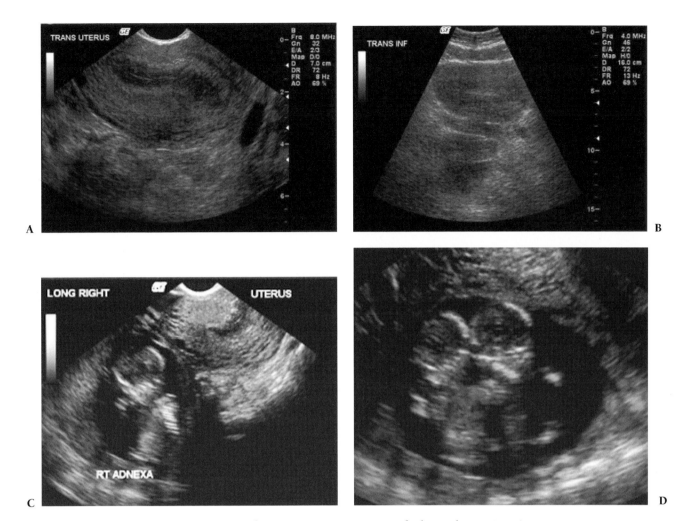

Figure 6.31. An unusual presentation of a twin ectopic pregnancy of advanced gestation. A transvaginal scan fails to demonstrate an IUP in either sagittal (**A**) or coronal (**B**) views. A scan of the right adnexa reveals a well-formed fetus (**C**). On closer inspection, a twin ectopic is seen (**D**). Although interesting, most ectopics fail to reach such an advanced gestational age. Images courtesy of David Greenberg, MD and Karen Cosby, MD.

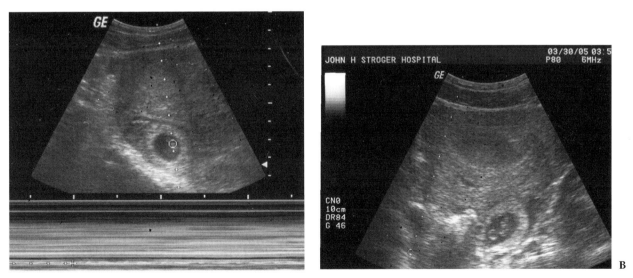

Figure 6.32. Ectopic Pregnancy. A live fetus is visualized in **A**, initially thought to be an IUP. In a transverse view of the uterus, the fetus is actually noted to be extrauterine. When an ectopic pregnancy is adjacent to the uterus it can be mistaken for an IUP. This is a good example of why it is essential to always obtain two views perpendicular to an object of interest to determine its exact location. Image courtesy of Karen Cosby, MD.

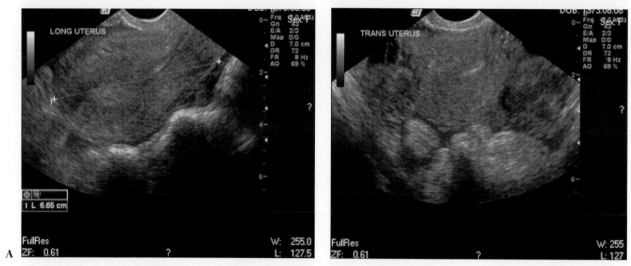

Figure 6.33. Free fluid seen outlining the uterus in both sagittal (**A**) and coronal (**B**) views in a patient with an ectopic pregnancy.

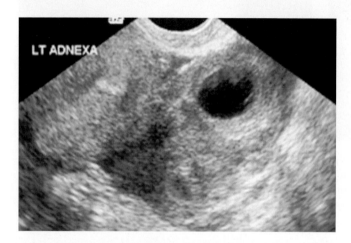

Figure 6.34. Complex adnexal mass and empty uterus in a pregnant patient found to have an ectopic pregnancy.

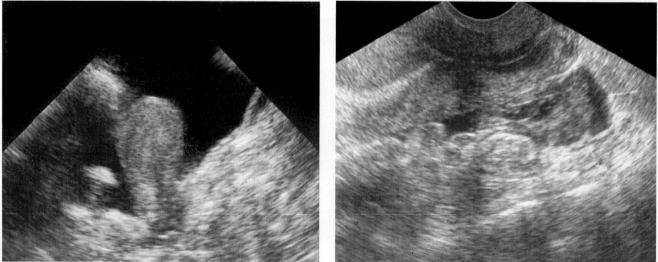

Figure 6.35. Free fluid seen in transabdominal (**A**) and transvaginal (**B**) scans of a pregnant patient with an empty uterus found to have an ectopic pregnancy. Image courtesy of John Kendall, MD.

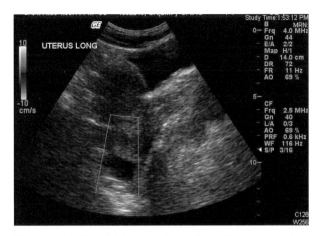

Figure 6.36. Transabdominal Scan. A small amount of free fluid is seen in the cul-de-sac in this patient who was found to have an ectopic pregnancy.

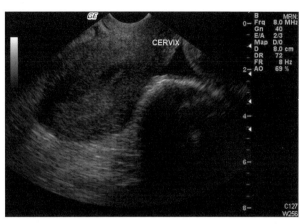

Figure 6.37. Transvaginal Scan. A small amount of free fluid is seen in the cul-de-sac in a patient found to have an ectopic pregnancy.

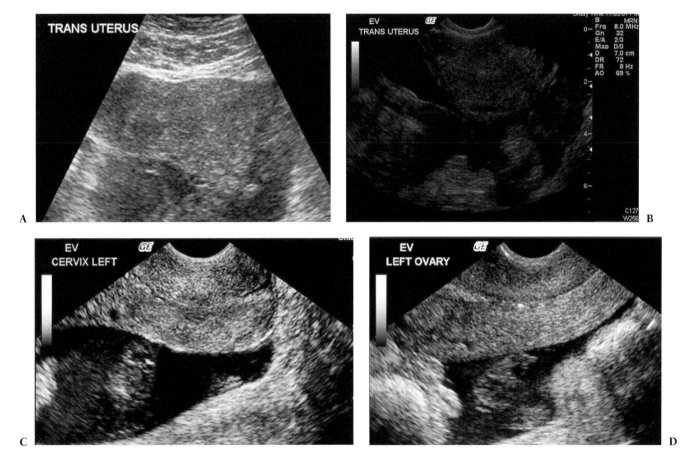

Figure 6.38. Large amount of free-flowing fluid in a patient with a ruptured ectopic pregnancy. Some of the blood has formed clots and appears echogenic. The fluid outlines loops of bowel (**B, D**).

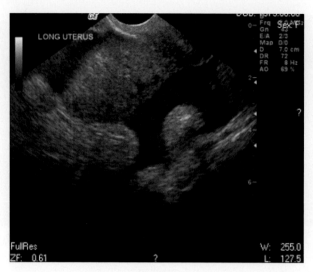

Figure 6.39. Large amount of free fluid in a patient with a ruptured ectopic pregnancy.

Patients with an empty uterus are 5 times more likely to have an ectopic pregnancy, compared to those with fluid or debris in the uterus (22). In the emergency medicine and obstetrical literature, detection of a nonovarian adnexal mass by transvaginal ultrasound or detection of free fluid is highly suspicious for ectopic pregnancy (23,24).

MOLAR PREGNANCY

Molar pregnancy is a complication of developing pregnancy in which chorionic villi proliferate in a disordered fashion, usually without the development of a fetus. Bleeding commonly is seen in the late first trimester or early second trimester, and β-hCG levels are markedly elevated. The diagnosis is suspected by the characteristic sonographic appearance of grapelike vesicles or "snowstorm" appearance of the endometrial cavity without an identifiable fetus at β-hCG levels considerably above the β-hCG thresholds to see an intrauterine pregnancy (Figs. 6.40–6.42). In two-thirds of cases, however, the sonographic findings are nonspecific, and include debris in the uterus or absence of a gestational sac and embryo at a high β-hCG level, with confirmation by histological examination. Neoplastic gestational disease develops in about 15% of molar pregnancies after dilatation and curettage (25,26).

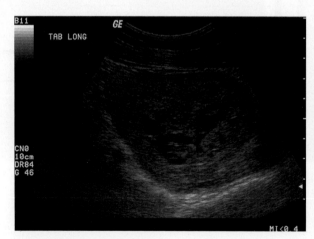

Figure 6.40. Molar Gestation.

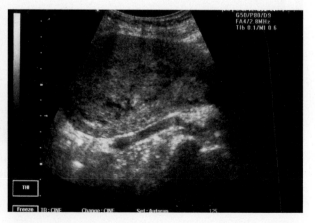

Figure 6.41. Molar Gestation. Image courtesy of John Kendall, MD.

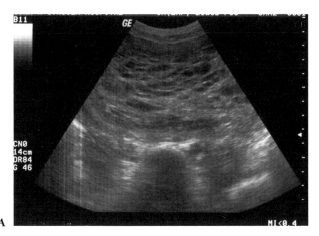 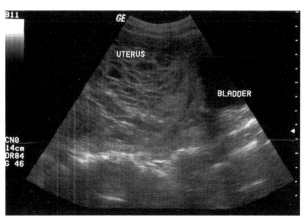

Figure 6.42. Molar Gestation. Image courtesy of Karen Cosby, MD.

OTHER PATHOLOGIC SONOGRAPHIC FINDINGS

Echogenic material within uterus

Echoes within the uterus must be distinguished from echoes within a gestational sac. Echogenic material in the uterus without a definite gestational sac is almost always abnormal. In a consecutive series over 6 years, Dart found 78 patients with intrauterine echogenic debris and found it to be nonspecific: seen in abnormal pregnancies, ectopic pregnancy, or molar pregnancy (27). Debris can also be seen in patients who have had elective or spontaneous abortions. It may resolve spontaneously, although an ectopic pregnancy must still be considered. Therefore a wide differential diagnosis and a low threshold for a consultative examination are necessary when nonspecific echoes are seen in the uterus (28,29).

Free fluid in the cul-de-sac

Fluid in the pelvic peritoneal cavity can be seen in the normal IUP, IUP with a ruptured corpus luteum cyst, or with a leaking or ruptured ectopic pregnancy. Echogenic fluid is particularly concerning for ectopic pregnancy (Figs. 6.38, 6.39).

PITFALLS AND ARTIFACTS OF IMAGE ACQUISITION

Common pitfalls include the following.

1. Failing to have a full urinary bladder in transabdominal pelvic ED ultrasound. This may limit the value of information obtained since the bladder provides an acoustic window and displaces the bowel.
2. Scanning past the uterus with the endovaginal probe. If the transducer is too deep within the vaginal canal, the uterus may not be visualized and only bowel is seen. If this occurs, it may be necessary to pull the transducer back until only a small fraction of the urinary bladder is seen.
3. Utilizing only the transvaginal modality to examine the first trimester uterus. The sonographer may miss cystic or complex ovarian masses, a large uterus, and other important findings if the transabdominal approach is not used first to obtain an overview.
4. Utilizing only the transabdominal modality without transvaginal scanning. Diagnosis of IUP is delayed by a week of gestational age using only the transabdominal approach

and adds technical challenges. In addition, in an obese patient or a patient with a retroverted uterus, the transvaginal scan enhances proximity to the uterus even more.

5. Using inadequate lubricant or having air bubbles at the ultrasound interface. Image quality is significantly compromised by the added acoustic noise.

6. Mistaking a large ovarian cyst or other fluid-filled structure for the urinary bladder may result in misdiagnosis.

PITFALLS OF IMAGE INTERPRETATION

Clinicians should avoid the following common pitfalls.

1. Considering history or examination indicating passage of tissue as evidence for a spontaneous abortion. Such tissue may represent sloughing of organized clot or uterine decidual tissue as the β-hCG levels decline with an ectopic pregnancy. (See recognition of chorionic villi below.)

2. Diagnosing an IUP when a gestational sac is seen without embryonic echoes. An early sac is difficult to distinguish from a pseudogestational sac, which is sometimes seen due to endometrial hypertrophy from an adjacent ectopic pregnancy.

3. Mistaking uterine artery or iliac vessel flow for cardiac activity of the embryo. At five weeks gestation, fetal heart rates can be as slow as 70 to 100 beats per minute and mimic the maternal heart rate (14).

4. Not measuring a definite 5 mm rim of myometrium around the entire gestational sac to locate the pregnancy within the body of the uterus. A gestational sac with a thin myometrial mantle can be seen with a cervical or even tubal gestation.

5. Detecting an IUP and completely discarding ectopic pregnancy from the differential when a heterotopic pregnancy (i.e., coexisting IUP and ectopic pregnancy) should still be considered (Fig. 6.43). While the chances of this occurring spontaneously are low (about 1 in 4,000 pregnancies), the incidence in women with multiple gestations from stimulated fertility or implantation procedures can be as high as 1:100 or less (30).

6. Detecting fetal heart tones and assuming that an IUP is present. While traditionally auscultation of fetal heart tones has implied an intrauterine location, newer sonographic techniques detect fetal heart activity in up to 20% of ectopics (20,31). The sonographer must complete the screening ultrasound examination by identifying myometrium with a minimum 5 mm rim surrounding the gestation to assure that the beating embryo is not in an ectopic location.

7. Failing to recognize that a small amount of cul-de-sac fluid can be normal. Echogenic fluid and larger volumes of peritoneal fluid correlate more with ectopic pregnancy than smaller volume and anechoic fluid.

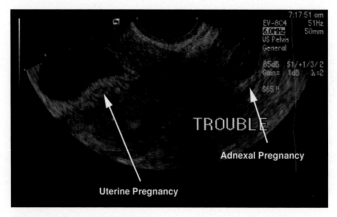

Figure 6.43. A heterotopic pregnancy is seen in the adnexa. Note the normal IUP. Image courtesy of Diku Mandavia, MD.

8. Mistaking an extrauterine gestational sac that lacks an embryo for a simple ovarian cyst.
9. Relying on subtle signs of ectopic pregnancy, such as complex adnexal masses, to diagnose ectopic pregnancy. While this should increase suspicion for ectopic pregnancy, no signs other than a gestational sac with embryonic structures in an extrauterine location are pathognomonic of ectopic pregnancy.
10. Assuming that debris in the uterus excludes an ectopic pregnancy. Heterogeneous debris in the uterus can either represent retained products of conception or endometrial sloughing associated with ectopic pregnancy (32).
11. Failure to recognize that infertility patients may have multiple gestations, and that the likelihood of heterotopic pregnancy is markedly increased in this patient group.
12. Assuming that an empty uterus implies a completed spontaneous abortion. This finding is reported commonly with ectopic pregnancy also (22).

USE OF THE IMAGE IN CLINICAL DECISION MAKING

THE GENERAL APPROACH

The approach to the patient with symptoms of bleeding or pain in early pregnancy should be systematic and aimed at early exclusion or diagnosis of ectopic pregnancy, and diagnosis of early pregnancy failure. Ultrasound has emerged as the best first ancillary study (6). The primary question in a first trimester pregnancy is the location of the pregnancy; thus the primary ED ultrasound question is, "Is there an IUP?" For emergency medicine sites where only transabdominal examinations are performed, a consultative examination including transvaginal ultrasound is probably the most useful next step if an IUP is not seen by transabdominal scans, because about twice as many IUPs can be identified with transvaginal scans (33). Likewise, if no IUP is seen on the ED transvaginal scan, a consultative examination is also a reasonable next step, since ED accuracy has not yet been robustly reported. The radiology or obstetric sonographer may be better able to detect subtle or indirect clues suspicious for ectopic pregnancy, like complex masses, echogenic fluid, etc. If transvaginal ultrasound is not immediately available, a quantitative β-hCG in addition to an obstetrical consultation will help prioritize patients and interpret the eventual ultrasound results. Figure 6.44 describes a recommended approach to evaluation of the first-trimester patient who presents with bleeding or pain to the ED.

THE PREGNANT PATIENT WITH HEMODYNAMIC INSTABILITY OR AN ACUTE ABDOMEN

The pregnant patient with hypotension or peritoneal findings requires a FAST examination to detect free fluid in the abdomen. During resuscitation, a transabdominal pelvic ultrasound, followed by a transvaginal scan if not definitive, should be performed to rapidly diagnose intrauterine pregnancy and detect free cul-de-sac fluid. About 20% of ectopic pregnancies present with emergent signs and symptoms (15). When an IUP can be identified at the bedside, the differential leans more towards nongynecologic causes of abdominal catastrophe, though a rare severe hemorrhagic corpus luteum cyst rupture or heterotopic pregnancy cannot be completely excluded.

IUP DETECTED

In the stable patient, pelvic ultrasound is used to detect an embryo within the gestational sac in the uterus, assuring that there is an IUP. When the pitfalls noted above are avoided and a definitive diagnosis of an IUP can be made, the risk of ectopic pregnancy decreases to the risk of heterotopic pregnancy to about 1 in 4,000. The risk of heterotopic pregnancy

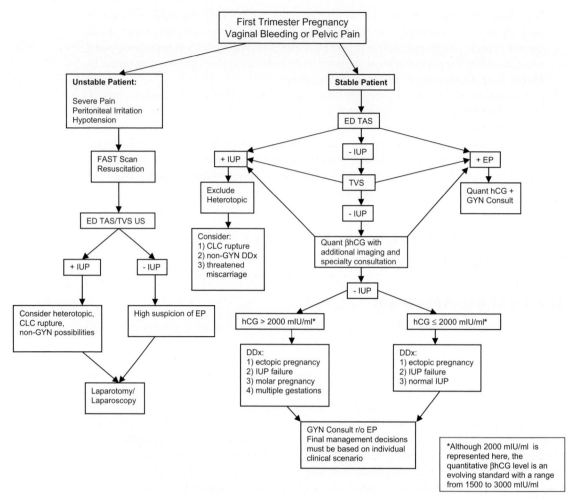

Figure 6.44. Approach to a first trimester pregnancy presenting with vaginal bleeding or pelvic pain.

is strikingly high, however, in patients undergoing pregnancy induction by embryo transfer techniques; in these patients consultative pelvic sonography and close specialty follow-up is required, even after an IUP is diagnosed (30).

For patients in whom an IUP is definitely visualized and in whom examination demonstrates a closed cervical os with bleeding, "threatened abortion" is diagnosed. Patients should be counseled that although an IUP with heartbeat is documented at this time, there is still about a 10 to15% risk of miscarriage. Quantitative serum β-hCG levels are less useful if an embryo is definitively seen on ultrasound, since viability and gestational age are determined by sonographic landmarks and serial studies once an embryo is seen. Serum β-hCG levels plateau after about 8 weeks gestation, rendering them uninterpretable at the gestational age that sonography becomes definitive.

Optimum ED care consists of primary care follow-up, discussion of the risks and symptoms of abortion, and pursuit of an alternative cause of symptoms, particularly if this is a clinical consideration due to significant pain. Alternative diagnoses, including appendicitis, molar pregnancy, ruptured corpus luteum cyst, ovarian torsion, or other intra-abdominal process are important, but are rendered easier by the exclusion of ectopic pregnancy.

ECTOPIC PREGNANCY DETECTED

Sonographic diagnosis of ectopic pregnancy is definitive if an embryo is seen within a gestational sac outside of the normal endometrial location. The accuracy of bedside sonography to visualize an ectopic pregnancy is not well-defined, but it is clear that current sonographic hardware detects fetal heart activity or a fetal pole in a significant minority of patients with ectopic pregnancies. Thus it is mandatory that the physician performing bedside sonography be able to recognize the signs that a living early embryo is within the uterus, as well as appreciate secondary findings suggesting an ectopic pregnancy.

No Definite IUP or Ectopic Pregnancy Detected (Indeterminant Scan)

If the ED ultrasound study is "indeterminant," i.e., an IUP is not found, it is most efficient to obtain a quantitative serum β-hCG and specialty consultation with radiology or obstetrics. The risk of an extrauterine pregnancy can be assessed by identifying each individual's ectopic risk factors; correlating gestational age with dates, physical exam, β-hCG, and sonographic findings; and assessing clinical suspicion based on the patient's presentation and physical findings. In a recent large prospective cohort study, 20% of all ED first trimester pelvic ultrasound examinations resulted in an "indeterminate" classification. Of these only 29% were ultimately diagnosed as IUP; the remaining patients either had ultimate diagnoses of embryonic demise (53%), ectopic pregnancy (15%), or "unknown" (3%) (8).

The management of suspected ectopic pregnancy in the face of a nondiagnostic or indeterminant ultrasound is largely based on the quantitative serum β-hCG. The "discriminatory zone" is a term developed to denote the quantitative β-hCG level at which a gestational sac or an embryo can almost always be seen if the pregnancy is developing normally. (This is in contrast to "threshold levels," which are the lowest β-hCG levels at which a finding may be detected.) Early work with transabdominal ultrasound determined that the gestational sac should be visible at β-hCG levels of 6500 mIU/ml (34). Transvaginal ultrasound discriminatory levels are lower (1000 to 2000 mIU/ml), but vary depending on the vaginal probe equipment used, operator skills, and patient population. A clear discriminatory threshold for ED transvaginal ultrasound has not been determined (17). For that reason, ED ultrasound should be used to demonstrate an IUP and to suspect, but not to definitively act on, possible fetal demise. The limited ED ultrasound still significantly narrows the number of women with concern for ectopic pregnancy to those with no sonographic evidence of IUP (Table 6.2).

Indeterminant Scan with a β-hCG ≥ 2000

A consultative ultrasound should be used to confirm the pelvic ultrasound in the ED and avoid unnecessary loss of an early normal IUP (35). When the β-hCG is ≥ 2000 mIU/ml and the ultrasound is indeterminant, some obstetricians will consider a dilatation and curettage that can be both diagnostic and therapeutic. If chorionic villi are seen on curettings, a diagnosis of an abnormal IUP is confirmed. If chorionic villi are not seen, a presumptive diagnosis of ectopic pregnancy is strongly supported. The decision to pursue this intervention is highly individualized, based on the practitioner's judgment, the patient's risk of ectopic, and the patient's desire to keep the pregnancy. Some clinicians recommend setting a higher discriminatory zone (β-hCG of 3000 mIU/ml) to avoid unnecessary intervention and possible termination of an early viable IUP (35).

Indeterminant Scan with a β-hCG ≤ 2000

The more difficult situation occurs when an indeterminant scan is obtained in a patient with a β-hCG ≤ 2000 mIU/ml. In the low-risk patient who is stable and relatively asymptomatic, serial β-hCG levels can be followed every 48 hours. The interpretation of the rate of change of β-hCG levels has been evaluated by Barnhart and Dart as a means of risk stratifying patients with an indeterminate ultrasound. Normally β-hCG rises by at least 50% every 2 days for the first 6 weeks of gestation (35,36). In ectopic pregnancy, the expected increase in β-hCG is often less than expected, although in about 25% of ectopic pregnancies, the β-hCG rises normally for a time. (In such cases the rate of change does not discriminate between early healthy IUP and ectopic pregnancies.) Hormone levels that drop 50% or more over 48 hours are least likely to be ectopic pregnancies, and almost always represent spontaneous abortions (36). Intermediate but abnormal β-hCG changes are seen in both abnormal IUPs and ectopic pregnancy.

Sonography is the primary assessment modality for first trimester pregnancy because it is useful at all quantitative β-hCG levels. The quantitative β-hCG level and size of the embryo do not correlate well with risk of ectopic rupture. In addition, useful findings by ultrasound are not infrequent, even if the β-hCG is below the discriminatory threshold. A majority of ectopic pregnancies present to the ED with a β-hCG less than 3000 mIU/ml, and many never rise above the discriminatory zone where an IUP or gestational sac should be seen (37). At the same time, patients with a β-hCG less than 1000 mIU/ml have a four time relative risk of ectopic pregnancy. (4). In one radiologic study, intrauterine gestational sacs were seen in up to half of women with β-hCG levels less than 1000 mIU/ml (38). In another study, 39% (9 of 23) of women ultimately diagnosed with ectopic pregnancy who had β-hCG levels less than 1000 mIU/ml had diagnostic ultrasounds for ectopic embryo or complex adnexal mass in studies performed by radiology (18).

In addition, clinicians may be misled when women give a history of passing tissue, presumed products of conception. If tissue is seen in the vault or brought to the ED by the patient, it can be rinsed and inspected for the white feathery appearance of villi or visual evidence of a gestational sac with a fetus, thus definitively diagnosing a failed pregnancy. However, nonspecific tissue, by history or examination, may represent organized blood clots, products of conception, or sloughed decidual lining, all compatible with an ectopic pregnancy. Thus, caution should be used in interpreting the passage of tissue.

A woman with an indeterminate bedside ultrasound, regardless of β-hCG level, should receive a consultative study relatively expeditiously. Whether this is done at the time of the initial ED visit or an early follow-up will depend on risk assessment after clinical evaluation and her access to a follow-up visit.

THE UTILITY OF EMERGENCY ULTRASOUND IN REACHING TREATMENT DECISIONS

About 75% of first trimester symptomatic patients can be determined at the time of the visit to have an intrauterine pregnancy with a consultative pelvic ultrasound that includes both transabdominal and transvaginal imaging (4). The efficiency of sonography by emergency physicians is not as well known, and probably varies considerably depending on machine, operator experience, and whether transabdominal ultrasound is used alone or in combination with transvaginal ultrasound. In one emergency medicine study, an IUP with embryonic structures was seen in 70% of women using transabdominal and transvaginal scanning. There were no false-positives in 87 women in whom emergency physicians detected an IUP, and overall 96% (CI 91–97%) of pelvic ultrasound results were consistent with the radiology department findings (7).

When an IUP can be correctly recognized, efficiency is clearly increased by rapid bedside ultrasound. Two studies have shown that pelvic ultrasound performed by emergency physicians reduces the time of the patient encounter by at least 60 minutes, and decreases the need for consultations in the ED by 85% (39,40). More recently, Blaivas et al showed that when an ED patient has a live IUP diagnosed by an emergency physician the ED length of stay was 21% less than if the diagnosis was made by radiology, and if those patients presented between 6PM and 6AM, they spent about an hour less in the ED (41).

INCIDENTAL FINDINGS

In the course of scanning pregnant patients, a number of incidental findings may be encountered. Many of these are not yet considered within the domain of emergency ultrasound. However, frequent use of bedside ultrasound will probably result in recognition of many of these findings and enhance image interpretation.

OVARIAN CYSTS

Ovarian cysts are common. There are a wide variety of ovarian cysts and masses with differing sonographic appearances (Figs. 6.45, 6.46). The expertise to distinguish between these is beyond the scope of ED ultrasound, although it is important to recognize ovarian cysts as problems that should eventually be addressed and referred. Ovarian cyst rupture can present with sudden pain and peritoneal irritation in the first trimester, and can result in free fluid in the pelvis. The cyst itself may collapse, making diagnosis less straightforward.

CORPUS LUTEUM

The corpus luteum cyst specifically develops from the ovarian follicle following ovulation and normally involutes after 14 days. In pregnancy the corpus luteum is maintained and supports the pregnancy for the first 6 to 7 weeks. It may become cystic and may rupture or torse. Some corpus luteum cysts fail to involute and continue into the second or third trimester. Rupture of the corpus luteum cyst in the first trimester results in pelvic pain and free fluid in the cul-de-sac and confounds first trimester differential diagnosis.

SUBCHORIONIC HEMORRHAGE

Subchorionic hemorrhage, intrauterine hematomas, or subchorionic blood collections may be seen on ultrasound and are not necessarily poor prognostic signs (42). The association with embryonic loss is strongest with large fluid collections (43). Subchorionic hemorrhage is a common cause of first-trimester vaginal bleeding. It appears as a wedge-shaped or crescent-shaped fluid collection between the chorion and the uterine myometrium (Figs. 6.47, 6.48).

ANATOMICAL VARIANTS: BICORNATE UTERUS

A bicornate uterus is an anatomic variant of the uterus where a septum divides the uterus into two "horns" to a varying degree. Spontaneous abortion is more common with a bicornate uterus and, rarely, the pregnancy may behave like an ectopic pregnancy, with erosion into the peritoneum. On ultrasound the separate horns can often be visualized, but this can also be a subtle finding (Fig. 6.25).

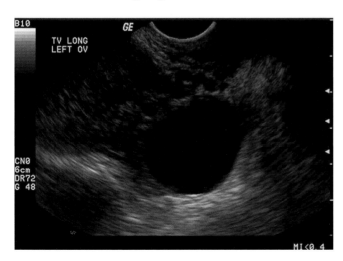

Figure 6.45. Left Ovarian Cyst.

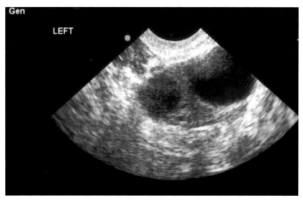

Figure 6.46. Ovarian Cyst. Image courtesy of Mark Deutchman, MD.

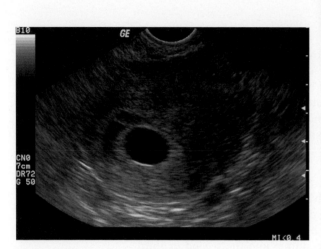

Figure 6.47. Subchorionic Hemorrhage.

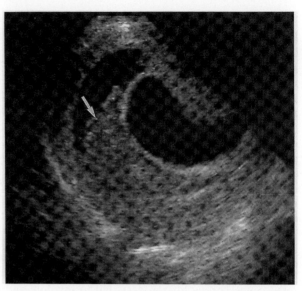

Figure 6.48. Subchorionic Hemorrhage. Reprinted from Brant WE. *Ultrasound. The Core Curriculum.* Philadelphia: Lippincott Williams & Wilkins 2001:240, with permission.

MULTIPLE GESTATIONS

Dichorionic twins will have two chorionic sacs (gestational sacs) and two yolk sacs, whereas monochorionic twins will only have one chorionic sac and either one or two yolk sacs depending on mono- or diamnionicity.

LEIOMYOMATA

Leiomyomata are also known as uterine fibroids. They are benign nodules or tumors that originate in the uterine wall. Myomata frequently grow during pregnancy secondary to the hormonal influences and can distort the normal contours of the uterus. They are common, especially in older women, and can be hyper- or hypoechoic. They occasionally calcify (Figs. 6.49, 6.50).

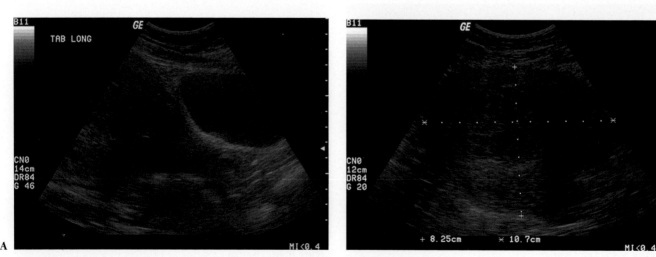

A   B

Figure 6.49. A large fibroid can be seen to arise from the uterine fundus.

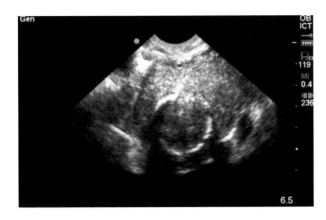

Figure 6.50. Calcified Fibroid.

ADNEXAL MASSES

Complex masses raise the suspicion for ectopic pregnancy, especially when no IUP is seen. Patients should be referred for a consultative ultrasound and specialty consultation. The differential diagnosis includes incidental ovarian pathology (Fig. 6.51).

CLINICAL CASE

A 25-year-old woman presents to the ED with vaginal bleeding beginning the day before her visit. She thinks her last menstrual period was about 28 days earlier, but admits it was an unusually short period, lasting only two days. She denies any pelvic pain or other complaints. Her blood pressure is 100/60 mm Hg, pulse is 77 beats per minute, respirations are 18 per minute, and temperature is 37.4°C. Pelvic exam reveals bleeding coming from an otherwise normal cervical os and slight tenderness and fullness in the left adnexa, but is otherwise normal.

A rapid urine pregnancy test is positive. A transabdominal ultrasound is performed by the ED physician, and the uterus is visualized and appears to have within it a discrete fluid collection in addition to a small amount of free fluid in the cul-de-sac (Fig. 6.52). An ED transvaginal ultrasound is then performed. An empty sac is visualized within the uterus, and a moderate amount of free fluid of mixed echogenicity is noted in the cul-de-sac, measuring up to half of the length of the posterior uterine wall. A quantitative β-hCG is 3500 mIU/ml.

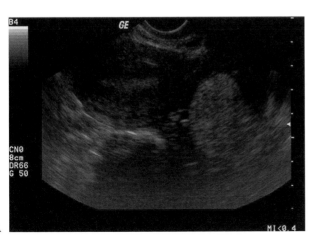
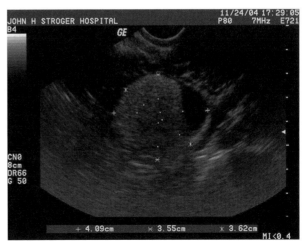

Figure 6.51. A complex left adnexal mass, found to be a dermoid tumor. Image courtesy of Karen Cosby, MD.

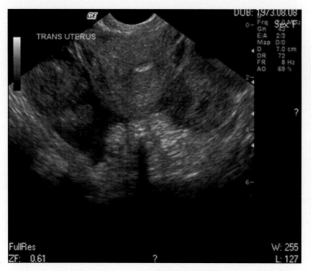
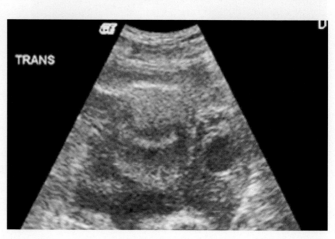

Figure 6.52. Ectopic Pregnancy. Free fluid and a complex left adnexal mass are very suspicious for an ectopic pregnancy.

Since no IUP is seen, obstetrical consultation is requested and a second transvaginal ultrasound is performed that confirms free fluid of mixed echogenicity in the cul-de-sac and a complex mass in the left adnexa. Given the β-hCG level of 3500 mIU/ml, lack of an IUP, and indirect evidence suspicious for ectopic pregnancy, the clinical picture is consistent with an ectopic pregnancy. There are a number of important points illustrated in this case.

1. Many symptomatic patients do not realize that they are pregnant and may give a history of recent menses which is in fact early bleeding from an abnormal pregnancy.
2. The "sac" identified within the uterus did not demonstrate a double decidual sign, did not contain a yolk sac, and was thus concerning for a pseudogestational sac of an ectopic pregnancy.
3. Identification of free echogenic cul-de-sac fluid, especially coupled with the findings of an absent yolk sac at this β-hCG level, along with mild tenderness in the left adnexa, appropriately mandated immediate specialty consultation (44).

REFERENCES

1. Abbott J, Emmans LS, Lowenstein SR. Ectopic pregnancy: ten common pitfalls in diagnosis. *Am J Emerg Med.* 1990;8:515–522.
2. Dart RG, Kaplan B, Varaklis K. Predictive value of history and physical examination in patients with suspected ectopic pregnancy. *Ann Emerg Med.* 1999;33:283–290.
3. Hick JL, Rodgerson JD, Heegaard WG, et al. Vital signs fail to correlate with hemoperitoneum from ruptured ectopic pregnancy. *Am J Emerg Med.* 2001;19:488–491.
4. Kaplan BC, Dart RG, Moskos M, et al. Ectopic pregnancy: prospective study with improved diagnostic accuracy. *Ann Emerg Med.* 1996;28:10–17.
5. Mateer JR, Valley VT, Aiman EJ, et al. Outcome analysis of a protocol including bedside endovaginal sonography in patients at risk for ectopic pregnancy. *Ann Emerg Med.* 1996;27: 283–289.
6. Gracia CR, Barnhart KT. Diagnosing ectopic pregnancy: decision analysis comparing six strategies. *Obstet Gynecol.* 2001;97:464–470.
7. Durham B, Lane B, Burbridge L, et al. Pelvic ultrasound performed by emergency physicians for the detection of ectopic pregnancy in complicated first-trimester pregnancies. *Ann Emerg Med.* 1997;29:338–347.
8. Tayal VS, Cohen H, Norton HJ. Outcome of patients with an indeterminate emergency department first-trimester pelvic ultrasound to rule out ectopic pregnancy. *Acad Emerg Med.* 2004; 11: 912–917.

9. Dart RG. Role of pelvic ultrasonography in evaluation of symptomatic first-trimester pregnancy. *Ann Emerg Med.* 1999;33:310–320.

10. Nyberg DA, Hughes MP, Mack LA, et al. Extrauterine findings of ectopic pregnancy of transvaginal US: importance of echogenic fluid. *Radiology.* 1991;178:823–826.

11. Ball RH. The sonography of pregnancy loss. *Semin Reprod Med.* 2000;18:351–355.

12. Laing FC, Frates MC. Ultrasound Evaluation During the First Trimester. In: Callen PW, ed. *Ultrasonography in Obstetrics and Gynecology, 4th ed.* Philadelphia: WB Saunders; 2000: 105–145.

13. Filly RA, Hadlock FP. Sonographic Determination of Menstrual Age. In: Callen PW, ed. *Ultrasonography in Obstetrics and Gynecology, 4th ed.* Philadelphia: W. B. Saunders; 2000:146–153.

14. Merchiers EH, Dhont M, De Sutter PA, et al. Predictive value of early embryonic cardiac activity for pregnancy outcome. Am J Obstet Gynecol. 1991;165:11–14.

15. Barnhart K, Mennuti MT, Benjamin I, et al. Prompt diagnosis of ectopic pregnancy in an emergency department setting. *Obstet Gynecol.* 1994;84:1010–1015.

16. Kohn MA, Kerr K, Malkevich D, et al. Beta-human chorionic gonadotropin levels and the likelihood of ectopic pregnancy in emergency department patients with abdominal pain or vaginal bleeding. *Acad Emerg Med.* 2003;10:119–126.

17. Goldstein SR. Early detection of pathologic pregnancy by transvaginal sonography. *J Clin Ultrasound.* 1990;18:262–273.

18. Dart RG, Kaplan B, Cox C. Transvaginal ultrasound in patients with low beta-human chorionic gonadotropin values: how often is the study diagnostic? *Ann Emerg Med.* 1997;30:135–140.

19. DeWitt C, Abbott J. Interstitial pregnancy: a potential for misdiagnosis of ectopic pregnancy with emergency department ultrasonography. *Ann Emerg Med.* 2002;40:106–109.

20. Athey PA, Lamki N, Matyas MA, et al. Comparison of transvaginal and transabdominal ultrasonography in ectopic pregnancy. *Can Assoc Radiol J.* 1991;42:349–352.

21. Dashefsky SM, Lyons EA, Levi CS, et al. Suspected ectopic pregnancy: endovaginal and transvesical US. *Radiology.* 1988;169:181–184.

22. Dart RG, Burke G, Dart L. Subclassification of indeterminate pelvic ultrasonography: prospective evaluation of the risk of ectopic pregnancy. *Ann Emerg Med.* 2002;39:382–388.

23. Cacciatore B, Stenman UH, Ylostalo P. Diagnosis of ectopic pregnancy by vaginal ultrasonography in combination with a discriminatory serum hCG level of 1000 IU/l (IRP). *Br J Obstet Gynaecol.* 1990;97:904–908.

24. Sadek AL, Schiotz HA. Transvaginal sonography in the management of ectopic pregnancy. *Acta Obstet Gynecol Scand.* 1995;74:293–296.

25. Mungan T, Kuscu E, Dabakoglu T, et al. Hydatidiform mole: clinical analysis of 310 patients. *Int J Gynaecol Obstet.* 1996;52:233–236.

26. Sebire NJ, Rees H, Paradinas F, et al. The diagnostic implications of routine ultrasound examination in histologically confirmed early molar pregnancies. *Ultrasound Obstet Gynecol.* 2001; 18:662–665.

27. Dart R, Dart L, Mitchell P. Normal intrauterine pregnancy is unlikely in patients who have echogenic material identified within the endometrial cavity at transvaginal ultrasonography. *Acad Emerg Med.* 1999;6:116–120.

28. Dillon EH, Case CQ, Ramos IM, et al. Endovaginal US and Doppler findings after first-trimester abortion. *Radiology.* 1993;186:87–91.

29. Rulin MC, Bornstein SB, Campbell JD. The reliability of ultrasonography in the management of spontaneous abortion, clinically thought to be complete: a prospective study. *Am J Obstet Gynecol.* 1993;168:12–15.

30. Braude P, Rowell P. Assisted conception. III–problems with assisted conception. *BMJ.* 2003; 327:920–923.

31. Fleischer AC, Pennell RG, McKee MS, et al. Ectopic pregnancy: features at transvaginal sonography. *Radiology.* 1990;174:375–378.

32. Yip SK, Sahota D, Cheung LP, et al. Accuracy of clinical diagnostic methods of threatened abortion. *Gynecol Obstet Invest.* 2003;56:38–42. Epub 2003 Jul 22.

33. Thorsen MK, Lawson TL, Aiman EJ, et al. Diagnosis of ectopic pregnancy: endovaginal vs transabdominal sonography. *AJR Am J Roentgenol.* 1990;155:307–310.

34. Kadar N, DeVore G, Romero R. Discriminatory hCG zone: its use in the sonographic evaluation for ectopic pregnancy. *Obstet Gynecol.* 1981;58:156–161.

35. Barnhart KT, Sammel MD, Rinaudo PF, et al. Symptomatic patients with an early viable intrauterine pregnancy: HCG curves redefined. *Obstet Gynecol.* 2004;104:50–55.

36. Dart RG, Mitterando J, Dart LM. Rate of change of serial beta-human chorionic gonadotropin values as a predictor of ectopic pregnancy in patients with indeterminate transvaginal ultrasound findings. *Ann Emerg Med.* 1999;34:703–710.
37. Buckley RG, King KJ, Disney JD, et al. Derivation of a clinical prediction model for the emergency department diagnosis of ectopic pregnancy. *Acad Emerg Med.* 1998;5:951–960.
38. Enk L, Wikland M, Hammarberg K, et al. The value of endovaginal sonography and urinary human chorionic gonadotropin tests for differentiation between intrauterine and ectopic pregnancy. *J Clin Ultrasound.* 1990;18:73–78.
39. Burgher SW, Tandy TK, Dawdy MR. Transvaginal ultrasonography by emergency physicians decreases patient time in the emergency department. *Acad Emerg Med.* 1998;5:802–807.
40. Shih CH. Effect of emergency physician-performed pelvic sonography on length of stay in the emergency department. *Ann Emerg Med.* 1997;29:348–352.
41. Blaivas M, Sierzenski P, Plecque D, et al. Do emergency physicians save time when locating a live intrauterine pregnancy with bedside ultrasonography? *Acad Emerg Med.* 2000;7:988–993.
42. Johns J, Hyett J, Jauniaux E. Obstetric outcome after threatened miscarriage with and without a hematoma on ultrasound. *Obstet Gynecol.* 2003;102:483–487.
43. Dickey RP, Olar TT, Curole DN, et al. Relationship of first-trimester subchorionic bleeding detected by color Doppler ultrasound to subchorionic fluid, clinical bleeding, and pregnancy outcome. *Obstet Gynecol.* 1992;80:415–420.
44. Dart R, Kaplan B, Ortiz L, et al. Normal intrauterine pregnancy is unlikely in emergency department patients with either menstrual day >38 days or beta- hCG >3,000 mIU/mL, but without a gestational sac on ultrasonography. *Acad Emerg Med.* 1997;4:967–71.

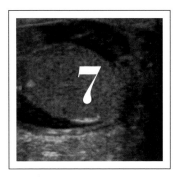

GENERAL GYNECOLOGY

Jeanne Jacoby
Michael Heller

INTRODUCTION

Although the use of pelvic ultrasound for the threatened first trimester pregnancy is well accepted in emergency department (ED) practice, its application to the nonpregnant patient has been less well defined. However, the ability of pelvic ultrasound (both transvaginal and transabdominal) to characterize solid and cystic masses and to identify abnormal fluid collections makes it well-suited for the investigation of many types of pelvic pathology. The purpose of this chapter is to describe both the normal and abnormal anatomy of the nongravid female, identify common variants, and to outline how pelvic ultrasound may be incorporated into routine ED practice.

CLINICAL APPLICATIONS: PELVIC PAIN AND PELVIC MASS

The pelvic ultrasound examination may be performed as part of the evaluation of pelvic pain or masses reported by the patient, found on physical exam, or visualized by other imaging modalities. Indeed, many clinicians have found that performing pelvic ultrasounds contemporaneously with each pelvic exam, regardless of pregnancy status, increases skill level and appreciation for normal anatomy and provides additional valuable clinical information. Once comfortable with the sonographic appearance of normal pelvic anatomy, the emergency sonographer should be able to recognize the findings discussed in this chapter.

IMAGE ACQUISITION: TRANSABDOMINAL AND TRANSVAGINAL

Transabdominal sonography (TAS) and transvaginal sonography (TVS) complement each other; each offers unique advantages and disadvantages in terms of visualizing pelvic anatomy. Transabdominal sonography (Fig. 7.1) is noninvasive and affords a broad view of all of the pelvic structures (including the uterus, cervix, vagina, and ovaries) and their relative relationship to each other and any mass seen. A full bladder is advantageous for TAS; a relatively empty bladder is optimal for TVS. A full bladder optimizes transabdominal scanning for two reasons. First, it provides an excellent acoustic window which allows for greater resolution of the pelvic structures in question. And second, the full bladder displaces bowel loops from the pelvis and acts as a spacer between the transducer and the pelvic organs allowing the areas of interest to be more optimally aligned with the focal length of the usual transabdominal probe (3.5 to 5 MHz). Occasionally an overfilled bladder may cause difficulty in visualizing the uterus if it displaces the uterus posteriorly to a retroverted position. In contrast to TVS, visualization of pelvic anatomy with TAS may be limited somewhat by marked obesity due to the attenuation that occurs as the ultrasound beam passes through the anterior abdominal wall and subcutaneous fat (1–6).

Transvaginal sonography offers the emergency physician several advantages over TAS. The transvaginal approach places the probe in closer proximity to the object of interest and allows for the use of a higher frequency probe (5 to 7.5MHz) with better

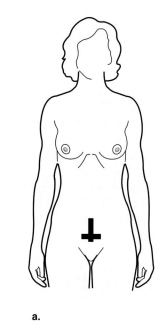

a.

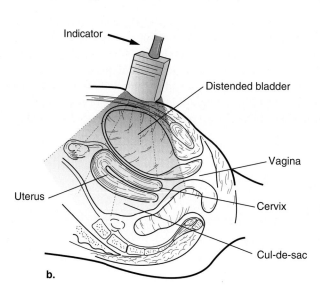

b.

Figure 7.1. Transabdominal Scan. Place the transducer in the midline just above the pubis (**A**). Place the transducer indicator to project the patient's head to the left of the screen to obtain a sagittal view. Rotate the transducer 90 degrees counterclockwise to obtain a transverse view. In each view, gently rock the transducer to obtain a 3-dimensional view of the uterus and adnexa. When possible, scan with a distended bladder to optimize the acoustic window to the pelvis (**B**). The internal landmarks of the TAS are visualized (**B**). (Figure **A** is redrawn from Simon and Snoey, eds. Ultrasound in Emergency and Ambulatory Medicine. St. Louis: Mosby-Yearbook; 1997.)

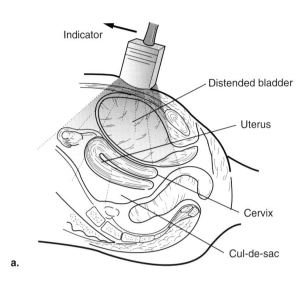

a.

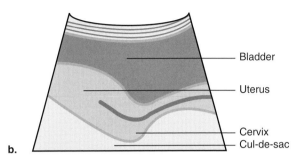

b.

Figure 7.2. Transabdominal Scan of the Female Pelvis, Sagittal View. The transducer is placed in the midline, just above the pubis, using the bladder as an acoustic window (**A**). The arrow notes the indicator positioned toward the patient's head to obtain a sagittal orientation (**A**). A schematic of the anatomy of the normal female pelvis (**B**). Ultrasound of the normal female pelvis (**C**). The vaginal stripe is visible. The angle between the cervix and the uterine fundus approximates 90 degrees. (Figure **A** is redrawn from Simon and Snoey, eds. Ultrasound in Emergency and Ambulatory Medicine. St. Louis: Mosby-Yearbook; 1997.)

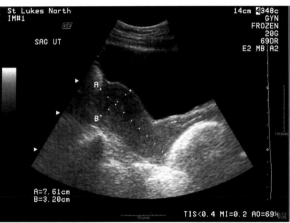

c.

resolution. Because it does not allow for an all-inclusive picture of the pelvic organs, the transvaginal approach is most useful when directed at a small area of interest, such as an area of tenderness or mass found previously on pelvic exam or TAS. As with other applications of ultrasound, there is an interactive component when scanning transvaginally that is lost when the scan is not performed by the emergency physician. The examiner can determine whether a visualized mass or cyst is the source of the patient's pain by applying gentle pressure to the structure and asking if that reproduces the pain. With the transvaginal approach it is best to have the bladder recently emptied, although a small amount of residual urine is used by many sonographers as a convenient landmark. In this approach, a bladder that is too full may displace the uterus outside the range of the higher-frequency probes. Another advantage of TVS versus TAS is the ability to assess pelvic anatomy in a patient of any size because interposing adipose tissue does not impact image quality (1–6). However, TVS is typically not performed by emergency physicians in premenarchal or virginal patients, and may be uncomfortable for some postmenopausal women, though it can be performed in any patient in whom a bimanual exam is appropriate (1,3,6).

The TAS exam is begun with a 3.5-MHz transducer placed just above the pubic symphysis, which is easily palpated in the midline, well below the umbilicus (Fig. 7.1). The bladder is an easily identified anechoic cystic structure through which the uterus and adnexa can be visualized. The area should be scanned in both the sagittal and, after rotating the probe 90 degrees, transverse planes (Figs. 7.2, 7.3). While in each plane, angling the probe on its point of contact allows the pelvic organs to be fully visualized (1).

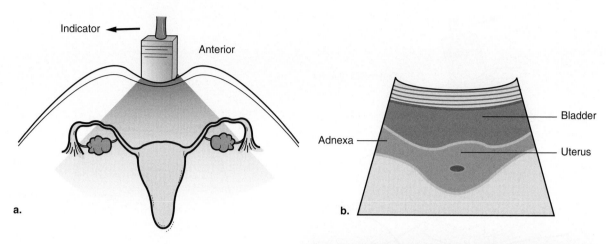

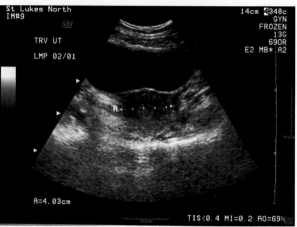

Figure 7.3. Transabdominal Scan of the Female Pelvis, Transverse View. The transducer is placed in the midline just above the pelvis in a transverse orientation (**A**). The indicator points to the patient's right (**A**). A schematic of the anatomy of the normal female pelvis is seen in transverse orientation (**B**). Ultrasound of the normal female pelvis in transverse orientation (**C**). (Figure **A** is redrawn from Simon and Snoey, eds. Ultrasound in Emergency and Ambulatory Medicine. St. Louis: Mosby-Yearbook; 1997.)

In nonemergency medicine practice, TAS is performed first, and then the bladder is emptied to facilitate TVS. An adequate explanation of the TVS procedure is important, including informing the patient that only part of the transducer, usually 3 to 4 cm, will be inserted. In the ED, a pelvic exam is often performed initially with TVS immediately following. The clean vaginal transducer is prepared by placing a small amount of conductive ultrasound gel on the tip of the probe which is then covered with a condom. It should be noted that if the condom has a reservoir tip, the tip should be completely filled with gel in order to avoid artifacts that occur when ultrasound waves pass through gas. Nonlubricated plain-end latex condoms work best, but the finger of a latex examining glove will do if none are available. The examiner then applies lubricating gel to the covered tip of the probe and inserts it into the vagina (Fig. 7.4). As is the convention for pelvic examinations, two medical personnel should be present in the room during the transvaginal examination, at least one of whom is female. It is easiest to perform the exam with the patient on a gynecologic exam table in the dorsal lithotomy position, but if this is not possible, a support such as an overturned bedpan or a rolled blanket may be placed beneath the buttocks in order to tilt the pelvic floor anteriorly (1,2,6).

The transducer should be advanced slowly into the vagina until there is optimal visualization of the pelvic organs. During insertion the orientation of the transducer and identification of pelvic structures is facilitated by noting the position of the bladder, which is easily identified with even a small amount of residual urine. There are four basic scanning maneuvers in TVS. The transducer is placed in the vagina with the transducer indicator oriented vertically, and then slowly moved on its long axis right and left, allowing for continuous sagittal slices (Fig. 7.5). The transducer should sweep slowly from the

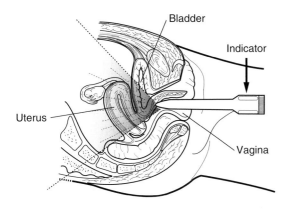

Figure 7.4. The Transvaginal Scan of the Female Pelvis. Place the endovaginal transducer in the vaginal vault, just as you would a speculum. Begin in the sagittal plane with the transducer indicator pointed up. Advance only as far as necessary to visualize the uterus. Find the endometrial stripe to identify the midline of the uterus. Rotate the transducer 90 degrees counterclockwise (indicator pointing toward the patient's right side) to obtain a coronal view. In each orientation, gently rock the transducer in all planes to obtain a 3-dimensional view of the uterus and adnexa. (Redrawn from Simon and Snoey, eds. Ultrasound in Emergency and Ambulatory Medicine. St. Louis: Mosby-Yearbook; 1997.)

midline through the uterus, through each adnexa and out to the lateral pelvic walls. The transducer is then rotated from 0 to 90 degrees on its long axis in order to obtain coronal views of the uterus and ovaries (Fig. 7.6). In this orientation the transducer is then angled superiorly and inferiorly in order to obtain coronal slices through the entire uterus (from the fundus through the cervix) and adnexa. The transducer can be inserted further or withdrawn to allow structures to be placed in the optimal range of the transducer. It can also be angled or pointed in any direction (within the limitations of patient comfort) in order to evaluate an area of interest. Between uses the transducer should be cleansed with the method and solution recommended by the manufacturer (1,2,6).

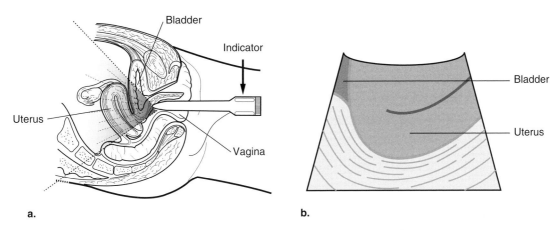

a.

b.

Figure 7.5. Transvaginal Ultrasound of the Normal Female Pelvis, Sagittal Orientation. The transducer is placed in the vaginal vault and advanced until the uterus is seen (**A**). The indicator is placed up to obtain a sagittal orientation (**A**). A schematic of the anatomy of the normal female pelvis (**B**). An ultrasound of a normal anteverted uterus as seen in sagittal orientation (**C**). Compare (**C**) to Figure 7.2 **C** (same patient). Note the improved visualization of the endometrial echo complex with the higher resolution transvaginal transducer. (Figure **A** is redrawn from Simon and Snoey, eds. Ultrasound in Emergency and Ambulatory Medicine. St. Louis: Mosby-Yearbook; 1997.)

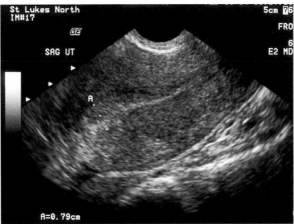

c.

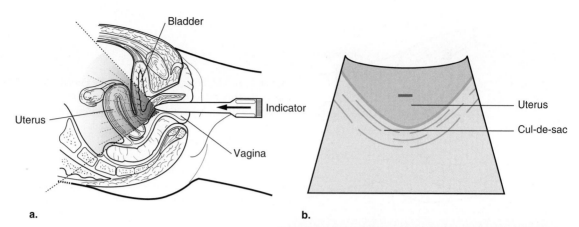

a.   b.

Figure 7.6. Transvaginal Ultrasound of the Normal Female Pelvis, Coronal Orientation. The transducer is placed in the vaginal vault and advanced until the uterus is seen (**A**). The indicator is placed on the patient's right side to obtain a coronal view (**A**). A schematic of the anatomy of the female pelvis (**B**). An ultrasound of a normal anteverted uterus (**C**). Compare Figure **C** to Figure 7.3 **C** (same patient). Note the improved visualization with the transvaginal view. In this coronal view of the uterus, the endometrial echo complex appears as a core in the center of the image. (Figure **A** is redrawn from Simon and Snoey, eds. Ultrasound in Emergency and Ambulatory Medicine. St. Louis: Mosby-Yearbook; 1997.)

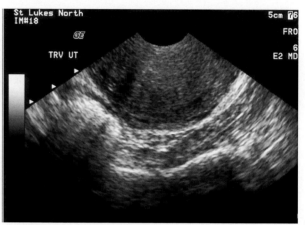

c.

Normal Anatomy and Landmarks

Uterine Anatomy

The uterus is a muscular, hollow organ with an average size of 7 × 4 cm in nulliparous and 8.5 × 5.5 cm in multiparous women. It is bounded by the rectum posteriorly, the bladder anteriorly, and the two bands of the broad ligament laterally (7). In TAS, the bladder acts as an acoustic window through which the uterus can be visualized. The position of the uterus

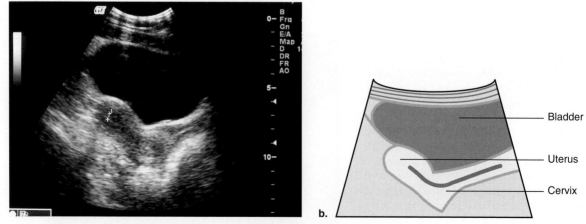

a.   b.

Figure 7.7. Transabdominal Scan of the Uterus—Anteflexion. The uterine fundus (left) usually forms a right angle with the cervix (right), called anteflexion.

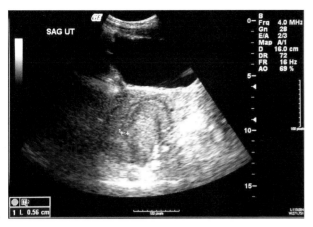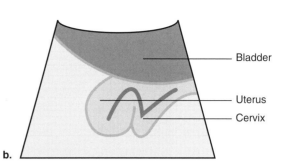

a. b.

Bladder

Uterus
Cervix

Figure 7.8. Transabdominal Scan of the Uterus—Retroflexion. The uterine fundus is "tipped" and is seen almost immediately below the cervix. This is called retroflexion.

can vary with the relative state of distention of the bladder and rectum. Except when displaced by a distended bladder, the uterus usually forms a right angle with the cervix; this is also called "anteflexion" (Fig. 7.7). "Version" refers to the axis of the cervix relative to the vagina, and "flexion," the axis of the uterine body to the cervix. The uterus may be retroflexed (Fig. 7.8), making it difficult to visualize the uterine fundus. This is a normal variant in some women and occurs in others when performing TAS with a full bladder (6).

The deep layer of the endometrium (the stratum basale) does not change significantly during menses, unlike the mucosal lining of the uterine canal (the stratum functionale) whose function and appearance varies throughout the menstrual cycle. The opposing surfaces of the endometrial lining form a hyperechoic line that is referred to as the "endometrial stripe" or "endometrial echo complex." The proliferative phase immediately follows menses and begins with a thin, 1- to 2-mm lining that grows under the influence of estrogen in preparation for implantation of the fertilized ovum (Fig. 7.9). Ovulation occurs on day 14 of the menstrual cycle and is followed by the secretory phase. Under the influence of progesterone secreted by the corpus luteum, the endometrium develops protein-rich secretory products and grows to up to 12 mm in width (Fig. 7.10) (8–10).

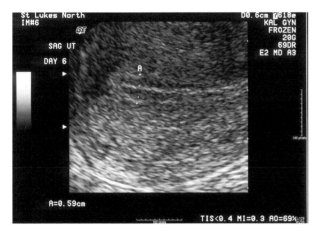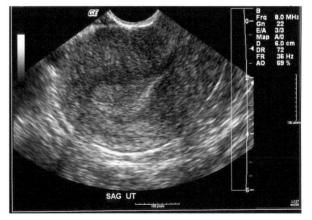

Figure 7.9. Transvaginal Scan of the Uterus – Proliferative Endometrium. During the proliferative phase of the menstrual cycle, the endometrial echo complex grows in preparation for ovulation (usually occurring on day 14 of the cycle). One should expect to see variations in the width and echogenic texture of the endometrium during different phases of the menstrual cycle.

Figure 7.10. Transvaginal Scan of the Uterus – Secretory Endometrium. During the secretory phase of the menstrual cycle, the endometrium develops protein-rich secretory products and may reach 12 mm in width.

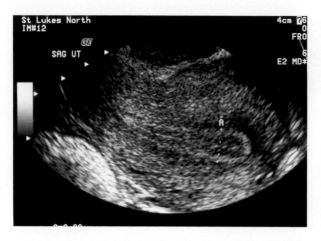

Figure 7.11. Transvaginal Scan of the Uterus. The endometrial echo complex should be measured in the sagittal plane between the two hyperechoic lines surrounding the hypoechoic functional layer.

Given the pear-shaped structure of the uterus, it follows that the endometrial echo complex is best visualized in the sagittal plane. The central canal, when viewed in the coronal plane, appears as an echogenic "core" (Fig. 7.6). The thickness of the endometrial lining should be measured between the basal layers which appear as hyperechoic lines surrounding the hypoechoic functional layer (Fig. 7.11) (1–6,11).

OVARIAN ANATOMY

The ovaries are paired oval-shaped organs that are approximately 3 cm long, 1.5 cm wide, and 1 cm thick. The ovaries lie anterior and medial to the internal iliac vessels which can serve as a useful landmark when attempting to locate the ovary (Fig. 7.12, 7.13). The ovaries effectively have a dual arterial blood supply; the ovarian artery arises from the lateral aorta and runs in the suspensory ligament of the ovaries, where it anastamoses with branches of the uterine artery (6,7). This additional blood supply becomes important when evaluating a patient for ovarian torsion as evidence of some blood flow to the ovaries does not rule out torsion.

On ultrasound examination of the premenopausal woman, ovaries often appear as foamy structures secondary to the presence of multiple follicles (Fig. 7.14) (1). Prior to the onset of menses, fluid accumulates in a cohort of follicles that increase in size. When they reach 1 to 2 mm in size, they can be visualized on TVS. Multiple small follicles are seen at day 5 to 7 and by day 8 to 12 one or more dominant follicles can be seen. Although up to

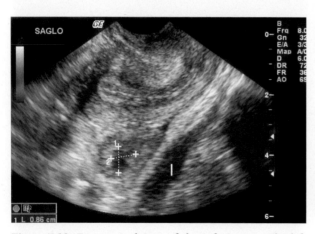

Figure 7.12. Transvaginal Scan of the Left Ovary – The left ovary is visible just medial to the internal iliac vein (*I*). This vessel is a useful landmark when attempting to locate the ovary.

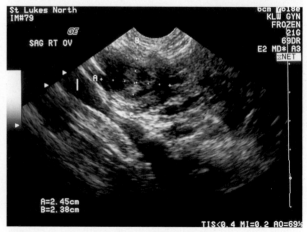

Figure 7.13. Transvaginal Scan of the Right Ovary – The right ovary (2.5 × 2.4 cm) is visible just medial to the internal iliac vessels (*I*).

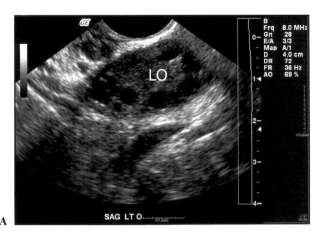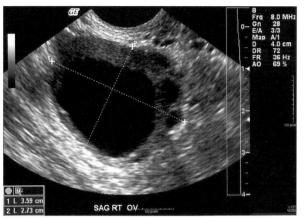

A

B

Figure 7.14. Transvaginal Scan – Left Ovary (**A**). Note the multiple small follicles seen in this normal ovary (*LO*). Right Ovary (**B**). Note the large dominant follicle on the right ovary of the same patient in A. In most patients a single unilateral dominant follicle is seen by midcycle.

10% of patients have two dominant follicles, each month there is usually only one follicle that achieves complete maturation (Fig. 7.14). Nondominant follicles are usually <14 mm in diameter. In the 4 to 5 days prior to ovulation (usually day 14 of the menstrual cycle), the dominant follicle grows 2 to 3 mm per day, reaching a maximum diameter of 16 to 28 mm. At the time of ovulation bleeding occurs into the follicle, which decreases in size and may become filled with echogenic debris. The follicle, now called the "corpus luteum," may retain fluid over the next 4 to 5 days and increase in size to 2 to 3 cm. If pregnancy does not occur, the corpus luteum gradually involutes and atrophies to become the "corpus albicans" which cannot be seen with ultrasound (2,6).

UTERINE PATHOLOGY

LEIOMYOMAS (FIBROIDS)

The uterine appearance can be distorted by leiomyomas (fibroids) which are composed of bundles of smooth muscle. Fibroids are not uncommon; 25% of women older than 30 have at least one. Risk factors include African American race, early menarche, nulliparity, and obesity. Leiomyomas can be subserosal, intramucosal, or submucosal; in the uterus or cervix, within the broad ligament, or outside of the uterus attached by a pedicle (Figs. 7.15–7.17). They may occur singly or as multiples. Although the majority of leiomyomas

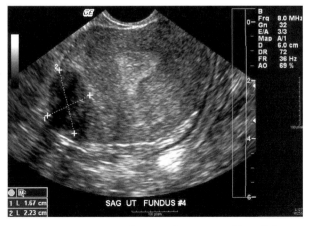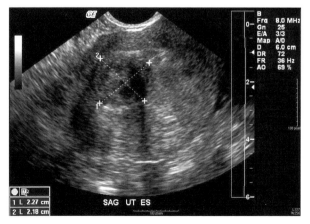

Figure 7.15. Transvaginal Scan. A leiomyoma (fibroid) (2.2 × 1.7 × 1.7 cm) seen in the fundus of the uterus.

Figure 7.16. Transvaginal Scan. Note the fibroid (2.3 × 2.2 × 2 cm) projecting into the endometrial cavity.

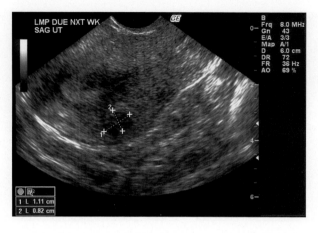

Figure 7.17. Transvaginal Scan. There is an intramural fibroid (1.1 × 0.8 × 1.3 cm) seen within the myometrium.

are asymptomatic, presenting only as incidental findings, fibroids may cause symptoms of pelvic pain and pressure. Fibroids tend to enlarge during pregnancy and regress after menopause (5,12–14).

ENDOMETRIAL CANCER

Eighty-one percent of postmenopausal women have an endometrial thickness of <8 mm. A postmenopausal woman with an endometrium >8 mm should be referred for further evaluation whether or not she has vaginal bleeding (Fig. 7.18). When a patient presents with postmenopausal bleeding the clinical suspicion for endometrial cancer is high, and evaluation is recommended for an endometrial echo complex >5 mm. Patients taking cyclic hormone replacement therapy or tamoxifen, used as adjunctive therapy after breast cancer, have more variation in endometrial thickness, however, the threshold for evaluation of these women is also 5 mm (2,11,15–18). No one would fault the emergency physician for referring all such cases for further evaluation regardless of the width of the endometrial stripe.

INTRAUTERINE DEVICES

Intrauterine devices (IUDs) inserted to prevent pregnancy are highly echogenic and are therefore easily identified on ultrasound examination. IUDs are widely used internationally but are less frequently seen in the United States (19). Identification of an IUD is especially useful when a female with a history of IUD use does not have a string visible in the cervical os. Ultrasound can be easily utilized to determine whether the device is actually in place

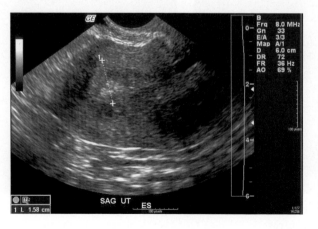

Figure 7.18. Transvaginal Scan. This 1.6-cm endometrial echo complex is abnormal for this postmenopausal female. When the endometrial echo complex exceeds 5 mm in width, especially when accompanied by vaginal bleeding, the patient should be referred for evaluation for endometrial cancer.

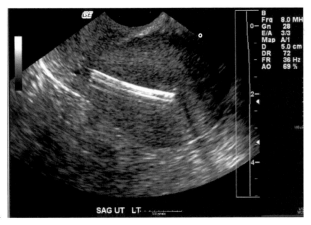 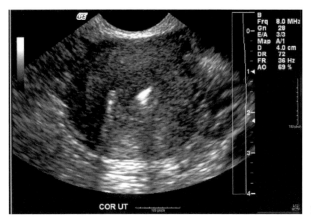

Figure 7.19. Transvaginal Scan – IUD. (**A**) Sagittal view. The highly echogenic IUD can be easily seen within the endometrial cavity of this sagittal section of the uterus. (**B**) Coronal view. The highly echogenic IUD can be seen in the center of this coronal section of the uterus.

(Fig. 7.19). If clinically indicated, e.g., in the presence of pelvic inflammatory disease (PID), the IUD may easily be removed by the emergency physician simply by applying gentle traction to the string.

OVARIAN PATHOLOGY

SIMPLE CYSTS

Simple (functional) cysts include follicular cysts, corpus luteum cysts, and theca lutein cysts (which result from high levels of β-hCG in trophoblastic disease or from iatrogenic stimulation with exogenous β-hCG). Simple cysts are most common during the reproductive years and are usually asymptomatic. Causes include increases in anterior pituitary gonadotrophins, low-dose contraceptives, and exogenous gonadotrophin-releasing hormones. Most regress within two months. Functional cysts have thin walls, are unilocular, and range from 3 to 8 cm in diameter (Fig. 7.20) (6,14,20,21). After a follicular cyst (>3 cm) is diagnosed, a 6-week follow-up ultrasound is recommended to ensure that the cyst is resolving (3). Emergency physicians should remember that ovarian cysts are very common in women of reproductive age; therefore simply finding a cyst does not establish that the cyst is the cause of the patient's abdominal or pelvic pain.

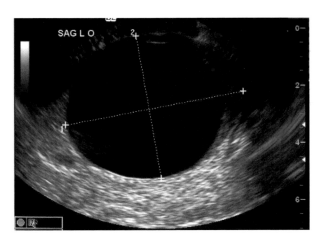

Figure 7.20. Transvaginal Scan – Simple Ovarian Cyst. This is a 5 × 6-cm simple cyst (anechoic, unilocular and without septations) which should be followed by a repeat ultrasound in 6 weeks to assess for resolution.

COMPLEX CYSTS

During the reproductive years, most (up to 85%) ovarian masses are benign. Ovarian tumors are usually asymptomatic; when present, the symptoms they produce are characteristically abdominal distention, pain, or pressure. A complex ovarian cyst is a cyst with one or more of the following characteristics: septations, irregular wall thickening, and shadowing echodensity. Septations and or a cyst wall > 2 to 3 mm are worrisome and considered by some to be a sign of malignancy (Fig. 7.21) (5,14,20–23).

DERMOID CYSTS

Mature cystic teratomas (dermoid cysts) are the most common benign germ cell tumor and the most common ovarian neoplasm. More than 80% of dermoid cysts occur during the reproductive years (although they can occur from infancy to old age) and malignant transformation occurs in less than 2%. Dermoids are composed of three germ cell layers: ectoderm, mesoderm, and endoderm, and often contain hair, fat, and even teeth. The sonographic appearance is usually that of a hyperechoic solid mass (Fig. 7.22 A and B); hyperechoic lines and dots and fluid-fluid levels may also be seen. When a dermoid is suspected, further evaluation by computed tomograhy (CT) or magnetic resonance imaging (MRI) is recommended for confirmation (Fig. 7.22 C and D) (6,14,20,24–27).

CHOCOLATE CYSTS

Endometriosis is defined as the presence of endometrial tissue outside of the uterus. Although endometriosis may be found in a wide variety of locations, the ovaries, uterine

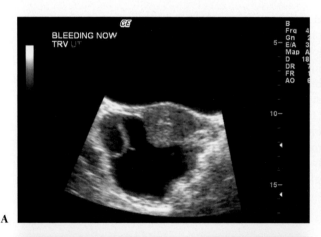

A

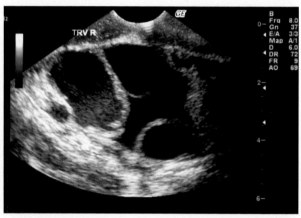

B

C

Figure 7.21. Complex Ovarian Cyst. (A) TAS. This large complex ovarian cyst is easily seen on TAS and is suspicious for malignancy because of its size, thick walls, and echogenic solid-appearing components. (B) TVS. This is the same patient as in A; note the improved resolution of the complex features of this cyst with the TVS technique. (C) TVS. Another view of the cyst seen in figures A and B.

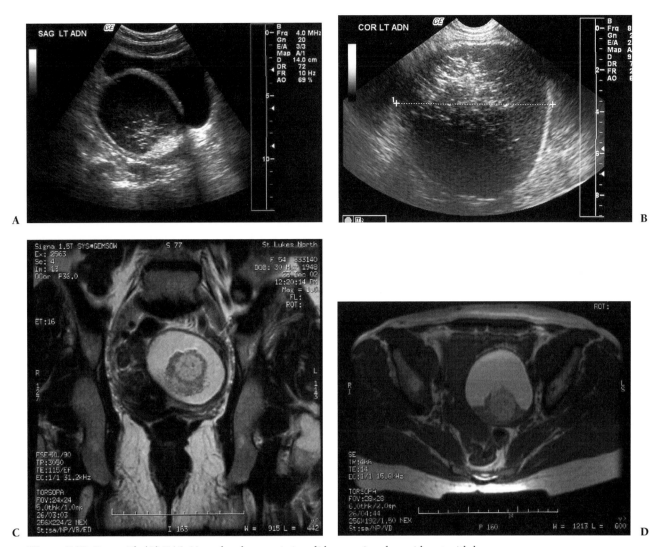

Figure 7.22. Dermoid. (**A**) TAS. Note the characteristic solid-appearing dermoid cyst with hyperechoic lines and dots. (**B**) TVS. Note the improved resolution by TVS. (**C**) MRI. Coronal section of the dermoid as seen by MRI. (**D**) MRI. Transverse section of the dermoid as seen by MRI.

ligaments, rectovaginal septum, cul-de-sac, and pelvic peritoneum are the most common sites. Most cases are asymptomatic, but the recurrent, cyclic, hormone-dependent changes that occur in endometrial tissue within the uterus also occur in the ectopic tissue, and are considered to be the cause of symptoms. Endometrial rests on the ovary are often covered with dense adhesions, resulting in fixation to adjacent structures; they are thick and fibrotic, and are often called chocolate cysts because they contain semifluid chocolate-colored material. Such cysts vary widely in size and often have a sonographic appearance of homogenous hypoechoic low-level echoes (Figs. 7.23, 7.24) (6,20,28–29).

POLYCYSTIC OVARIAN SYNDROME

Polycystic Ovarian Syndrome (PCOS) is an endocrine disorder associated with chronic anovulation and is found in a wide spectrum of patients, from lean hyperandrogenic women who menstruate normally to patients with classic Stein-Leventhal syndrome, associated with obesity, hirsutism, and oligo- or amenorrhea (30). The disease is not uncommon, occurring in up to 27% of reproductive age women (31,32). Polycystic ovaries

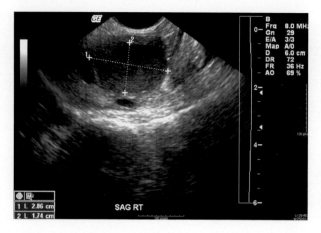

Figure 7.23. Transvaginal Scan. Endometrial (chocolate) cyst: Note the characteristic homogenous echogenic material within this cyst.

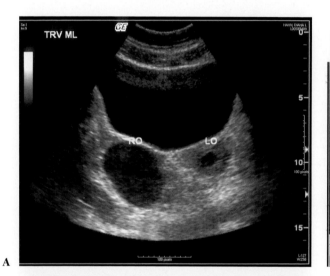

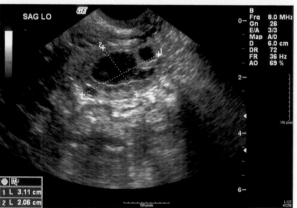

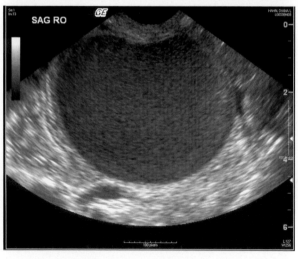

Figure 7.24. Endometrial cyst (right ovary). (**A**) Transabdominal Scan: A chocolate cyst is seen on the right ovary (RO); a normal ovary is also seen on the left side (*LO*). (**B**) Transvaginal Scan: The normal appearing left ovary of the patient in figure A. Note the improved resolution with TVS. (**C**) Transvaginal Scan: Right ovary with endometrioma. Note the homogenous solid-appearing characteristic appearance of this chocolate cyst and the improved resolution with Transvaginal Scan.

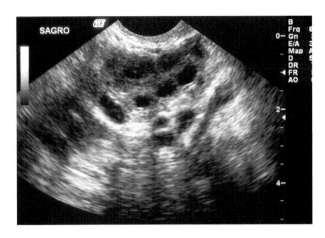

Figure 7.25. Transvaginal Scan: Polycystic Ovarian Syndrome. This patient with polycystic ovarian syndrome has ten small follicles visible on this Transvaginal Scan.

are generally 2 to 5 times normal size and are described as having more than five microcysts (ranging from 0.5–0.8 cm in diameter) in each ovary which usually occur in the periphery but can occur within the parenchyma (Fig. 7.25) (11,20,30).

OVARIAN HYPERSTIMULATION SYNDROME

Ovarian Hyperstimulation Syndrome (OHS) occurs in as many as 65% of women undergoing ovulation induction, and is an entirely iatrogenic disease. In mild OHS, patients complain of mild abdominal distention, nausea and vomiting, and ovaries can enlarge to 5 to 12 cm (Fig. 7.26). Moderate disease is characterized by abdominal ascites on ultrasound examination. Severe disease occurs when there are signs of tense ascites, hydrothorax, dyspnea, hemoconcentration due to massive third-spacing of fluids, or any of the complications of OHS; including renal failure, thromboembolism, and acute respiratory distress syndrome. In all but the mildest cases, inpatient management is recommended and care includes intravenous hydration, treatment of oliguria, and thromboembolic prophylaxis. Even with mild disease, these patients should only be discharged with very close follow-up as the severity of OHS may change at any time (33,34). OHS is important to the emergency physician as it may be confused with ruptured ectopic pregnancy and ruptured ovarian cysts.

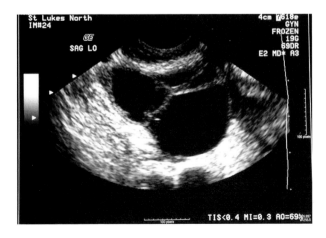

Figure 7.26. Transvaginal Scan: Ovarian Hyperstimulation Syndrome. Note the enlarged ovary and multiple large cysts visible in this patient with ovarian hyperstimulation syndrome.

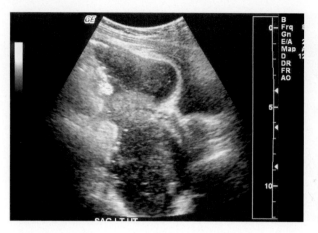

Figure 7.27. Transvaginal Scan: Tubo-ovarian abscess (TOA). Note the breakdown of defined ovarian borders. This mass, in a patient with a history of PID, proved to be a TOA.

TUBO-OVARIAN ABSCESS AND HYDROSALPINX

Ascending infection in the genital tract progresses from the cervix (cervicitis), up the fallopian tube (salpingitis), to the peritoneal cavity (PID). There are no distinct ultrasound findings of cervicitis or salpingitis, but at least three complications of PID have been described that may be seen on ultrasound. Tubo-ovarian abscess (TOA) is diagnosed when a true abscess develops, which is often noted as a tender heterogeneous mass in the adnexa (Fig. 7.27). Hydrosalpinx is a condition in which the normally very thin fallopian tubes become greatly enlarged (>5 mm) and fluid-filled, presenting a characteristic appearance that has been likened to that of a winding river (Fig. 7.28). Pyosalpinx is said to exist when the tube is thickened and filled with nonsonolucent material (11,20,35–39).

OVARIAN TORSION

Ovarian torsion is a difficult diagnosis to make. It is suggested when there is acute unilateral pelvic pain; but is quite rare, accounting for only 3% of emergent gynecologic surgeries. Torsion occurs when the ovary either partially or completely twists on its axis with the fallopian tube. Ovarian torsion usually occurs in the first three decades of life. Ultrasound is the initial imaging modality and must be done emergently as torsion requires surgical repair. The most common ultrasound finding of a torsed ovary is

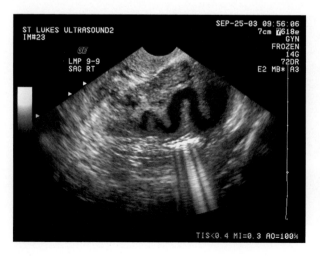

Figure 7.28. Transvaginal Scan: Hydrosalpinx. Note the dilated fallopian tube (not usually visible on ultrasound); it has the characteristic appearance of a meandering river.

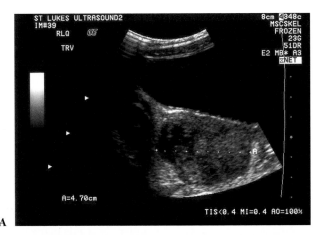

A

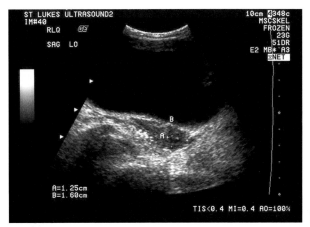

B

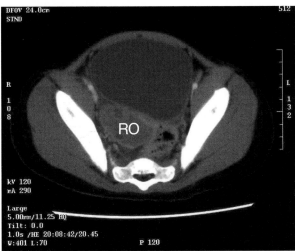

C

Figure 7.29. Ovarian Torsion. A. This patient (8-year-old female), has the finding of a unilaterally enlarged right ovary. B. The left ovary is normal contrasted to the right. C. MRI reveals an abnormally enlarged right ovary. Subsequent laparotomy revealed a right ovarian torsion.

unilateral enlargement and increased volume secondary to edema from venous and lymphatic congestion (Fig. 7.29). Other less common findings are engorged blood vessels at the periphery and multiple enlarged follicles from transudation of fluid into the follicles. As the ovary has a dual blood supply, ultrasound is not 100% sensitive even with the addition of Doppler to gray-scale ultrasound imaging. In women of reproductive age, ovarian torsion is usually precipitated by ovarian masses including both complex and large functional cysts, OHS, and PCOS. Primary ovarian torsion is more common in children (3,5,11,20,39).

CORRELATION WITH OTHER IMAGING MODALITIES

Computed tomography has several uses in gynecologic practice, including further definition of pelvic masses, staging of pelvic cancer, and evaluation of tumor recurrence; it is also useful for guided aspiration and biopsy. In the ED, CT is utilized for better definition of pelvic masses when the ultrasound exam has not clarified the cause of the pelvic symptoms (36, 39–40). In such cases the use of oral, intravenous, and even rectal contrast may be very helpful in defining the nature and scope of the mass in question.

Magnetic resonance imaging provides excellent soft tissue imaging without artifact, but is not indicated emergently for gynecologic conditions except possibly in the evaluation of ovarian vein thrombosis (OVT). OVT usually occurs postpartum and occurs in approximately 1 in 600 deliveries. OVT is potentially fatal as embolization can occur. Importantly, given the limited availability of MRI, the diagnosis of OVT can also be made by CT scan. Examples of gynecologic cases which can be nonemergently imaged by MRI are: congenital abnormalities of the uterus, leiomyomas, endometrial and cervical carcinoma diagnosis and staging, and evaluation of ovarian masses (2,39).

ARTIFACTS AND PITFALLS

Both TAS and TVS are subject to the usual pitfalls encountered with any sonographic examination, e.g., the inability to visualize anatomy with poor skin contact or in the presence of free air. However, several artifacts and pitfalls are specific to the sonographic exam of the pelvis.

1. Bladder fullness: TAS is best performed with a relatively full bladder. This aids in image acquisition as it serves as an acoustic window through which pelvic structures can be visualized. In contrast, when performing TVS, a relatively empty bladder greatly improves visualization of the uterus and adnexa.
2. Bowel: In both TAS and TVS, fluid in the bowel can be mistaken for free fluid in the pelvis.
3. Physiologic free fluid: In many reproductive age women, a small amount of physiologic free fluid is often seen on TVS; a less-experienced sonographer could mistake this as pathologic.
4. Limited field of view: TVS offers a focused view of the uterus and adnexa, but when used without TAS, may miss pelvic masses outside of its limited field of view.
5. Ovaries: Despite their characteristic follicular appearance, it is possible to mistake other pelvic structures, such as vessels on end, for ovaries.
6. Endovaginal probe preparation: The sonographer must be careful to put an adequate amount of conductive gel in the tip of the condom prior to placing it on the endovaginal probe, and must be sure to get any air bubbles out of the tip, as ultrasound waves are not conducted through air.

INCIDENTAL FINDINGS

UTERINE ANOMALIES

Congenital variations of the uterus and vagina are not uncommon, generally occurring secondary to failure of fusion of the mullerian ducts, which normally fuse caudally in the midline with the unfused cranial portions of the ducts giving rise to the fallopian tubes. Failure of fusion, or failure to resorb septae, can result in several variations of uterine anatomy. The mildest version results in an arcuate uterus, a variant of normal characterized by a concave portion of the fundus. Other congenital anomalies include bicornuate, septate, didelphic (two complete uteri which can extend down to include the cervix and involve a septated vagina), and unicornuate uteri (Fig. 7.30). In women with septate, didelphic, and unicornuate uteri, rates of miscarriage and preterm delivery are increased. Uterovaginal failure of septal resorption can result in hematometra and hematometrocolpos (Fig. 7.31). This can present as an otherwise healthy young female with abdominal pain who has begun to ovulate but has not yet manifested menstrual bleeding because of an imperforate hymen (9,33,41).

VAGINAL AND CERVICAL FINDINGS

On occasion, more commonly during TVS, cysts may be seen in the cervix and vagina. Numerous cervical glands extend from the endocervical mucosa into the cervix. When

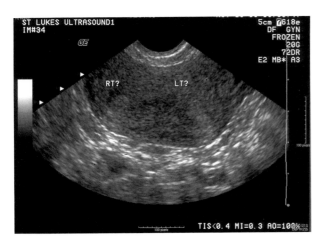

Figure 7.30. Transvaginal Scan: Transverse view, Bicornuate Uterus. Both horns of this bicornuate uterus are labeled.

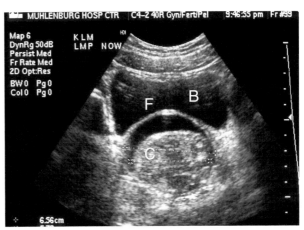

Figure 7.31. Transabdominal Scan: Transverse view, Hydrometrocolpus. The bladder (*B*) is seen above the dilated vagina which is seen with a large clot (*C*) above which an anechoic fluid stripe (*F*) is seen. This represents blood and clot in the vagina of a patient with an imperforate hymen.

these glands become occluded, they result in the formation of retention cysts within the cervix. These are known as nabothian cysts; this condition is benign and no treatment is required (Fig. 7.32). Gartner's cysts are found in the lateral wall of the vagina; they are of mesonephric origin, are rarely symptomatic and do not require treatment (Fig. 7.33) (9,14,41).

FREE FLUID

When TVS is used, it is not uncommon and not abnormal to visualize a small amount of free fluid in the rectouterine space or posterior cul-de-sac (also called the pouch of Douglas) (Fig. 7.34). However, when fluid is demonstrated in the anterior cul-de-sac (uterovesical space) or lateral pelvic recesses, or a large amount of fluid is seen in the posterior cul-de-sac, a Focused Assessment with Sonography for Trauma (FAST) exam may be performed in order to assess the volume of intraperitoneal free fluid.

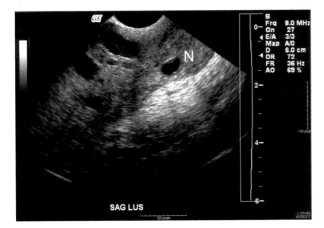

Figure 7.32. Transvaginal Scan: Nabothian cyst. A Nabothian cyst is demonstrated in the cervix; there are also multiple endometrial cysts seen within the uterus of this patient.

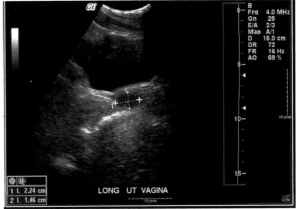

Figure 7.33. Transabdominal Scan: Gartner's cyst. A Gartner's cyst is demonstrated in the vagina; these are benign and require no treatment.

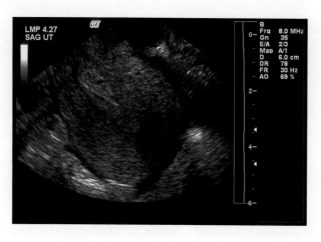

Figure 7.34. Transvaginal Scan: Free fluid. A small amount of physiologic free fluid is seen on this TVS; this is normally seen in many women during the course of a menstrual cycle.

USE OF THE IMAGE IN CLINICAL DECISION MAKING

Management of ovarian cysts relates to the size and characteristics of the cyst. In a premenopausal female with a simple cyst (either with or without hemorrhage), a cyst ≤ 3 mm is functional and no follow-up is needed. If a simple cyst is ≥ 3 mm, it is probably functional, but a follow-up TVS is recommended in 6 weeks, preferably during the first week of a cycle. Postmenopausal cysts ≤ 5 mm are usually benign, but follow-up is recommended, and when ≥ 5 mm surgical removal or very close follow-up is recommended because there is an increased risk of malignancy. Complex ovarian cysts and solid or predominantly solid-appearing ovarian masses are evaluated further with CT or MRI as certain findings such as dermoids, endometriomas, and fibroids permit conservative follow-up. Persistent or malignant-appearing masses are removed surgically (5,20).

CLINICAL CASE

A 37-year-old white female presents with a six-hour history of left-sided pelvic pain and vaginal bleeding. She is gravida 2, para 2 and her last menses 3 weeks prior to arrival is described as shorter than usual. She is sexually active and uses oral contraceptives. She denies previous sexually transmitted diseases but admits to multiple sexual partners currently. There is no surgical history. She is in mild distress. She has a blood pressure of 117/60 mm Hg, heart rate of 96 beats per minute, temperature is 98.6° F, and oxygen saturation of 99% on room air. The general physical exam is normal except for mild tenderness in the left lower quadrant with no rebound, guarding, or rigidity. The pelvic exam is normal except for scant blood oozing from cervix and pooling in the vaginal canal. The urine β-hCG is negative. The hemoglobin is 13; hematocrit is 39. Her transvaginal ultrasound is shown in figure 7.35 A. TVS of the adnexa reveals a 4 × 6 cm mass which is heterogeneously echogenic. Her pelvic pain is reproduced with probe pressure on the mass. These findings are confirmed on TAS (Fig. 7.35 B) which reveals no other masses and no free fluid. She was referred to her gynecologist and confirmatory imaging with MRI revealed an ovarian cyst suspicious for ovarian carcinoma. Subsequent laparoscopy revealed the mass to be a papillary serous cystadenofibroma of borderline malignancy.

Although the final diagnosis was essentially benign, this case demonstrates the utility of ED-performed ultrasound as an adjunct to the clinical exam. The presenting complaints of pelvic pain and bleeding in the absence of pregnancy and peritoneal findings could be dismissed as one of many common benign problems including dysfunctional uterine bleeding. When used routinely as part of the pelvic exam, TVS may often identify findings that would otherwise go undetected.

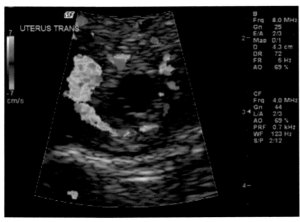

Figure 6.24. A ring of fire is seen by Doppler indicating hypervascularity around the gestational sac (**D**). Images courtesy of Cory Cunningham, PA-C, and Karen Cosby, MD.

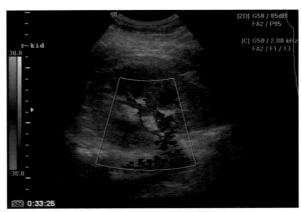

Figure 10.22. Color Doppler through the hilium of the kidney shows that an apparent enlarged ureter is actually vascular structures superimposed on the collecting system.

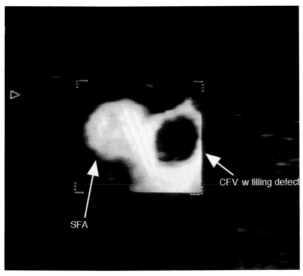

Figure 11.11. A filling defect is seen during augmentation. (CFV, Common Femoral Vein; SFA, Superficial Femoral Artery)

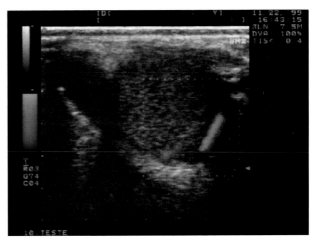

Figure 12.7. Color Doppler imaging (CDI). Power Doppler showing testicular blood flow. Power Doppler displays color-coding in one color that can vary with the velocity of flow but is not directionally dependent.

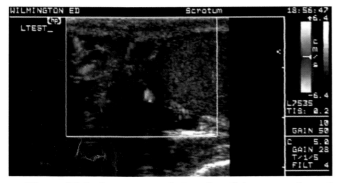

Figure 12.8. Spermatic cord. Doppler of the spermatic cord as well as the upper pole of the testicle.

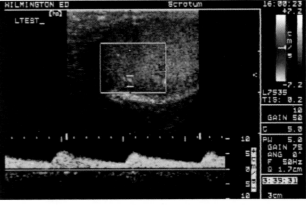

Figure 12.9. Arterial spectral Doppler. Directional color and spectral Doppler waveform is displayed. A normal arterial spectral waveform is demonstrated.

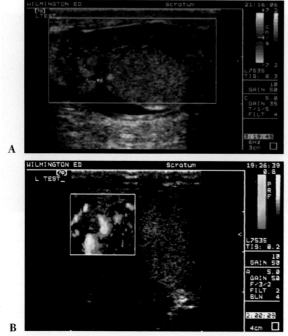

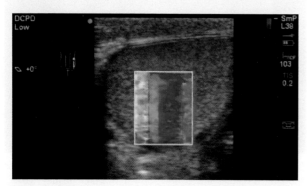

Figure 12.12. (A) Epididymitis with orchitis. Sagittal image from a 13-year-old who presented with a painful swollen testicle. Note the enlarged epididymis superior to the testicle. (B) Epididymitis. Power Doppler showing increased flow within and around the epididymis.

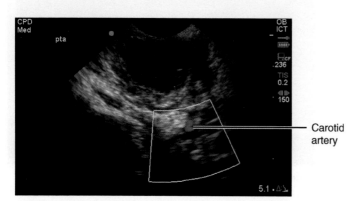

Figure 12.19. Color Doppler "flash" artifact. This image shows color filling within the sample volume that results from the Doppler shift caused by either the patient or the transducer moving. Though this is an extreme example, it is critical that Doppler signals be clearly identified resulting from true venous and arterial flow rather than from either patient movement or transducer movement artifacts.

Carotid artery

Figure 14.15. (B) With color Doppler, revealing location of the internal carotid artery.

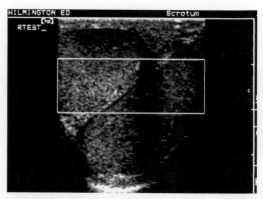

Figure 12.13. Acute left testicular torsion. Note absence of color power Doppler flow compared to right testicle. An edge artifact obscures a portion of the left testicle.

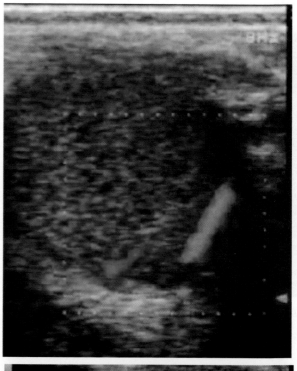

A

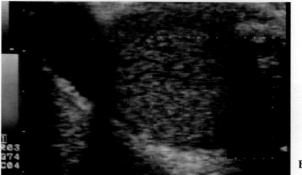

B

Figures 12.24. Acute left testicle torsion. Sagittal images of patient's testicles 3 hours after onset of acute left testicular pain. Note power color Doppler flow in the unaffected right testicle (A) compared to the absence of flow in the color gate for the left testicle with superior reactive hydrocele (B).

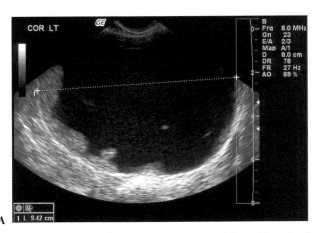
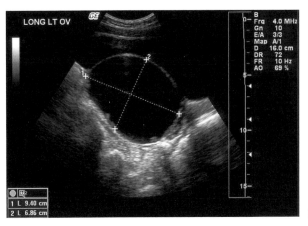

Figure 7.35. Complex cyst. **A.** Transvaginal Scan. Note the frondlike projections in this 10 × 7-cm complex cyst; this is suspicious for malignancy. **B.** Transabdominal Scan. Appearance of the cyst by a transabdominal approach.

ACKNOWLEDGMENTS

The authors would like to acknowledge the work of Mary Whitsett, RT, AS, RVT, RDMS and Kerri Lyn Wheeler, RT, BS, RDMS whose assistance in image acquisition was invaluable.

REFERENCES

1. Heller M, Jehle D, eds. *Ultrasound in Emergency Medicine*. 2nd ed. Philadelphia: W. B. Saunders; 2001.
2. Levi CS, Holt SC, Lyons EA, et al. Normal Anatomy of the Female Pelvis. In: Callen, ed. *Ultrasonography in Obstetrics and Gynecology*. 4th ed. Philadelphia: W. B. Saunders; 2000:781–813.
3. Bau A, Atri M. Acute female pelvic pain: ultrasound evaluation. *Semin Ultrasound CT MR*. 2000;21:78–93.
4. Sivyer P. Pelvic ultrasound in women. *World J Surg*. 2000;24:188–197.
5. Laing FC, Brown DL, DiSalvo DN. Gynecologic ultrasound. *Radiol Clin North Am*. 2001; 39:523–540.
6. Salem S. The Uterus and Adnexa. In: Rumack CM, Wilson SR, Charboneau JW. *Diagnostic Ultrasound*. 2nd ed. St. Louis: Mosby; 1998:521–573.
7. Grays Anatomy. 36th British ed. Williams P and Warwick R, eds. Philadelphia: W. B. Saunders; 1980:1423–1433.
8. Palter SF, Olive DL. Reproductive Physiology. In: *Novak's Gynecology*. 13th ed. Philadelphia: Lippincott Williams & Wilkins; 2002:149–171.
9. Richenberg J, Cooperberg P. Ultrasound of the Uterus. In: Callen, ed. *Ultrasonography in Obstetrics and Gynecology*. 4th ed. Philadelphia: WB Saunders; 2000:814–846.
10. Bakos O, Lundkvist O, Wide L, et al. Ultrasonographical and hormonal description of the normal ovulatory menstrual cycle. *Acta Obstet Gynecol Scand*. 1994;73:790–796.
11. Goldstein RB, Bree RL, Benson CB, et al. Evaluation of the woman with postmenopausal bleeding: Society of Radiologists in Ultrasound-Sponsored Consensus Conference Statement. *J Ultrasound Med*. 2001;20:1025–1036.
12. Robboy SJ, Duggan MA, Kurman RJ, et al. Gynecologic Pathology. In: Rubin E, Farber JL, eds. *Pathology*. Philadelphia: JB Lippincott Co; 1988; 942–989.
13. Flake GP, Anderson J, Dixon D. Etiology and pathogenesis of uterine leiomyomas: A review. *Environ Health Perspect*. 2003;111:1037–1054.
14. Adams Hillard PJ. Benign Diseases of the Female Reproductive Tract: Symptoms and Signs. In: *Novak's Gynecology*. 13th ed. Philadelphia: Lippincott Williams & Wilkins; 2002:351–420.
15. Lin MC, Gosink BB, Wolf SI, et al. Endometrial thickness after menopause: effect of hormone replacement. *Radiology*. 1991;180:427–432.
16. Karlsson B, Granberg S, Wikland M, et al. Transvaginal ultrasonography of the endometrium in women with postmenopausal bleeding: a Nordic multicenter study. *Am J Obstet Gynecol*. 1995;172:1488–1494.

17. Smith-Bindman R, Kerlikowske K, Feldstein VA, et al. Endovaginal ultrasound to exclude endometrial cancer and other endometrial abnormalities. *JAMA*. 1998;280:1510–1517.

18. Merz E, Miric-Tesanic D, Bahlman F, et al. Sonographic size of uterus and ovaries in pre- and postmenopausal women. *Ultrasound Obstet Gynecol*. 1996;7:38–42.

19. Stubblefield, PG. Family Planning. In: *Novak's Gynecology*. 13th ed. Philadelphia: Lippincott Williams & Wilkins; 2002:242–245.

20. Dill-Macky MJ, Atri M. Ovarian Sonography. In: Callen, ed. *Ultrasonography in Obstetrics and Gynecology*. 4th ed. Philadelphia: W. B. Saunders; 2000:857–896.

21. Clement PB. Nonneoplastic Lesions of the Ovary. In: Kurman RJ, ed. *Blaustein's Pathology of the Female Genital Tract*. 4th ed. New York: Springer-Verlag New York; 1994:597–645.

22. Atri M, Nazarnia S, Bret PM, et al. Endovaginal sonographic appearance of benign ovarian masses. *Radiographics*. 1994;14:747–760.

23. Osmers RG, Osmers M, von Maydell B, et al. Preoperative evaluation of ovarian tumors in the premenopause by transvaginosonography. *Am J Obstet Gynecol*. 1996;175:428–434.

24. Koonings PP, Campbell K, Mishell DR Jr, et al. Relative frequency of primary ovarian neoplasms: a 10-year review. *Obstet Gynecol*. 1989;74:921–926.

25. Sheth S, Fishman EK, Buck JL, et al. The variable sonographic appearances of ovarian teratomas: correlation with CT. AJR *Am J Roentgenol*. 1988;151:331–334.

26. Patel MD, Feldstein VA, Lipson SD, et al. Cystic teratomas of the ovary: diagnostic value of sonography. AJR *Am J Roentgenol*. 1998;171:1061–1065.

27. Talerman, A. Germ Cell Tumors of the Ovary. In: Kurman RJ, ed. *Blaustein's Pathology of the Female Genital Tract*. 4th ed. New York: Springer-Verlag New York; 1994:849–914.

28. Kupfer MC, Schwimer SR, Lebovic J. Transvaginal sonographic appearance of endometriomata: spectrum of findings. *J Ultrasound Med*. 1992;11:129–133.

29. Clement, PB. Diseases of the Peritoneum (Including Endometriosis). In: Kurman RJ, ed. *Blaustein's Pathology of the Female Genital Tract*. 4th ed. New York: Springer-Verlag New York; 1994:647–703.

30. Hershlag A, Peterson CM. Endocrine Disorders. In: *Novak's Gynecology*. 13th ed. Philadelphia: Lippincott Williams & Wilkins; 2002:871–930.

31. Botsis D, Kassanos C, Pyrgiotis E, et al. Sonographic incidence of polycystic ovaries in a gynecological population. *Ultrasound Obstet Gynecol*. 1995;6:182–185.

32. Farquhar CM, Birdsall M, Manning P, et al. Transabdominal versus transvaginal ultrasound in the diagnosis of polycystic ovaries in a population of randomly selected women. *Ultrasound Obstet Gynecol*. 1994;4:54–59.

33. Yao MW, Schust DJ. Infertility. In: *Novak's Gynecology*. 13th ed. Philadelphia: Lippincott Williams & Wilkins; 2002:973–1066.

34. Wiseman DA, Greene CA, Pierson RA. Infertility. In: Rumack CM, Wilson SR, Charboneau JW, eds. *Diagnostic Ultrasound*. 2nd ed. St. Louis: Mosby; 1998:1407–1439.

35. Timor-Tritsch IE, Lerner JP, Monteagudo A, et al. Transvaginal sonographic markers of tubal inflammatory disease. *Ultrasound Obstet Gynecol*. 1998;12:56–66.

36. Khan A, Muradali D. Imaging acute obstetric and gynecologic abnormalities. *Semin Roentgenol*. 2001;36:165–172.

37. Ignacio EA, Hill MC. Ultrasound of the acute female pelvis. *Ultrasound Q* 2003;19:86–98.

38. Kaakaji Y, Nghiem HV, Nodell C, et al. Sonography of obstetric and gynecologic emergencies: Part II, Gynecologic emergencies. AJR *Am J Roentgenol*. 2000;174:651–656.

39. Harrison BP, Crystal CS. Imaging modalities in obstetrics and gynecology. *Emerg Med Clin North Am*. 2003;21:711–735.

40. Togashi K. Ovarian cancer: the clinical role of US, CT, and MRI. *Eur Radiol*. 2003 Dec;13 Suppl 4:L87-104.

41. Robboy SF, Duggan MA, Kurman RJ, et al. Benign gynecologic lesions. In: Droegemueller W, Mishell DR, Stenchever MA, et al. (eds). *Comprehensive Gynecology*. 3rd ed. St. Louis: Mosby; 1997:467–516.

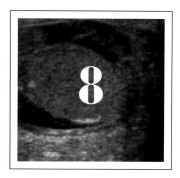

LIVER, GALLBLADDER, AND BILIARY TREE

Karen S. Cosby
John L. Kendall

INTRODUCTION

Abdominal pain is a leading cause for visits to the Emergency Department (ED). The evaluation of the abdomen frequently utilizes many resources, not the least of which is the time often invested in serial exams, use of consultants, and imaging procedures. Focused bedside ultrasound offers a valuable adjunct for the assessment of abdominal pain. With even a moderate amount of training and limited experience, emergency physicians can obtain sufficient skill to incorporate right upper quadrant (RUQ) ultrasound into their bedside exams and clinical decisions (1–4). Most studies can be completed in less than 10 minutes (3). The current literature verifies that emergency ultrasound of the RUQ is accurate, improves time to diagnosis and treatment, decreases ED length of stay, and improves patient satisfaction (1–6). Bedside ultrasound can facilitate rapid screening for life-threatening conditions and may prevent delays in detecting serious illness. Ultrasound of the RUQ is included in the list of six primary applications for emergency ultrasound and has been added to the standard curriculum of emergency medicine residency training programs.

CLINICAL APPLICATIONS

Right upper quadrant ultrasound is useful in assessing three common problems:

1. Right upper quadrant and epigastric pain
2. Jaundice
3. Ascites

There are four common practical applications for bedside ultrasound of the RUQ:

1. Detecting gallstones
2. Diagnosing cholecystitis
3. Imaging dilated bile ducts and diagnosing biliary obstruction
4. Visualizing ascites

These are the most commonly cited indications for ED ultrasound of the RUQ, however ultrasound can also potentially help in the search for a focal source of infection in patients who are septic, those with altered mental status and unreliable exams, and in the elderly or immunocompromised who may be less likely to have focal findings (7).

The liver is the major acoustic window to the abdomen. Familiarity with the liver and its surrounding structures will open up a variety of applications for abdominal scanning beyond those listed here. As clinicians become proficient in RUQ scans, they will become more confident and competent in the Focused Assessment by Sonography for Trauma (FAST) exam (to assess for free fluid in Morison's pouch) and in the scan of the proximal abdominal aorta (to detect aneurysms and dissections). Although RUQ ultrasound is primarily focused on the liver, gallbladder, and biliary tree, it may also detect disease in adjacent areas in the right kidney, pleural space, pancreas, and aorta.

GUIDE TO IMAGE ACQUISITION

The liver, gallbladder, and biliary tree can be imaged from a number of approaches (subcostal, intercostal, and flank) with the patient in a variety of positions (supine, semirecumbent, erect, left lateral decubitus, and prone). The optimal technique will vary based on differences in anatomy, body habitus, and bowel gas patterns. Ideally, the sonographer should begin with a few standard approaches, modified and guided by both external and internal landmarks (Fig. 8.1).

The subcostal approach is the most commonly used initial approach to imaging the gallbladder. Begin with the patient supine and place the transducer in the midline at the epigastrium with the transducer oriented in the sagittal plane (Fig. 8.1A). If there is a large left hepatic lobe the liver may be easily seen in this position. Leaving the transducer in the

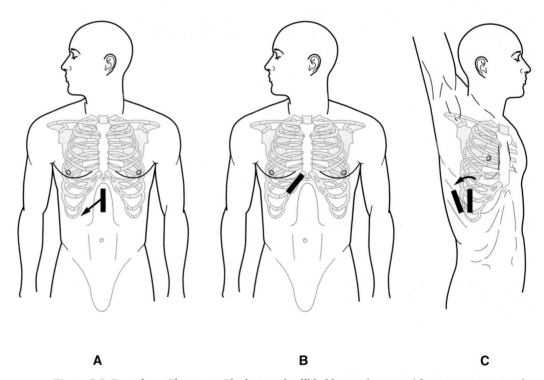

A　　　　　　　　**B**　　　　　　　　**C**

Figure 8.1. Transducer Placement. The liver and gallbladder can be imaged from an epigastric, subcostal (**A**), intercostal (**B**), or flank (**C**) approach with the patient in any of several positions, including supine, semirecumbent, erect, left lateral decubitus, or prone. Begin with the transducer in the epigastrium and scan below the right costal margin, moving from the epigastrium toward the right flank (**A**). A high liver can be imaged through the intercostal space (**B**). A flank approach (**C**) can minimize interference from bowel gas.

midline, tilt the transducer to project the sound wave toward the patient's right side. In some cases this will be sufficient to localize the gallbladder. If it is not, move the transducer down the costal margin while projecting it cephalad under the rib margin to scan through the dome of the liver. In many patients, the liver is mostly intrathoracic. In these patients, an improved image can be obtained by placing the transducer between the ribs (intercostal approach) (Fig. 8.1B). Alternatively, the patient can be positioned to bring the liver down below the costal margin. Have patients sit erect or semirecumbent and instruct them to breathe deeply with their "belly out." As the liver descends, the liver and gallbladder may be more easily imaged. If these maneuvers fail, move the patient to a left lateral decubitus position. This maneuver brings the liver and gallbladder more toward the midline and closer to the transducer. Scan again from the subcostal approach, then continue to move the transducer along the costal margin toward the right flank. If the anterior subcostal approach is unsuccessful, leave the patient in a left lateral decubitus position and scan through the right flank to identify the right kidney and Morison's pouch (Fig. 8.1C). Once the right kidney is in view, the transducer should be angled slightly cephalad and anterior. The fundus of the gallbladder lies in close proximity to the right kidney and will often pop into view with this maneuver. Occasionally it is useful to roll the patient from a left lateral decubitus position into a nearly prone position and scan from a subcostal approach. This position brings the gallbladder anterior. If heavy shadowing is seen from the gallbladder fossa, moving the patient prone may help the stones fall forward and make the echogenic stones more visible themselves, helping distinguish the shadows of a gallbladder packed with stones from artifact from bowel gas (8).

If these external landmarks do not produce a good image, focus on obtaining the best possible acoustic window of the liver and follow internal landmarks. The portal triad and main lobar fissure (MLF) are useful landmarks that can be used to locate the gallbladder fossa. If the portal triad is used to define the center of a clock face, the gallbladder is usually found around 2 o'clock. The MLF can be seen as an echogenic line joining the portal triad to the gallbladder. (See section on Anatomy.)

Regardless of how the image is obtained, once the gallbladder is identified the entire organ should be scanned to fully visualize it. Gently rocking the transducer right and left, then rotating it 90 degrees to view both the long and short axis will produce a three-dimensional perspective. It is often necessary to manipulate the transducer to fully define the anatomy and pick up stones that may be obscured by the twists and turns common to many gallbladders.

In general the best ultrasound images are obtained when sound waves are directed perpendicular to the organ of interest in as direct a path as possible. Unfortunately, this approach may not always work for the gallbladder. From patient to patient there is considerable variation in the location and orientation of the gallbladder and there are a number of acoustic barriers. For example, the transverse colon often rests immediately adjacent to the gallbladder, and the duodenum sweeps along its medial margin (Fig. 8.2). If the sound waves encounter bowel gas from either, shadowing will obscure the image. Most of the maneuvers described here are simply attempts to direct the ultrasound beam around these obstacles.

There are no consistent external landmarks or transducer positions that can adequately guide the emergency sonographer in reliably visualizing the gallbladder in all patients. These guides are a starting point. Ideally, sonographers should use a systematic approach for scanning and modify their approach based on their experience and success.

NORMAL ANATOMY

The primary indication for a bedside ED ultrasound of the RUQ is detecting gallbladder disease as a potential source of pain. The novice may be tempted to focus solely on identifying the gallbladder and then be satisfied once it's visualized. However, the RUQ is an anatomically complex area traversed by a number of vascular and ductal structures, most of which

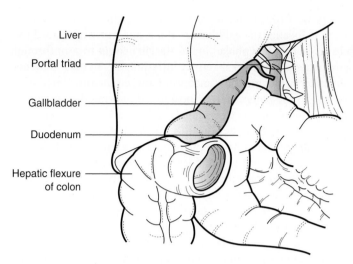

Figure 8.2. Structures Surrounding the Gallbladder. The gallbladder is surrounded by a number of structures that can interfere with acquiring a quality image. The right hepatic flexure and transverse colon lie just anterior and inferior to the gallbladder. The C-loop of the duodenum often crosses just medial to the gallbladder. Air in either structure can produce shadowing and create artifact.

are well visualized by ultrasound. Even if the sonographer does not initially desire to identify this anatomy, the busy network of vessels and structures in the area will likely be distracting, if not confusing. Some sonographers have found that this region is more difficult than many applications of ED bedside ultrasound, but once mastered, their ability to explore the abdomen and their confidence in their results are greatly enhanced. A thorough and methodical review of this anatomy will improve the diagnostic utility of RUQ ultrasound.

THE LIVER

The liver is a major solid organ that serves as a good acoustic window to image most of the upper abdominal structures. A cross section of the liver reveals organized hepatocytes punctuated by branches of the bile ducts, hepatic artery, and hepatic and portal veins. The liver has a gray echotexture typical of solid viscera; the numerous vessels coursing through the organ give it a "salt-and-pepper" appearance, with areas of increased and decreased echogenicity scattered uniformly throughout (Fig. 8.3). The capsule of the liver appears brightly echogenic, especially in its border with the diaphragm. The major structures that

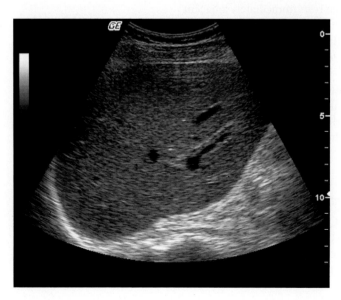

Figure 8.3. Sonographic Appearance of the Normal Liver. The liver has a uniform salt-and-pepper appearance created by the numerous vessels coursing through the parenchyma.

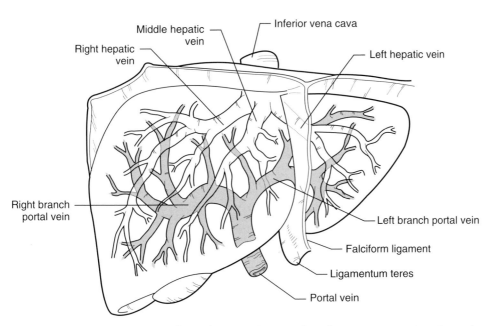

Figure 8.4. The Hepatic Veins and Portal Venous System. The inferior vena cava gives rise to three main hepatic veins that travel in the interlobar segments of the liver. The portal vein has two main branches that travel within the lobes of the liver.

are identifiable by ultrasound include the hepatic and portal veins, the hepatic arteries, and bile ducts (9). Figure 8.4 demonstrates a general outline of the major branches of the hepatic and portal venous structures.

HEPATIC VEINS

The liver is divided into anatomical lobes and segments by the hepatic veins (Fig. 8.4) (9). Three branches of hepatic veins arise from the inferior vena cava just after it enters the abdominal cavity near the diaphragm (Figs. 8.4, 8.5). The middle hepatic vein divides the liver into anatomical right and left lobes and courses through the MLF. The right hepatic

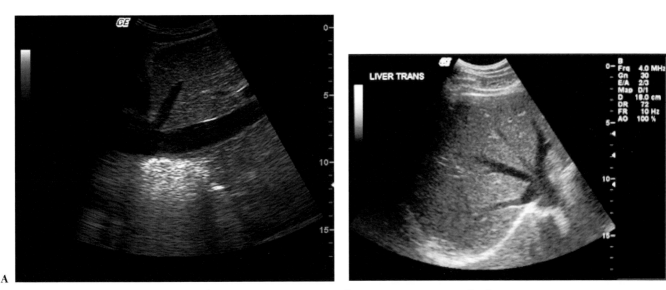

Figure 8.5. The Inferior Vena Cava and Hepatic Veins. **A:** The inferior vena cava pierces the diaphragm and enters the abdominal cavity where it can be seen posteriorly. **B:** It gives rise to three main hepatic veins that define the major lobes and segments of the liver.

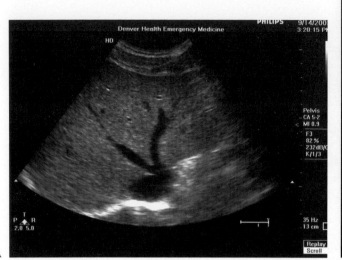

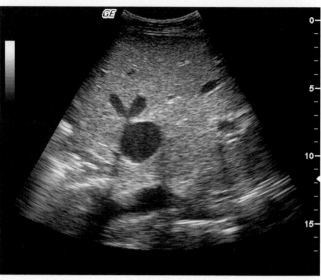

A
B

Figure 8.6. Playboy Bunny Sign. Sometimes the hepatic veins take on the appearance of bunny ears. In **A**, the bunny has long floppy ears. The appearance in **B** has been described as the "Playboy bunny sign." This description is an easy way to learn to recognize hepatic veins. (Image **B** courtesy of Mark Deutchman, MD.)

vein divides the right lobe of the liver into anterior and posterior segments; the left hepatic vein divides the left lobe of the liver into medial and lateral segments. The hepatic veins are thin, smooth-walled structures; the walls themselves are almost invisible to ultrasound. As the veins converge toward the vena cava, they sometimes look like rabbit ears; some have colorfully described their appearance as the "*Playboy* bunny sign" (Fig. 8.6). For the purposes of ED ultrasound, the middle hepatic vein serves as a landmark for the MLF, a valuable guide to the gallbladder. The appearance of the hepatic veins and inferior vena cava can give indirect evidence of fluid status and cardiac performance. The vessels may be engorged and especially prominent in the face of fluid overload and/or elevated right heart pressures (Fig. 8.7). For experienced sonographers, the hepatic veins can help localize pathology to specific lobes or segments.

PORTAL VEINS

The portal vein forms the most recognizable part of the portal triad and is usually an easy landmark to identify in the liver. For the emergent sonographer, it serves a role in helping to identify the common bile duct and gallbladder. The portal venous system returns blood from

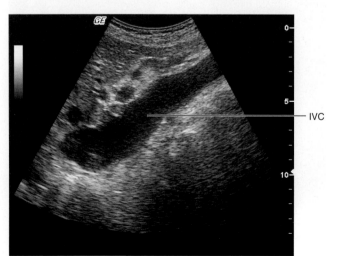

IVC

Figure 8.7. The Appearance of the Inferior Vena Cava and Hepatic Veins. An engorged inferior vena cava (IVC) is seen in a patient with congestive heart failure.

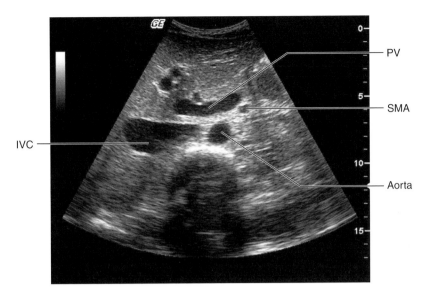

Figure 8.8. Origin of the Portal Vein. In a transverse section through the midline abdominal vasculature, the splenic vein is seen crossing anterior to the superior mesenteric artery (SMA). As it is joined by the inferior mesenteric artery (running perpendicular to this view, not imaged), the portal vein (PV) is formed. The portal vein then enters the hilum of the liver, just anterior to the inferior vena cava (IVC).

the intestines to the liver. The main portal vein is formed by the union of the splenic, inferior, and superior mesenteric veins. The splenic vein can be seen in a transverse section of the midline abdominal vasculature, where it courses just anterior to the superior mesenteric artery (Fig. 8.8). In a plane transverse to the body, the long axis of the splenic vein is seen as a regular tubular structure that suddenly balloons out at the portosplenic convergence, formed when the inferior mesenteric vein joins it (10). The portosplenic convergence defines the origin of the portal vein. As the portal vein enters the liver it lies just anterior to the inferior vena cava; this point defines the hilum of the liver (Fig. 8.9) (9). When the long axis of the main portal vein is viewed the common bile duct can be seen to accompany it toward the porta hepatis (Figs. 8.9, 8.10). The normal common bile duct is barely visible as an irregular structure just anterior to the portal vein. The portal vein rapidly gives rise to two main branches, the right and left portal veins (Figs. 8.4, 8.11). The right portal vein is the major landmark of the portal triad in the porta hepatis. The portal veins are characterized by bright echogenic walls that help distinguish them from other vessels in the liver. This peculiar echogenicity gives the appearance of a halo surrounding the portal venous vessels.

HEPATIC ARTERY

The hepatic artery (usually) originates as a branch off the celiac trunk. The main hepatic artery branches into the gastroduodenal artery and the proper hepatic artery. The gastroduodenal artery follows the course of the C-loop of the duodenum and defines the head of

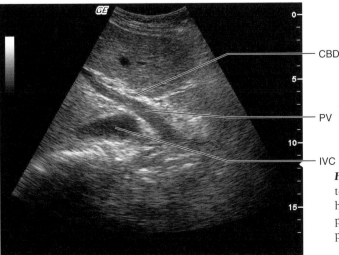

Figure 8.9. Portal Vein. The portal vein (PV) crosses just anterior to the inferior vena cava (IVC). It then travels toward the porta hepatis where it forms the most visible landmark in the liver, the portal triad. The common bile duct (CBD) lies just anterior to the portal vein.

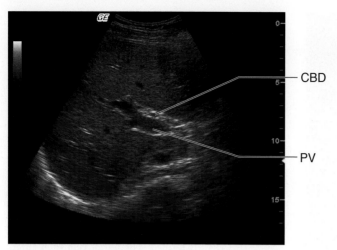

Figure 8.10. The Portal Vein and Common Bile Duct. In a long axis of the portal vein (PV), the common bile duct (CBD) is seen as an irregular beaded structure just anterior to the vein.

the pancreas. The proper hepatic artery ascends toward the porta hepatis to join the portal vein in the portal triad (Fig. 8.12). Its value in ED ultrasound is limited. For experienced sonographers it can be used to localize the pancreas (11).

BILE DUCTS

The hepatocytes are drained by tiny biliary radicles that converge toward the porta hepatis. Eventually they drain into the common hepatic duct. Just before the portal triad, the common hepatic and cystic ducts join to form the common bile duct. Common bile duct stones and pancreatic head tumors can obstruct outflow from the common bile duct, resulting in an enlarged duct. A dilated common bile duct is the hallmark of obstructive jaundice.

Bile ducts follow the path of the portal venous system throughout the liver. In routine scans of the liver the peripheral biliary radicles are typically not visualized unless they are enlarged. The larger common bile duct can be identified at the portal triad. If a transverse section is obtained through the portal triad, the common bile duct is seen just anterior to and to the right of the portal vein (Fig. 8.12). The diameter of the common bile duct is much smaller than the main portal vein, and is often almost imperceptible. When the portal vein is viewed in its long axis, the common duct can be seen to accompany it in its course toward the duodenum. It may be difficult to see if it is not enlarged, but it can be appreciated by the irregular beaded appearance it gives just anterior to the main portal vein (Fig. 8.10).

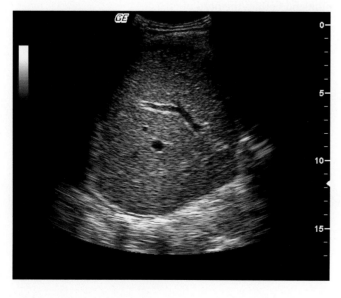

Figure 8.11. The Main Portal Vein Divides into Two Main Branches. Note the echogenic halo that surrounds the portal vessels, a characteristic that can be used to distinguish the portal veins from other structures.

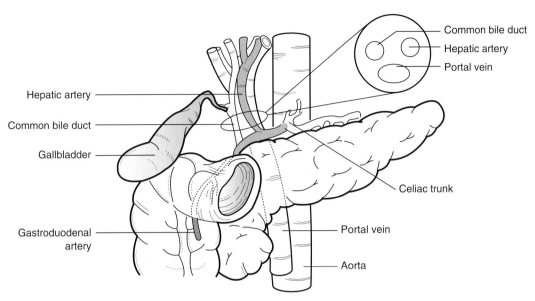

Figure 8.12. The Portal Triad. The hepatic artery, common bile duct, and the portal vein are seen together at the portal triad. The origin of the gastroduodenal artery is seen branching from the proper hepatic artery after its take-off from the celiac trunk. A short axis view of the portal triad has the appearance of a face with two ears, sometimes referred to as the "Mickey Mouse Sign."

GALLBLADDER

The gallbladder is a pear-shaped cystic structure that occupies the region between the right and left lobes of the liver and typically lies on the inferior surface of the liver (Fig. 8.13). The normal gallbladder has the typical sonographic features of a cyst:

1. The lumen is an echofree space, bounded by
2. Smooth regular walls, with
3. Posterior wall enhancement (more echogenic than surrounding tissue), and
4. Increased "through-transmission." (The region immediately behind a simple cyst appears more echogenic than surrounding tissue. This artifact is created as the sound waves hit the interface between liquid and solid media.)

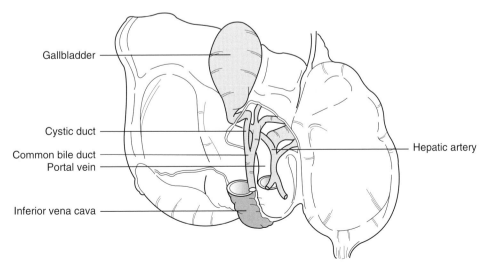

Figure 8.13. The Gallbladder and Portal Triad. The relative position of the gallbladder, portal vein, hepatic artery, and common bile duct is shown. (Redrawn from Simon and Snoey, eds. *Ultrasound in Emergency and Ambulatory Medicine.* St. Louis, MO: Mosby-Year Book; 1997.)

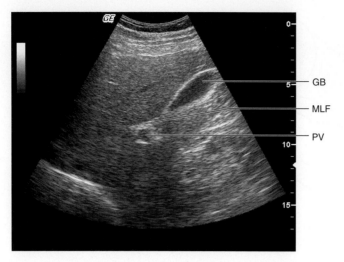

Figure 8.14. Normal Gallbladder. The gallbladder (GB), main lobar fissure (MLF), and portal vein (PV) are seen. A tear-shaped gallbladder points toward the MLF and portal triad. (Courtesy of EMH Bockenfeld.)

When a longitudinal or long axis view of the gallbladder is obtained, it appears to be connected to the portal triad by a visible echogenic line, the MLF. The MLF runs between the gallbladder and the inferior vena cava. The *MLF View* is a convenient view that defines much of the relevant anatomy for examinations of the gallbladder (Figs. 8.14, 8.15). In that one view, abnormalities of the gallbladder and common bile duct can be seen.

There are a number of congenital variants in gallbladders. Gallbladders may have folds, internal septums, and duplications. It is important to explore the full dimensions of the gallbladder and cystic duct to avoid missing stones. Folds, twists, turns, and septums complicate imaging of the gallbladder by creating shadows and artifacts that can mimic stones. Small stones can also hide in these regions as well. The sonographer will need to view each turn of the gallbladder in two dimensions to distinguish between shadows created by anatomical structures from those caused by stones (Figs. 8.16–8.18).

Occasionally the gallbladder may not be visualized. Agenesis of the gallbladder has been described but is rare. Most likely, the scan is simply inadequate. Formal ultrasound protocols request a fasting state to minimize bowel gas and optimize gallbladder distention. The sonographer should recognize the limitations of bedside scans in the unprepped patient and be willing to declare the exam indeterminant.

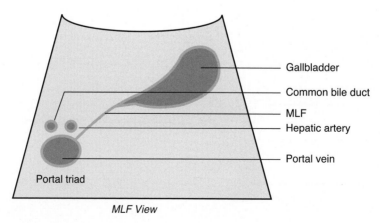

Figure 8.15. The *MLF View* of the Gallbladder and Portal Triad. The gallbladder, main lobar fissure (MLF), and portal triad are all seen in this view.

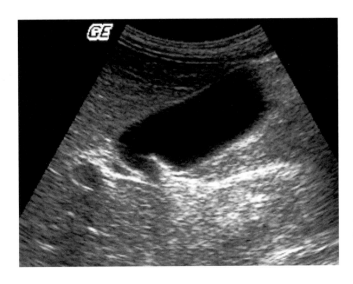

Figure 8.16. Normal Gallbladder. This normal gallbladder takes a sharp turn as it empties into the cystic duct. Such curves and twists can create shadows, as well as serve as sites where stones can become lodged.

MORISON'S POUCH

The interface between the liver and the right kidney can be visualized from a flank approach. This potential space, Morison's pouch, is an area where free fluid may accumulate. A view of Morison's pouch is useful when looking for free intra-abdominal fluid, either from ascites or intra-abdominal hemorrhage (Fig. 8.19).

STANDARD VIEWS OF THE RIGHT UPPER QUADRANT

A few specific views define most of the anatomy relevant for the focused bedside exam of the RUQ. A longitudinal cut through the long axis of the gallbladder should include a view of the MLF and portal triad (Figs. 8.14, 8.15). A second view through the short axis of the gallbladder should be obtained. The emergency sonographer should acquire a minimum of two views perpendicular to each other for any organ of interest, then scan from side to side. This creates a three-dimensional view of the object in the mind's eye.

Before completing the examination of the gallbladder, the portal triad should be examined. The portal vein, hepatic artery, and common bile duct are all viewed in their transverse orientation in the portal triad, as shown in Figure 8.15. The normal portal triad looks something like Mickey Mouse, with the portal vein making up Mickey's face, his ears formed anteriorly by the hepatic artery on the left, the common bile duct on the

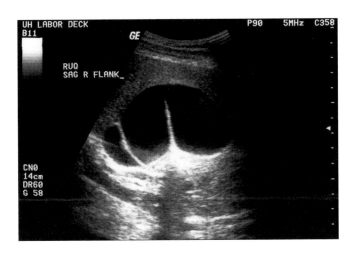

Figure 8.17. Normal but Tortuous Gallbladder. Normal gallbladders can have septums and unsuspecting twists. (Courtesy of Mark Deutchman, MD.)

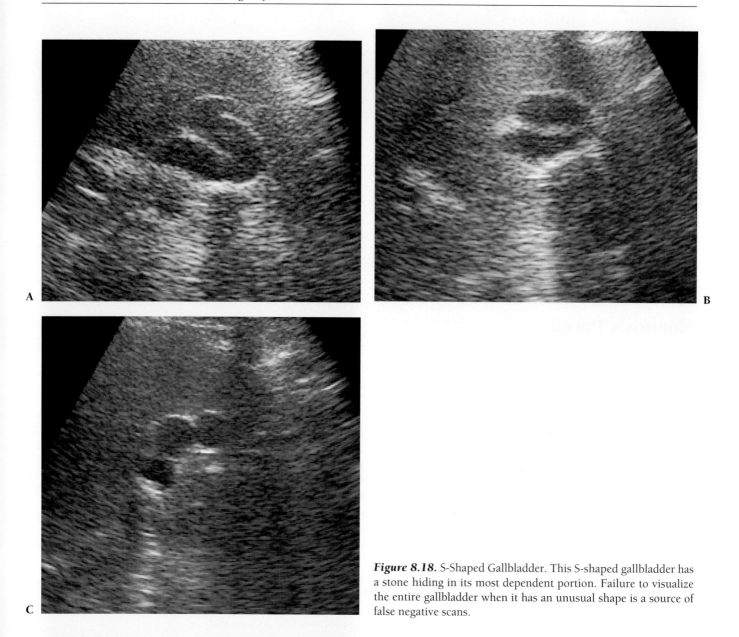

A

B

C

Figure 8.18. S-Shaped Gallbladder. This S-shaped gallbladder has a stone hiding in its most dependent portion. Failure to visualize the entire gallbladder when it has an unusual shape is a source of false negative scans.

Liver

Morison's Pouch

Right Kidney

Figure 8.19. Morison's Pouch. This potential space is a common site for free fluid to collect.

right (Fig. 8.12). In the normal portal triad, the "ears" are symmetrical. If they are not symmetrical, a more detailed exam should be done to measure the common bile duct and trace its path back toward the duodenum looking for a source and site of obstruction. In order to better visualize the common bile duct, the sonographer first identifies the portal vein in transverse orientation, then twists the probe to obtain a longitudinal view. When the portal vein is viewed in its long axis, the common bile duct should be seen just anterior to it. The normal common duct will be barely visible as it travels alongside the portal vein and has a beaded irregular appearance (Fig. 8.10). The normal common bile duct measures less than 6 mm in cross-sectional diameter. Although the hepatic artery occupies the portal triad, it ascends in a different plane than the portal vein and bile duct and tends to disappear when the long axis of the portal vein is viewed. Sometimes the common duct can be seen to loop over the hepatic artery in its course toward the duodenum.

Although it is helpful to recognize the major structures of the liver described above, it is not necessary to identify each of them in every exam. The ability to recognize the normal hepatic architecture can help to improve the quality of the study. Sonographers who are familiar with the anatomy of the liver, biliary tract, and abdominal vasculature will likely be less distracted or confused by anatomical details, able to recognize subtle variations from normal, and better able to complete definitive exams in a timely manner.

PATHOLOGY

CHOLELITHIASIS

The most common ED application for a scan of the RUQ is for detection of gallstones in patients suspected of having biliary colic or cholecystitis. With a sensitivity of more than 96% for the detection of stones, ultrasound is ideally suited for the detection for gallstones and is the imaging modality of choice for the gallbladder (12–15). Emergency sonographers have demonstrated the ability to accurately detect gallstones after moderate training, achieving sensitivities of 86 to 96%, and specificities of 78 to 97% (1–3). Gallstones have four sonographic features (7,16).

1. They are echogenic structures within the usual echo-free gallbladder lumen. Most are round, curvilinear, or multifaceted in shape. They range in shape from just a few millimeters to over a centimeter in size.
2. They create acoustic shadows. The typical gallstone shadow is described as "clean," meaning black with well-defined, discrete margins. Since the usual space behind the gallbladder has enhanced echogenicity, the shadow created by a stone is pronounced. In contrast, shadows created by artifact and bowel gas are described as "dirty," meaning they are grayish and poorly delineated. Bowel gas in particular scatters the ultrasound beam, creating a snowstorm of grayish artifact with poorly defined margins. Classically, stones were believed to create shadows because they contain calcium. In fact, the shadow created by a stone is more dependent upon the size of the stone than on its mineral content. Very small (1 to 3 mm) stones may not create shadows and are one source of false-negative scans (17).
3. They are dependent. They seek the most dependent portion of the gallbladder. Cholesterol stones are an exception; they are known to float (17).
4. They are typically mobile and move with changes in body position. Some stones may be embedded and fail to move; if they have the other three characteristics of stones, failure to move suggests chronic inflammation or impaction. An important caveat is that a stone impacted in the neck of the gallbladder may not move.

Gallstones may be single or multiple; they have a variety of sizes and shapes and may lodge in a variety of positions within the gallbladder (Figs. 8.20–8.29).

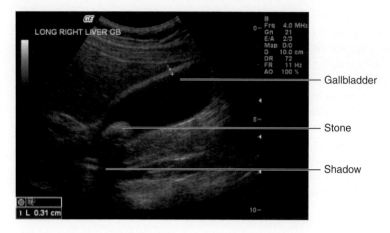

— Gallbladder

— Stone

— Shadow

Figure 8.20. Gallstone. A single stone is seen in the dependent portion of the gallbladder. Note the clean black shadow behind the stone.

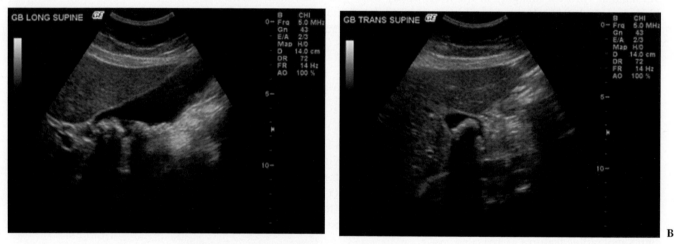

A   B

Figure 8.21. Gallstones. Multiple stones are seen as they layer out in the dependent portion of the gallbladder. Longitudinal (A) and transverse (B) images.

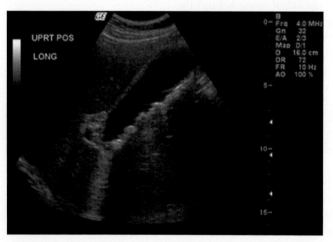

Figure 8.22. Gallstones. Multiple mobile and dependent stones are seen in this long axis view of the gallbladder.

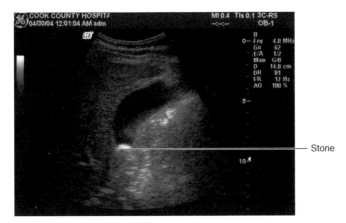

Figure 8.23. Gallstone. The echogenic outline is seen of a single stone impacted in the neck of the gallbladder.

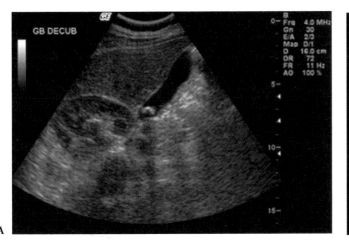

A

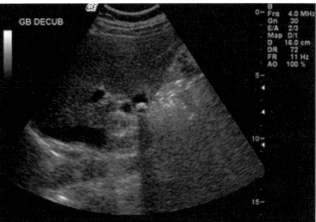

B

Figure 8.24. Gallstone. A stone is seen in the dependent part of the gallbladder in both longitudinal (A) and transverse (B) views.

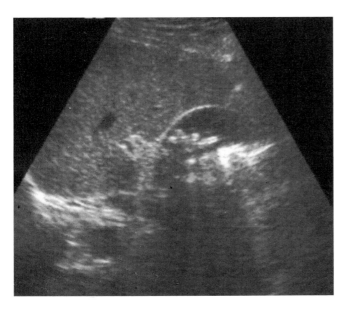

Figure 8.25. Gallstones. Multiple stones are seen casting a broad shadow. These stones appear to float, and probably contain cholesterol.

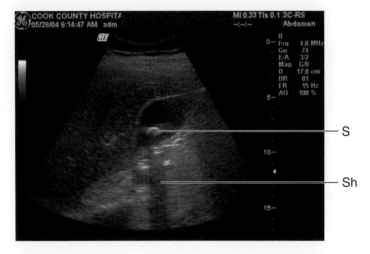

Figure 8.26. Gallstone. A single stone (S) with a shadow (Sh) is seen. The shadow contrasts sharply with the more echogenic region that is typically behind cystic structures created by increased through transmission.

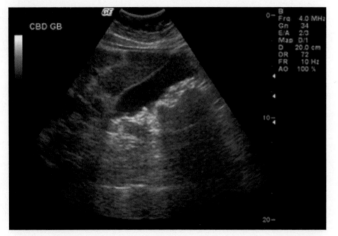

Figure 8.27. Gallstones. Multiple small stones create a broad shadow.

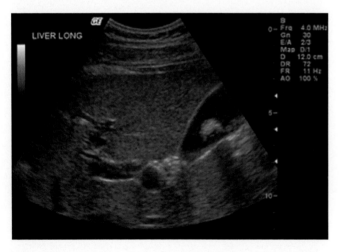

Figure 8.28. Gallstone. A single stone with shadowing is seen.

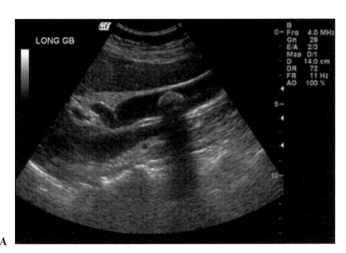 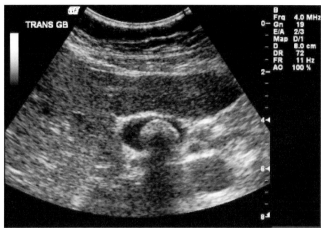

A   B

Figure 8.29. Gallstone. A large stone and its shadow are seen in longitudinal (A) and transverse (B) views of the gallbladder.

The lumen of the gallbladder may contain lithogenic bile, known as "sludge" (Figs. 8.30–8.32). Sludge has low-level echogenicity (it appears less "white" than stones), tends to layer out in the dependent portion of the gallbladder with a flat fluid:fluid interface, and fails to shadow. It is viscous and moves slowly with changes in position (13). When it co-exists with small stones, it may produce a gray shadow. The clinical relevance depends upon the patient's clinical signs and symptoms, associated stones, and secondary abnormalities of the gallbladder wall (7,13,15,16,18,19). Nonetheless, biliary sludge is not a normal finding and typically connotes a diseased gallbladder.

In some cases, heavy shadowing may obscure details of the gallbladder fossa. This may occur when the gallbladder is packed with stones, or when a contracted gallbladder encompasses a stone. Closer examination may reveal a gallbladder wall with heavy shadow; this "WES" (Wall-Echo-Shadow) phenomenon is well described for gallbladders filled with stones (Fig. 8.33) (13,16,20). A second possibility when heavy shadows come from the gallbladder fossa is a calcified, or porcelain gallbladder. Calcified gallbladders are associated with gallbladder cancer and require additional imaging and referral (21). The inexperienced scanner should beware when considering these possibilities. Bowel gas from the duodenum and adjacent colon can also create shadowing near the gallbladder fossa (Fig. 8.34). Distinguishing

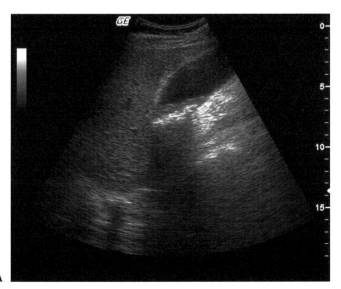 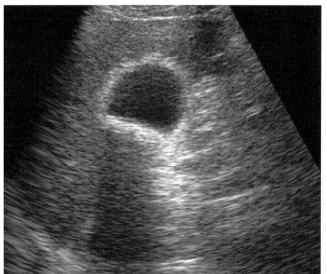

A   B

Figure 8.30. Stones and Sludge. The gray fluid level in this gallbladder is sludge accompanied by small stones, seen in longitudinal (A) and transverse (B) views.

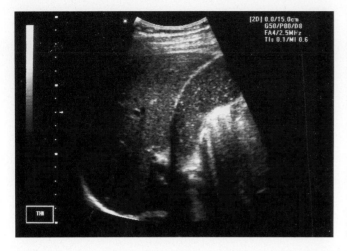

Figure 8.31. Sludge. The usual anechoic lumen of this gallbladder is replaced with gray material typical of sludge.

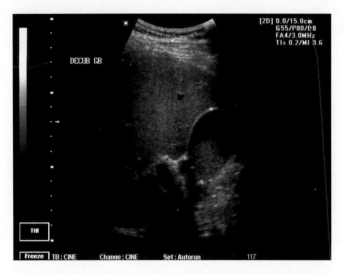

Figure 8.32. Sludge. The normal anechoic gallbladder lumen contrasts with the gray echotexture created by sludge in the dependent portion of this gallbladder.

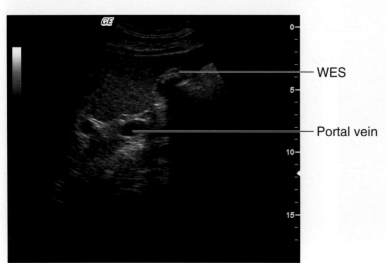

Figure 8.33. Gallbladder Fossa Obscurred by Shadow. Sometimes the gallbladder may be difficult to see when obscured by shadowing from large stones. The Wall-Echo-Shadow (*WES*) phenomenon is seen.

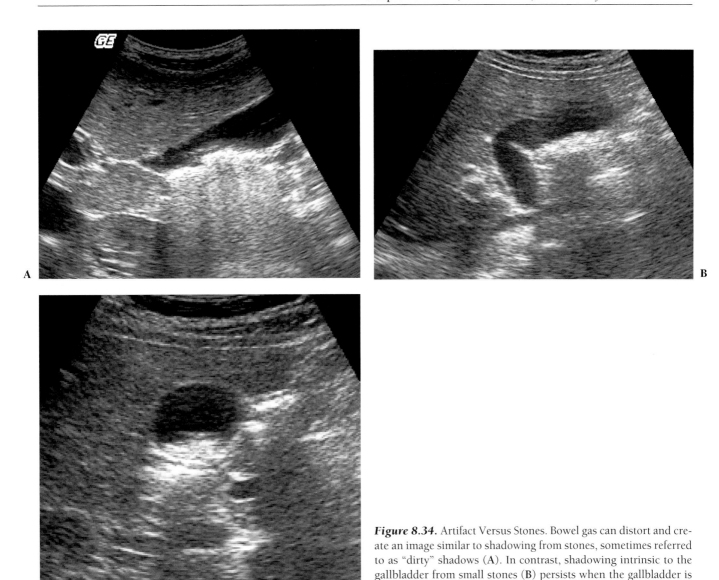

Figure 8.34. Artifact Versus Stones. Bowel gas can distort and create an image similar to shadowing from stones, sometimes referred to as "dirty" shadows (**A**). In contrast, shadowing intrinsic to the gallbladder from small stones (**B**) persists when the gallbladder is viewed in different orientations (**C**).

between these entities may be difficult. In general, shadowing from intrinsic gallbladder disease persists when viewed in different orientations and with changes in patient positioning, unlike shadowing from artifact, which disappears or changes with orientation (Fig. 8.34).

The sonographer may encounter echogenic structures within the gallbladder that do not meet the usual characteristics of stones. Gallbladder polyps are regular-appearing structures that may adhere to the gallbladder wall. They are less echogenic than stones, immobile, and are sometimes found on nondependent areas of the gallbladder. Although rare, irregular thickening or luminal masses may be the only sign of gallbladder cancers. If there is any suspicion of tumor, additional imaging is necessary.

CHOLECYSTITIS: ACUTE, CHRONIC, AND ACALCULOUS

There is a broad spectrum of gallstone-related disease, as well as a wide range of clinical presentations and sonographic findings. Gallstones may persist in asymptomatic patients for many years without apparent harm. Some patients with gallstones describe brief postprandial pain secondary to uncomplicated biliary colic. In others, the chronic presence of stones may set off an inflammatory process leading to hypertrophy of the muscular layer of the wall and fibrosis of the subserosa (22). These patients may have recurrent episodes of pain secondary to chronic cholecystitis. Once the gallbladder becomes obstructed, the severe inflammatory process characterizing acute cholecystitis is set up as the gallbladder becomes distended and the intraluminal pressure rises. The inflammation results in edema and inflammatory cells accumulating in and around the gallbladder wall. In the most severe cases, the mucosa may slough or the wall may become necrotic and perforate (22). These patients commonly present with fever, leukocytosis, and intractable pain and vomiting.

Ultrasound demonstrates a range of findings that parallels this spectrum of disease. Occasionally, gallstones may be detected that are of no clinical significance in the asymptomatic patient. When there is a history of postprandial pain, the diagnosis of biliary colic is supported by the presence of stones in an otherwise normal gallbladder. In the acutely ill patient with active pain and tenderness, the sonographic diagnosis of acute cholecystitis is based on the presence of stones or sludge with any of the following (13,16,19,22,23):

1. Sonographic Murphy's sign
2. Gallbladder distension
3. Gallbladder wall thickening
4. Intramural gallbladder wall edema
5. Pericholecystic fluid
6. Intraluminal material
7. Increased flow with color Doppler.

The likelihood of acute cholecystitis increases with each positive finding (13).

Sonographic Murphy's sign

The "sonographic Murphy's sign" is a variation of the classical "Murphy's sign" detected during the physical exam. It is elicited by localizing the gallbladder with the ultrasound transducer and then attempting to find the point of maximal tenderness. If the point of maximal tenderness corresponds to the area around the gallbladder, a sonographic Murphy's sign is noted (24). The literature reports a wide variation in the sensitivity and specificity of the Murphy's sign in cholecystitis, although in the hands of emergency physicians, it can be a valuable aid (3,25).

Gallbladder distension

The normal gallbladder is less than 10 cm in length and less than 5 cm in diameter. Gallbladder distension is taken as a sign of obstruction, suspicious for an obstructing stone, but this is a nonspecific finding (Fig. 8.35).

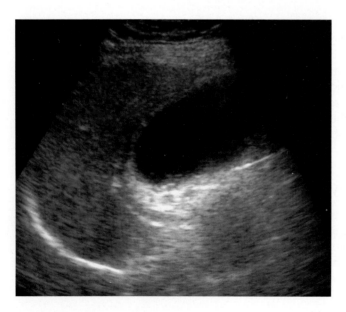

Figure 8.35. Distended Gallbladder. A distended gallbladder is a nonspecific finding, but may be one sign of an obstructing stone.

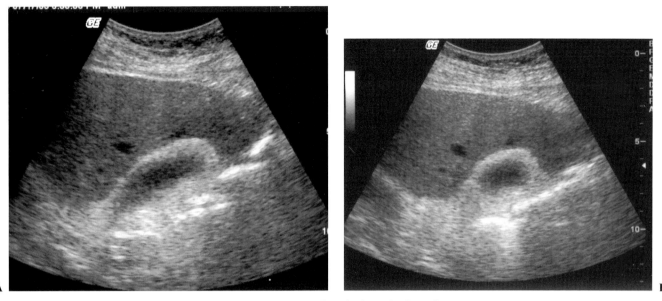

A   B

Figure 8.36. Thickened Gallbladder Wall. This gallbladder wall is thick in the face of congestive heart failure.

Gallbladder wall edema

The normal gallbladder wall is defined as less than 3 mm wide. When it is distended, the gallbladder has a smooth, regular thin wall. However, once the gallbladder contracts after a meal, the wall can be seen to be composed of three distinct layers that can exceed the "normal" thickness. The appearance of the gallbladder wall at any particular time is influenced by many factors, both local and systemic. The wall can be thickened in a variety of pathological conditions, including hypoalbuminemia, hepatitis, portal hypertension, congestive heart failure, and pancreatitis, as well as in the normal postprandial state (Figs. 8.36, 8.37) (13,16,23,26,27). In the face of biliary tract disease, the wall may be thickened by edema and hemorrhage (as in acute cholecystitis) or muscular hypertrophy and fibrosis (as in chronic cholecystitis). Thus, the absolute measurement of the gallbladder wall is neither sensitive nor specific for cholecystitis. The descriptive appearance of the thickness is more specific. In nonbiliary disease, the thickened wall is more typically uniform throughout with well-defined margins (Figs. 8.36, 8.37). In the face of acute inflammation, the wall tends to have focal collections of striated fluid that are irregular and somewhat less well-defined (Fig. 8.38) (13). In early cholecystitis, the development of gallbladder thick-

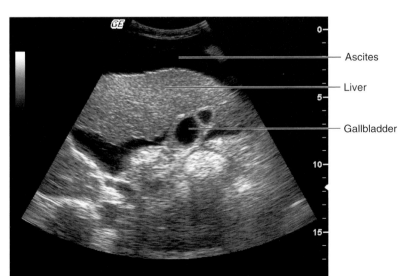

— Ascites

— Liver

— Gallbladder

Figure 8.37. Thickened Gallbladder Wall. This thick gallbladder wall occurs in a patient with hemachromatosis, hepatitis, and ascites. The diseased liver is more echogenic than normal. Ascites is present. The gallbladder wall is thickened, however there is no intrinsic gallbladder disease.

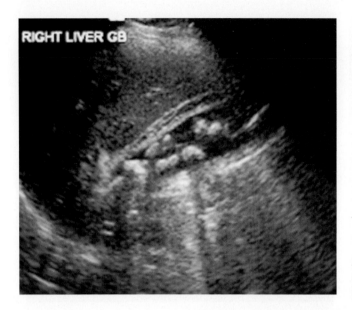

Figure 8.38. Thickened Gallbladder Wall. This diseased gallbladder has an irregular contour with streaking edema. This patient has acute cholecystitis.

ening and edema may be delayed; the absence of wall edema should not dissuade the clinician from considering the diagnosis of acute cholecystitis (28). Although the presence of gallbladder thickening and wall edema is considered an important finding consistent with cholecystitis, sonographers should cautiously interpret their findings and correlate the sonographic findings with the clinical setting.

Pericholecystic fluid

As the inflammation progresses, fluid may accumulate outside the gallbladder (Figs. 8.39, 8.40). If this pericholecystic fluid is loculated or focal, it may mark the beginning of an abscess or a perforation. In advanced cases, the gallbladder wall may appear disrupted, surrounded by complex pericholecystic fluid, consistent with a perforation or fistula formation. The sonographic appearance of the disrupted wall has been described as the "sonographic hole sign" (Fig. 8.41) (29,30).

Mucosal sloughing

In severe cases, the ischemic mucosal surface of the gallbladder may ulcerate and slough, sometimes leaving debris that can be seen to float in the gallbladder lumen (Figs. 8.41, 8.42). This typically represents advanced disease.

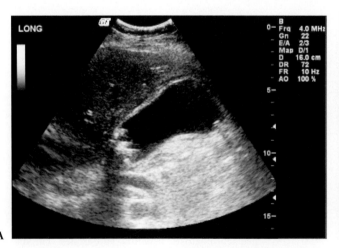
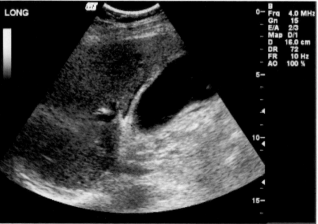

Figure 8.39. Acute Cholecystitis. This gallbladder has multiple stones (A), a thickened wall, and pericholecystic fluid (B).

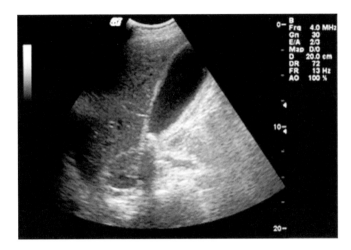

Figure 8.40. Acute Cholecystitis. A single stone is seen in the neck of this thickened, edematous gallbladder.

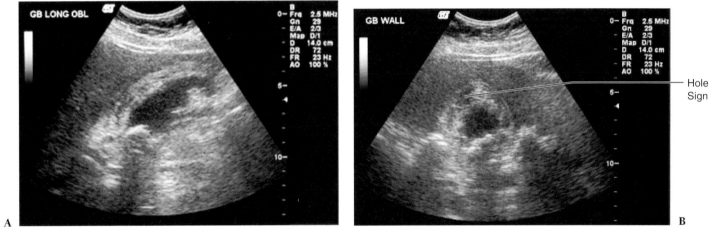

Hole Sign

Figure 8.41. Acute Cholecystitis. **A:** Marked changes consistent with acute cholecystitis are seen with an irregular thickened gallbladder wall, intramural edema, and stones. The mucosal surface appears ulcerated. In **B**, a "sonographic hole sign" suggests perforation.

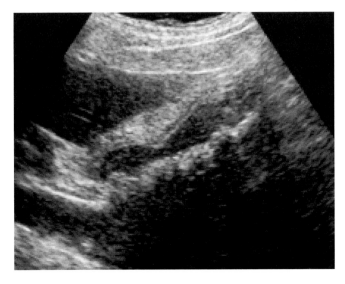

Figure 8.42. Acute Cholecystitis. Multiple stones are seen in this gallbladder. The gallbladder wall is thickened.

Increased vascularity

As with any inflammatory state, the inflamed gallbladder may be hypervascular. Power Doppler may demonstrate this increased vascularity. Typical findings in acute cholecystitis are seen in Figures 8.38–8.43. The most basic and practical criteria applied for the diagnosis of acute cholecystitis is the presence of stones in the face of a positive sonographic Murphy's sign. In the proper clinical setting, particularly in emergency medicine, this straightforward approach may be appropriate. The variety of secondary sonographic findings for acute cholecystitis described above has a wide range of sensitivity and specificity, probably reflecting the variety of clinical, laboratory, imaging, and pathology criteria used in the literature to define acute cholecystitis.

The variety of abnormal sonographic findings in acute cholecystitis may be difficult for the beginner trying to master bedside ultrasound. While relatively inexperienced emergency sonographers seem to pick up the skill to detect gallstones quickly, they are slower to detect and note the secondary findings of gallbladder wall edema and pericholecystic fluid (3). Gallstones are common; the more advanced findings of acute cholecystitis are relatively uncommon and thus less likely to fall within their range of experience. The use of the sonographic Murphy's sign provides important information of practical significance. Ralls, et al. reported that the presence of gallstones and a positive sonographic Murphy's sign had a positive predictive value of 92.2% for acute cholecystitis. The additional finding of gallbladder wall edema, a finding that is more difficult to appreciate and interpret by the beginning sonographer, improved the positive predictive value minimally to 95.2% (24). The accuracy of the sonographic Murphy's sign has been reported with variable results, with sensitivities ranging between 72 to 86% and specificities ranging between 35 to 94%. The emergency medicine literature has shown that emergency physicians' performance equals or exceeds this with a sensitivity of 75% for acute cholecystitis (3). Emergency sonographers should elicit and interpret the sonographic Murphy's sign early in their ultrasound training as they develop proficiency and expertise in detecting the more advanced secondary findings of acute cholecystitis. The presence of gallstones and a positive sonographic Murphy's sign is good evidence for symptomatic gallbladder disease. The absence of gallstones and a negative sonographic Murphy's sign strongly suggests an alternative diagnosis. Occasionally the signs, symptoms, and sonographic findings of acute cholecystitis occur in the absence of stones. Acalculous cholecystitis is described, although it is less common than calculous disease and typically occurs in seriously ill patients with biliary stasis. This is most likely to occur in hospitalized patients in critical care units.

Gallstones may make their way into the common bile duct and lodge at the ampulla of Vater. They can contribute to a clinical picture of cholangitis and pancreatitis. This is discussed more in the section on jaundice.

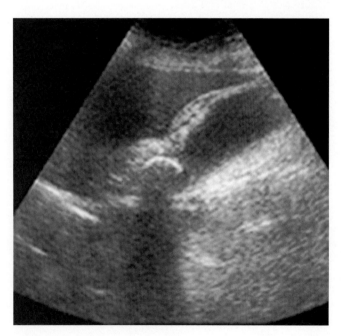

Figure 8.43. Acute Cholecystitis. Striated collections of fluid are seen in this irregular, thickened gallbladder wall consistent with acute cholecystitis. (Reused from *Ultrasound in Emergency Medicine and Trauma* © 2005, Challenger Corporation.)

JAUNDICE

One of the first steps in evaluating the patient with jaundice is distinguishing between obstructive and nonobstructive causes. This distinction frequently determines the need for specialty consultation and intervention and may dictate the pace at which the diagnostic workup and treatment should proceed. For the emergency physician it may determine the need for admission and the urgency of further treatment. The ability to make this determination at the bedside can avoid unnecessary tests in some, and facilitate appropriate aggressive care in others. Although this distinction has traditionally relied on historical and laboratory criteria, the clinical distinction often requires imaging. Right upper quadrant pain, fever, and jaundice can be a sign of viral hepatitis (a condition that can often be managed as an outpatient) or a presenting picture of cholangitis in obstructive jaundice (a condition requiring more aggressive intervention).

Ultrasound is a quick and noninvasive means to detect biliary obstruction (31,32). The normal common bile duct is easiest to identify at the portal triad. The normal common bile duct is less than 6 mm in diameter when measured adjacent to the right or main portal vein. As the common bile duct dilates, it gives the usual Mickey Mouse view of the portal triad the appearance of a swollen right ear (Fig. 8.44). When the portal vein and common bile duct are viewed in their long axis coursing toward the midline, the abnormal common bile duct becomes more prominent. When the common bile duct approximates or exceeds the diameter of the portal vein, the two vessels look like two parallel structures that resemble a "double barrel shotgun" (Figs. 8.45, 8.46) (33). As the obstruction persists and the peripheral biliary radicles dilate, they emanate outward from the portal triad like spokes of a wheel in a stellate pattern (Fig. 8.47) (34). Normally these peripheral biliary radicles are not visible by ultrasound (34). When they are seen, they are pathological. The formal rule of thumb is that any biliary radicle larger than 40% the diameter of its adjacent portal vein is pathological (27). As peripheral bile ducts enlarge they can be seen along with the branches of the portal veins; this gives the appearance of "parallel channels" of branching vessels in the parenchyma (Figs. 8.47, 8.48) (27). When biliary obstruction is noted, the gallbladder should be visualized to detect stones and the common bile duct carefully studied to determine the site of obstruction. Occasionally a source of obstruction can be seen within the lumen of the common bile duct or at the ampulla (Figs. 8.49, 8.50) (27,31,35). If a source of obstruction is not seen, additional imaging is necessary to find the source.

ASCITES

Patients may present with abdominal distension and suspected ascites. When the physical findings are indefinite, particularly in mild to moderate ascites, ultrasound can clarify if free fluid is present within the peritoneal cavity. A view of Morison's pouch, the flanks, or

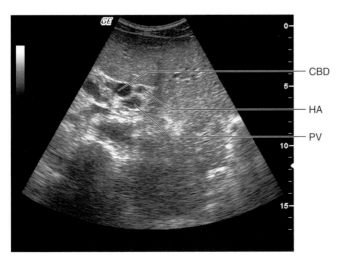

Figure 8.44. Dilated Common Bile Duct. When a dilated common bile duct (CBD) is visualized at the portal trial in transverse orientation, the typical "Mickey Mouse face" has a swollen right ear. The portal vein (PV) and hepatic artery (HA) are seen.

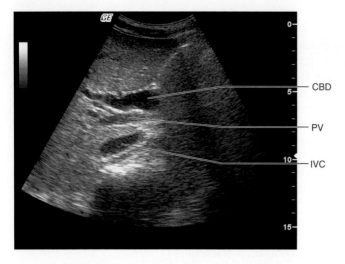

Figure 8.45. Dilated Common Bile Duct. The dilated common bile duct (CBD) and the portal vein (PV) look like a "double-barrel shotgun" as they course together toward the midline. The inferior vena cava (IVC) is seen posteriorly.

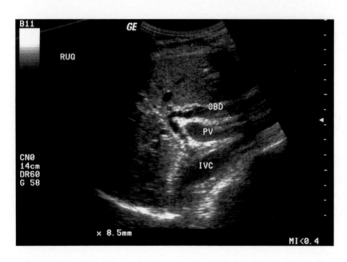

Figure 8.46. Dilated Common Bile Duct. The common bile duct (CBD) accompanies the portal vein (PV) toward the midline of the body. The inferior vena cava (IVC) is seen posteriorly. (Courtesy of Mark Deutchman, MD.)

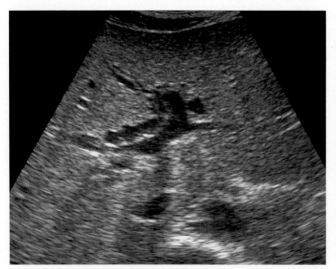

Figure 8.47. Dilated Bile Ducts. The dilated biliary ducts radiate outward from the portal triad in a stellate pattern.

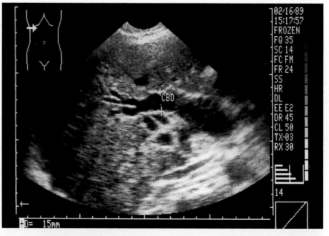

Figure 8.48. Dilated Bile Ducts. As biliary radicles dilate they form a series of branching channels in the hepatic parenchyma. (Courtesy of Mark Deutchman, MD.)

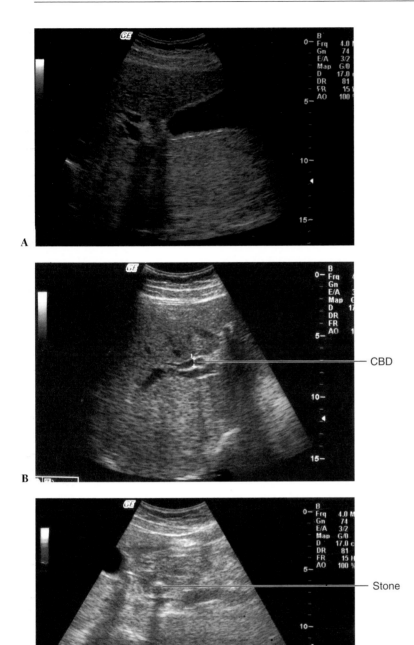

Figure 8.49. Biliary Obstruction. This patient developed right upper quadrant pain that spontaneously resolved. A few days later he noticed that he was jaundiced. The gallbladder is distended but without stones (A). Shadowing is seen coming from the cystic and common bile ducts (A). The common bile duct (CBD) is dilated (B). Multiple stones are seen in the common bile duct, one near the duodenum (C).

the pelvis is adequate to view ascites (Figs. 8.51–8.53). If necessary, ultrasound can help guide paracentesis for diagnosis and treatment of ascites and suspected spontaneous bacterial peritonitis. (See Chapter 13 for ultrasound-guided paracentesis).

OTHER PATHOLOGY

The occasional scan may encounter unsuspected findings. Changes in the usual character and organization of the hepatic parenchyma may occur with hepatitis. The architecture may be disrupted by liver masses. The recognition of hepatitis, cirrhosis, portal hypertension,

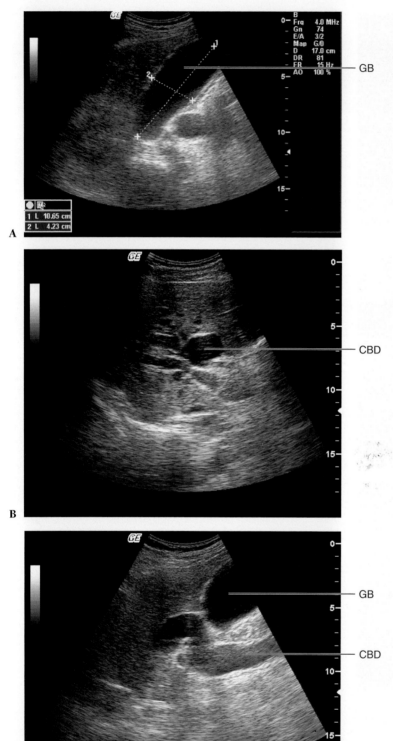

Figure 8.50. Biliary Obstruction. This patient presented with weight loss and painless jaundice. The gallbladder (GB) is distended, but without stones (**A**). The common bile duct (CBD) is markedly enlarged (more than 2 cm in diameter) throughout its length (**B**). The dilatation persists as the CBD is followed towards the ampulla (**C**). This patient was found to have a mass in the head of the pancreas.

and liver masses is generally beyond the scope of emergency physician–performed ultrasound. However, emergency sonographers will likely encounter these conditions and should recognize them as variations from normal (Figs. 8.54–8.56). Once they are detected, the physician should pursue additional imaging and appropriate follow-up.

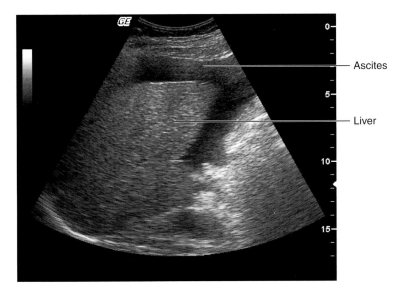

Figure 8.51. Ascites. Free fluid surrounds the liver bed.

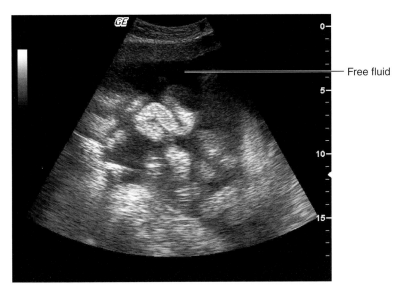

Figure 8.52. Ascites. Loops of bowel seem to float in free fluid.

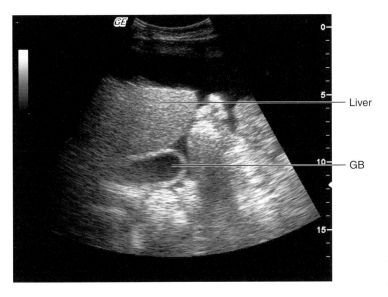

Figure 8.53. Ascites. Free fluid is seen about the liver and gallbladder (GB).

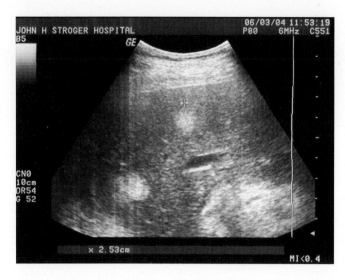

Figure 8.54. Liver Mass. Hyperechoic liver masses are noted, most consistent with a neoplasm.

ARTIFACTS AND PITFALLS

A variety of sources of artifacts is common in imaging gallbladders.

SIDE LOBE ARTIFACT

Sound waves travel in straight lines. When cysts with rounded edges (like the gallbladder) are imaged, an acoustically silent space is created around the curvature of the structure. This space creates a shadow simply because the sound waves never get there to generate a signal. Side lobe artifact should be recognized and not confused with shadowing from stones.

SHADOWING

A variety of shadows are generated by surrounding structures in the RUQ. When the intercostal approach is used to visualize the liver and gallbladder, the ribs create a dark shadow that traverses the entire image. Their shadows usually have a clear origin from the rib that

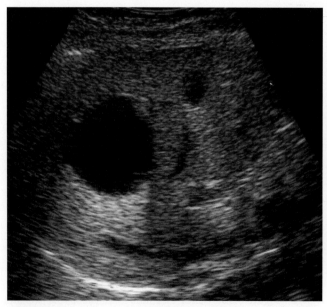

Figure 8.55. Liver Cyst. A simple but large cyst is noted in the liver.

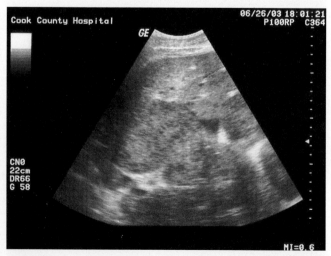

Figure 8.56. Renal cancer. A large renal neoplasm is seen invading the liver.

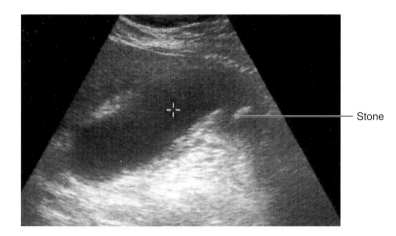

Stone

Figure 8.57. Phrygian cap. Stones can hide anywhere in the gallbladder. In this gallbladder, a stone is seen in a Phrygian cap at the fundus. The initial scan on this patient failed to visualize the cap and missed the stone.

is outside the margin of the gallbladder. Their appearance is typical of calcified structures, with an echogenic proximal surface and sharply marginated distal shadows as well.

Bowel gas commonly interferes with images of the gallbladder. When the gallbladder is viewed in its long axis, the medial margin lies in close proximity to the duodenum and colon. The scatter of bowel gas may produce shadows that create an appearance of stones (Fig. 8.34). The sonographer can evaluate the source of shadow by changing the orientation of the transducer and patient position. A shadow intrinsic to the gallbladder will remain; shadows created by other objects will change or disappear (Fig. 8.34).

Occasionally shadows will appear if the gallbladder or cystic duct is tortuous. This may represent side lobe artifact, but could arise from a small impacted stone. The best way to distinguish artifact from stone is to trace the structure distally, elongating each segment of the gallbladder neck or cystic duct by rotating the ultrasound transducer. Artifacts will disappear, while stones persist or become more apparent.

COMMON PITFALLS

1. Failing to visualize the entire gallbladder, missing hidden stones (Fig. 8.57).
2. Failing to visualize the gallbladder in two dimensions, in both its long and short axis.
3. Overreading artifact and misinterpreting shadows.
4. Overreading a poor-quality image.

USE OF THE IMAGE IN CLINICAL DECISION MAKING

Incorporating ultrasound in clinical practice requires skills in ultrasound as well as clinical judgment and sound decision making. A variety of mistakes can occur if caution and discretion are not used in applying this technology.

1. The presence of gallstones does not prove that they are the source of pain or fever. Gallstones are common, occurring in up to 10% of all adults, and 20% of patients over 50. As always, images should be interpreted in clinical context.
2. Patients present to the ED in a variety of stages in their disease. The sonographic clinical findings of acute cholecystitis take time to evolve; a lack of gallbladder wall edema or pericholecystic fluid should not eliminate the diagnosis of acute cholecystitis in the ill-appearing patient with RUQ pain and gallstones, especially in the presence of fever and leukocytosis.
3. The presence of gallstones in the face of a sonographic Murphy's sign is strong evidence of gallbladder disease.
4. The absence of gallstones and a negative sonographic Murphy's sign is good evidence against acute gallbladder disease.

5. Ultrasound should rarely be used as an isolated diagnostic modality. In many instances, laboratory values can add valuable information to an emergency ultrasound exam. Consequently, sonographic findings should be interpreted with results of laboratory tests.

6. Sometimes, the unprepped bedside exam is simply inadequate. If the image is incomplete or has significant shadowing and artifact, it is wise to consider it an inadequate exam and seek an alternative test. Sound clinical decisions need quality data.

CORRELATION WITH OTHER IMAGING MODALITIES

Ultrasound is the imaging modality of choice for the detection of gallstones and cholecystitis; it may also detect other causes of RUQ pain, including aortic pathology and renal stones. It offers a noninvasive and rapid means to establish a specific diagnosis in many cases of isolated RUQ pain. Computed tomography (CT) is a valuable adjunct in the assessment of abdominal pain but, unlike ultrasound, requires a stable patient who can be transported outside the ED and tolerate administration of contrast. In the workup for biliary colic and cholecystitis, CT is less sensitive than ultrasound and can miss stones. In the ideal setting, the two tests do not compete; they are complementary. A bedside ultrasound can be used to image the gallbladder, biliary system, and right kidney. In cases of biliary colic, cholecystitis, cholangitis, and even renal colic, the sonogram may be sufficient to reach diagnostic and treatment endpoints. When the findings are inconclusive, or when concern persists for other diagnostic possibilities, CT can be added as a second study. Rather than argue for one test over the other, most clinicians find that ultrasound serves as a reasonable first-line screen that may be sufficient by itself. CT can serve as a second-line study when additional information is needed.

Historically, ultrasound has been compared with plain radiography for the detection of gallstones; ultrasound is clearly superior. In some settings, nuclear medicine scans are used to detect cholecystitis; however, these studies are time-consuming and not readily available around the clock in most EDs. There is no alternative imaging choice that competes with the sensitivity, ease, and availability of bedside ultrasound in the diagnosis of gallbladder and biliary tract disease.

INCIDENTAL FINDINGS

Right upper quadrant ultrasound is useful to detect gallbladder and biliary disease. However, in the absence of liver or biliary tract disease, it may reveal unsuspected pathology and suggest an alternative diagnosis in a significant number of cases. In one report, ultrasound done for RUQ pain identified an alternative nonbiliary source of pain in 21% of cases (36). In the authors' experience alone, RUQ scans have picked up unexpected diagnoses in adjacent areas, including pleural effusion, empyema, liver masses, hepatic abscess, renal cell cancer, infected renal cyst, hydronephrosis, aortic dissection, pancreatic mass, and pancreatic pseudocyst. Once bedside ultrasound is widely used in daily practice, the sonogram can be a useful tool that greatly improves bedside diagnosis of a variety of conditions.

CLINICAL CASE

A 55-year-old woman presented with painless jaundice. She denied a history of abdominal pain, weight loss, fever, or other systemic illness. On exam, she was a well-appearing but icteric woman. Her vital signs, including her temperature, were normal. She had mild RUQ tenderness but no guarding or rebound. Her bedside ultrasound is shown in Figure 8.58. The scans demonstrate a distended gallbladder with a thickened wall, the absence of

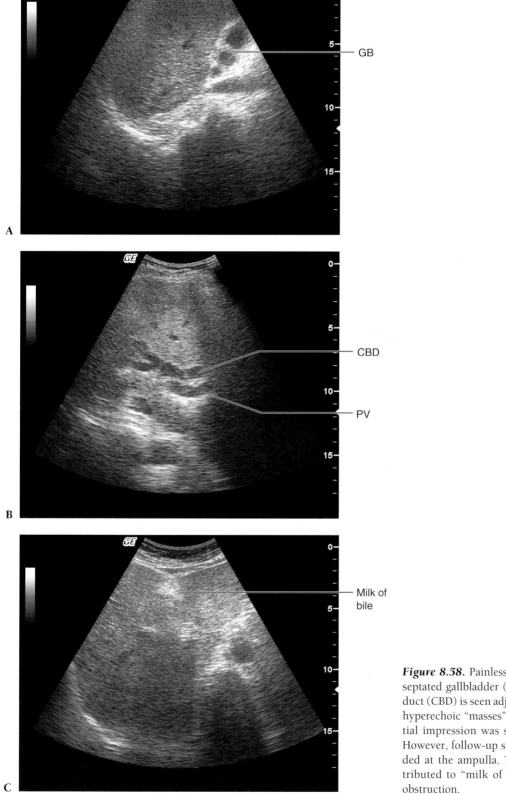

Figure 8.58. Painless Jaundice. In **A**, note a thickened, septated gallbladder (GB). In **B**, a dilated common bile duct (CBD) is seen adjacent to the portal vein (PV). In **C**, hyperechoic "masses" are seen within the liver. The initial impression was suspicious for a pancreatic mass. However, follow-up studies found a large stone embedded at the ampulla. The hyperechoic masses were attributed to "milk of bile reflux" from chronic biliary obstruction.

gallstones, a dilated common bile duct, and several echogenic focal areas within her liver that produced shadows. A CT scan confirmed an obstructed common bile duct with a single large multilaminated gallstone impacted at the ampulla of Vater. The liver lesions noted by ultrasound were found to be due to "milk of bile reflux" secondary to chronic obstruction. She was admitted for surgical management.

REFERENCES

1. Rosen CL, Brown DF, Chang Y, et al. Ultrasonography by emergency physicians in patients with suspected cholecystitis. *Am J Emerg Med.* 2001;19:32–36.
2. Schlager D, Lazzareschi G, Whitten D, et al. A prospective study of ultrasonography in the ED by emergency physicians. *Am J Emerg Med.* 1994;12:185–189.
3. Kendall JL, Shimp RJ. Performance and interpretation of focused right upper quadrant ultrasound by emergency physicians. *J Emerg Med.* 2001;21:7–13.
4. Jehle D, Davis E, Evans T, et al. Emergency department sonography by emergency physicians. *Am J Emerg Med.* 1989;7:605–611.
5. Blaivas M, Harwood RA, Lambert MJ. Decreasing length of stay with emergency ultrasound examination of the gallbladder. *Acad Emerg Med.* 1999;6:1020–1023.
6. Durston W, Carl ML, Guerra W. Patient satisfaction and diagnostic accuracy with ultrasound by emergency physicians. *Am J Emerg Med.* 1999;17:642–646.
7. Romano WM, Platt JF. Ultrasound of the abdomen. *Crit Care Clin.* 1994;10:297–319.
8. Hough DM, Glazebrook KN, Paulson EK, et al. Value of prone positioning in the ultrasonographic diagnosis of gallstones: prospective study. *J Ultrasound Med.* 2000;19:633–638.
9. Marks WM, Filly RA, Callen PW. Ultrasonic anatomy of the liver: a review with new applications. *J Clin Ultrasound.* 1979;7:137–146.
10. Filly RA, Laing FC. Anatomic variation of portal venous anatomy in the porta hepatis: ultrasonographic evaluation. *J Clin Ultrasound.* 1978;6:83–89.
11. Ralls PW, Quinn MF, Rogers W, et al. Sonographic anatomy of the hepatic artery. *AJR Am J Roentgenol* 1981;136:1059–1063.
12. Cooperberg PL, Burhenne HJ. Real-time ultrasonography. Diagnostic technique of choice in calculous gallbladder disease. *N Engl J Med.* 1980;302:1277–1279.
13. Gore RM, Yaghmai V, Newmark GM, et al. Imaging benign and malignant disease of the gallbladder. *Radiol Clin North Am.* 2002;40:1307–1323.
14. Shea JA, Berlin JA, Escarce JJ, et al. Revised estimates of diagnostic test sensitivity and specificity in suspected biliary tract disease. *Arch Intern Med.* 1994;154:2573–2581.
15. Johnston DE, Kaplan MM. Pathogenesis and treatment of gallstones. *N Engl J Med.* 1993; 328:412–421.
16. Zeman RK, Garra BS. Gallbladder imaging. The state of the art. *Gastroenterol Clin North Am.* 1991;2:127–156.
17. Good LI, Edell SL, Soloway RD, et al. Ultrasonic properties of gallstones. Effect of stone size and composition. *Gastroenterology.* 1979;77:258–263.
18. Angelico M, De Santis A, Capocaccia L. Biliary sludge: a critical update. *J Clin Gastroenterol.* 1990;12:656–662.
19. Laing FC. Ultrasonography of the acute abdomen. *Radiol Clin North Am.* 1992;30:389–404.
20. Rybicki FJ. The WES sign. *Radiology.* 2000;214:881–882.
21. Kane RA, Jacobs R, Katz J, et al. Porcelain gallbladder: ultrasound and CT appearance. *Radiology.* 1984;152:137–141.
22. Lim JH, Ko YT, Kim SY. Ultrasound changes of the gallbladder wall in cholecystitis: a sonographic-pathological correlation. *Clin Radiol.* 1987;38:389–393.
23. Burrell MI, Zeman RK, Simeone JF, et al. The biliary tract: imaging for the 1990s. *AJR Am J Roentgenol.* 1991;157:223–233.
24. Ralls PW, Colletti PM, Lapin SA, et al. Real-time sonography in suspected acute cholecystitis. Prospective evaluation of primary and secondary signs. *Radiology.* 1985;155:767–771.
25. Bree RL. Further observations on the usefulness of the sonographic Murphy sign in the evaluation of suspected acute cholecystitis. *J Clin Ultrasound.* 1995;23:169–172.
26. Marchal G, Van de Voorde P, Van Dooren W, et al. Ultrasonic appearance of the filled and contracted normal gallbladder. *J Clin Ultrasound.* 1980;8:439–442.
27. Baron RL, Tublin ME, Peterson MS. Imaging the spectrum of biliary tract disease. *Radiol Clin North Am.* 2002;40:1325–1354.

28. Engel JM, Deitch EA, Sikkema W. Gallbladder wall thickness; sonographic accuracy and relation to disease. *AJR Am J Roentgenol.* 1980;134:907–909.
29. Sood BP, Kalra N, Gupta S, et al. Role of sonography in the diagnosis of gallbladder perforation. *J Clin Ultrasound.* 2002;30:270–274.
30. Chau WK, Wong KB, Chan SC, et al. Ultrasonic "hole sign": a reliable sign of perforation of the gallbladder? *J Clin Ultrasound.* 1992;20:294–299.
31. Haubek A, Pedersen JH, Burcharth F, et al. Dynamic sonography in the evaluation of jaundice. *AJR Am J Roentgenol.* 1981;136:1071–1074.
32. Sample WF, Sarti DA, Goldstein LI, et al. Gray-scale ultrasonography of the jaundiced patient. *Radiology.* 1978;128:719–725.
33. Weill F, Eisencher A, Zeltner F. Ultrasonic study of the normal and dilated biliary tree. The "shotgun" sign. *Radiology.* 1978;127:221–224.
34. Laing FC, London LA, Filly RA. Ultrasonographic identification of dilated intrahepatic bile ducts and their differentiation from portal venous structures. *J Clin Ultrasound.* 1978;6:90–94.
35. Laing FC, Jeffrey RB Jr. Choledocholithiasis and cystic duct obstruction: difficult ultrasonographic diagnosis. *Radiology.* 1983;146:475–479.
36. Shuman WP, Mack LA, Rudd TG, et al. Evaluation of acute right upper quadrant pain: sonography and 99mTc-PIPIDA cholescintigraphy. *AJR Am J Roentgenol.* 1982;139:61–64.

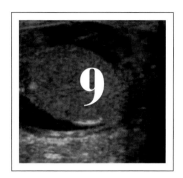

THE AORTA

Carrie Tibbles
Adam Barkin

INTRODUCTION

The timely diagnosis of an abdominal aortic aneurysm (AAA) is one the most important applications of ultrasound in the emergency department (ED). Rupture of an AAA is the 13th leading cause of death in the United States, yet many of these deaths could be prevented by early detection and repair of the aneurysm (1,2). Complications of AAA include rupture, which is often fatal; distal embolism or thrombosis; fistula formation; and dissection (3). Patients with an AAA present with a variety of symptoms, ranging from nonspecific back pain to full cardiac arrest. Unfortunately, the history is not always straightforward because up to 75% of patients are unaware they have an aneurysm before presenting with complications (4). As well, the physical exam has also been shown to be unreliable for the detection of AAA (5). In fact, the triad of hypotension, back pain, and a pulsatile mass is present in less than a third of cases of ruptured AAA (6). In a recent meta-analysis, Lederle and Simel concluded that some form of imaging is required to adequately exclude or diagnose an AAA because history and physical exam are so insensitive (7).

Compared to other imaging tests available to the emergency physician, bedside ultrasound has many advantages for the detection of an AAA. Ultrasound is portable, noninvasive, and readily accessible. ED ultrasound has been shown to be 100% sensitive in the detection of AAA when performed by emergency physicians with limited experience and is comparable or superior to other imaging modalities, such as computed tomography (CT), magnetic resonance imaging (MRI), and operative findings (laparatomy) (8–11).

CLINICAL APPLICATIONS

There are three principle clinical scenarios in which a bedside ultrasound examination of the aorta can be beneficial: (1) adult patients with abdominal pain and hypotension, (2) unexplained abdominal/ flank/ back pain in an adult patient, and (3) screening in adult patients for asymptomatic AAA.

Following rupture or leaking of the aneurysm, patients may present in hypovolemic shock. In these critical patients, the ultrasound exam can be performed rapidly in the ED while the patient is simultaneously being resuscitated. Many patients who present with a ruptured AAA are not stable enough to be transported to the radiology suite. While ultrasound does not usually demonstrate signs of rupture, the detection of an aneurysm in a hypotensive, critically ill patient can facilitate urgent vascular surgery consultation. In the patient who presents in pulseless electrical activity (PEA) arrest, the detection of an AAA directs the physician to a potentially treatable cause (12).

An ultrasound exam establishes the presence of an AAA in the hemodynamically stable patient who presents with flank or back pain, syncope, abdominal pain, or other symptoms suggestive of aortic dilatation. The diagnosis of an AAA may be missed up to 24% of the time. The most common misdiagnosis is renal colic, followed by diverticulitis, and gastrointestinal bleeding (13). The patient may present with atypical symptoms such as altered mental status or focal abdominal pain. The screening bedside ultrasound may pick up both typical and atypical symptomatic AAAs. If an AAA is detected, the physician can then expedite appropriate care and consultation. If an AAA is excluded from consideration by the screening ultrasound, the physician can continue the evaluation for other potential causes of the patient's symptoms.

A third application of ED ultrasound of the aorta is the screening of high-risk patients (14). It is estimated that over 5% of men above the age of 65 have an AAA. The elective repair of an aneurysm has a mortality of less than 5%, compared to over 50% in the patient who survives to surgery following rupture (15). A recent study demonstrated that screening of this high-risk population can be effectively accomplished in the ED (16).

IMAGE ACQUISITION

The patient is initially and almost exclusively examined in the supine position (Fig. 9.1). For the majority of adults, a 2.5- to 3.5-MHz curved array transducer provides adequate tissue penetration and sufficient resolution to examine the aorta. The depth should be set at 20 cm to begin the exam, but may be adjusted to optimize the image after the aorta is located. If the patient is morbidly obese, a lower-frequency transducer may be needed to adequately visualize the deeper structures in the abdomen, including the aorta. The exam begins with the transducer in the midepigastrium in the transverse plane with the patient in a supine position (Figs. 9.1, 9.2A). This position is similar to the subxiphoid window used to visualize the heart and pericardium (17). Standard transverse abdominal ultrasound orientation has the indicator on the transducer pointing toward the patient's right. The liver is visualized in the upper left corner of the monitor screen and acts as an acoustic window to view other structures (Figs. 9.2B, 9.2C). The anterior aspect of the vertebral body is often the first visible landmark. This appears as a hyperechoic, shadow-casting arch (Fig. 9.3). The aorta lies just anterior to the vertebral body, and appears as an anechoic cylinder. The inferior vena cava (IVC) lies just to the right of the aorta (Fig. 9.4). Once a midline view is obtained, the identity of the aorta should be confirmed by visualizing either the celiac trunk or the superior mesenteric artery, and the IVC should be located to confirm its identity. Once the aorta has been identified in the epigastrium, it can be traced caudad most easily in the longitudinal orientation. The longitudinal orientation is obtained by rotating the transducer to move the indicator to a 12-o'clock position; this projects the head of the patient toward the left of the monitor screen (Fig. 9.5). Whenever possible, it is ideal to maintain the transducer at the epigastrium in order to take full advantage of the liver as an acoustic window. It can then be projected caudad without actually moving the transducer from the epigastrium, and the aorta can be followed as inferiorly as possible. Because 95% of AAAs are distal to the renal arteries, it is important to visualize the abdominal aorta in its entirety from the diaphragm to the bifurcation (Fig. 9.6)(18).

Bowel gas or obesity may obscure images of the aorta (Fig. 9.7A). Gentle, constant pressure with the transducer may displace the bowel gas (Fig. 9.7B). In fact, one of the pitfalls in imaging the aorta is moving the transducer away from an area of bowel gas too quickly. Usually, peristalsis combined with gentle pressure from the transducer will dissipate most problematic bowel gas. Other techniques to improve visualization include modifying the angle of the transducer, and displacing the panniculus away from the area that is being imaged.

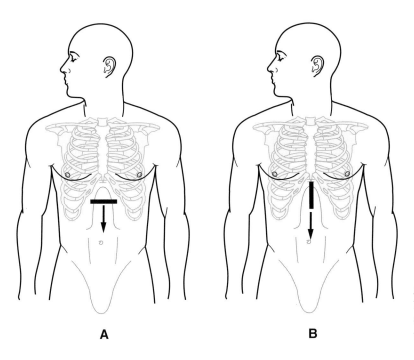

A   **B**

Figure 9.1. Guide to Image Acquisition: The Aorta. Begin in the midline of the epigastrium and scan down the abdomen to the umbilicus in both transverse (**A**) and longitudinal (**B**) orientations.

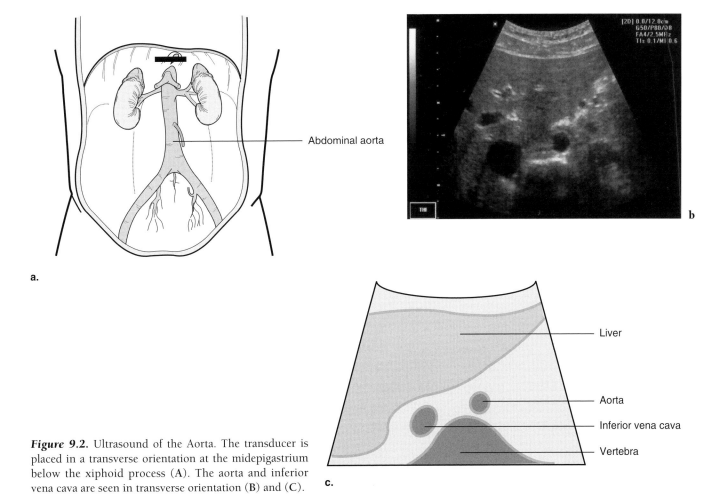

Abdominal aorta

a.

b

Liver

Aorta

Inferior vena cava

Vertebra

c.

Figure 9.2. Ultrasound of the Aorta. The transducer is placed in a transverse orientation at the midepigastrium below the xiphoid process (**A**). The aorta and inferior vena cava are seen in transverse orientation (**B**) and (**C**).

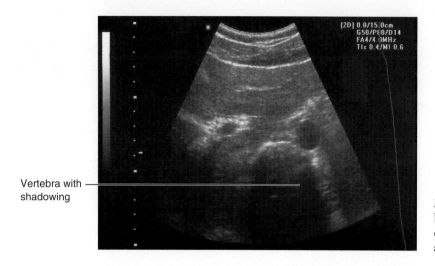

Figure 9.3. Sonographic appearance of a vertebral body in the transverse orientation. Note the echogenic proximal surface and the distal attenuation shadow of the vertebra.

Vertebra with shadowing

Eventually, the sonographer will have to move the transducer from the epigastrium to trace the aorta distally. Even if the image is temporarily lost, efforts to continue distally can often pick it up again. An alternative to the supine position is placing the patient in the left lateral decubitus position and scanning in the midaxillary line. This approach takes advantage of the liver as an acoustic window and provides a longitudinal image of the aorta (Fig. 9.8).

The aorta should be visualized in both the transverse and longitudinal orientations. As much of the aorta as possible should be visualized in the longitudinal views. Transverse views should be obtained of the aorta at the branches of the celiac trunk and/or superior mesenteric artery and the bifurcation. Three standard measurements of the aorta should be made including both anterior-posterior and transverse measurements of the aorta in transverse orientation, and the anterior-posterior measurement in the longitudinal orientation (Fig. 9.9). These measurements correct for deformations that can be created when pressure is applied by the transducer. Measurements should be made from outer wall to outer wall (12). The normal aorta is less than 2 cm at the epigastrium and gently tapers as it descends.

ULTRASOUND ANATOMY AND LANDMARKS

The aorta enters the abdomen through an opening in the posterior diaphragm and is located in the retroperitoneum immediately anterior to the lumbar spine (Fig. 9.2).

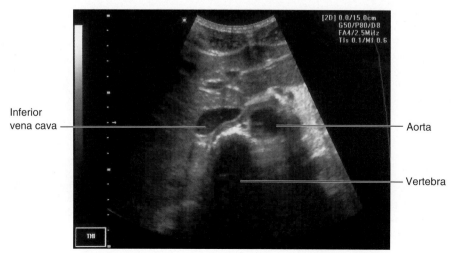

Inferior vena cava

Aorta

Vertebra

Figure 9.4. Ultrasound image of the inferior vena cava (IVC) and the aorta with the transducer oriented transversely.

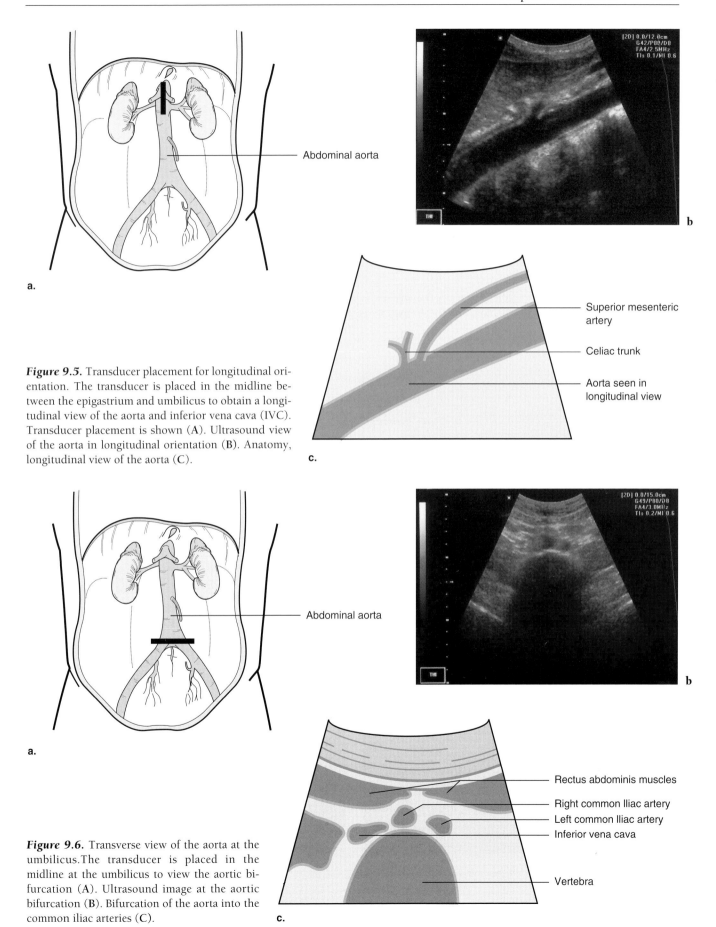

Figure 9.5. Transducer placement for longitudinal orientation. The transducer is placed in the midline between the epigastrium and umbilicus to obtain a longitudinal view of the aorta and inferior vena cava (IVC). Transducer placement is shown (**A**). Ultrasound view of the aorta in longitudinal orientation (**B**). Anatomy, longitudinal view of the aorta (**C**).

Figure 9.6. Transverse view of the aorta at the umbilicus. The transducer is placed in the midline at the umbilicus to view the aortic bifurcation (**A**). Ultrasound image at the aortic bifurcation (**B**). Bifurcation of the aorta into the common iliac arteries (**C**).

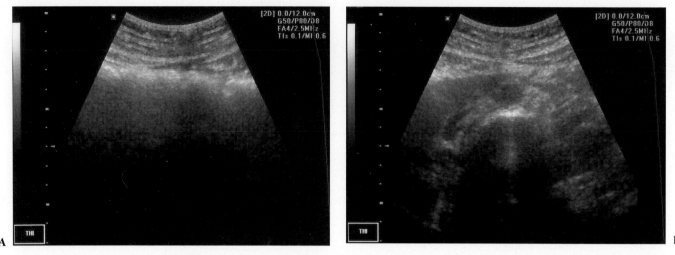

Figure 9.7. Ultrasound image of bowel gas obstructing views of the aorta (**A**). Ultrasound image of the same patient after gentle transducer pressure and peristalsis has decreased shadowing from bowel gas to allow visualization of the aorta (**B**).

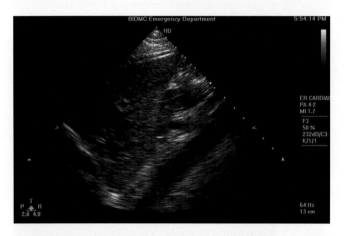

Figure 9.8. View of the aorta with the patient in a left lateral decubitus position with the transducer placed in the midaxillary line to use the liver as an acoustic window.

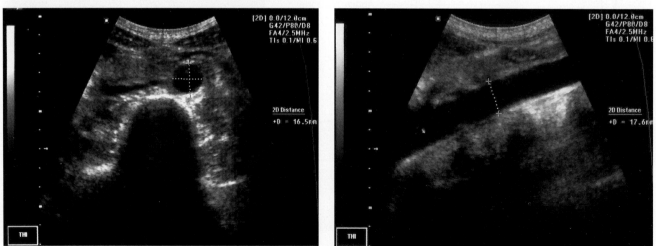

Figure 9.9. Measurements of the aorta taken in transverse (**A**) and longitudinal (**B**) views.

It is important to distinguish between the aorta and the IVC. The aorta lies in the midline and has a thickened, echogenic, and sometimes irregular wall. An atherosclerotic aorta may contain plaque and calcium and often creates shadows. In contrast, the IVC lies just to the right of midline and has a smooth, regular wall. The ultrasound appearance of the IVC depends largely upon the degree of hydration and is effected by volume and blood pressure. The normal IVC takes on a tear shape and tends to lie just to the right of the midline; sometimes it appears to drape over the vertebral column (Fig. 9.4). The IVC is the most posterior vascular structure in the retroperitoneum. The aorta has five major branches in the abdomen prior to its bifurcation (Fig. 9.10). The first is the celiac trunk.

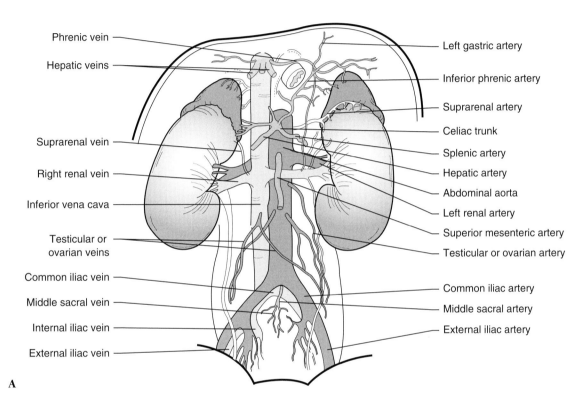

A

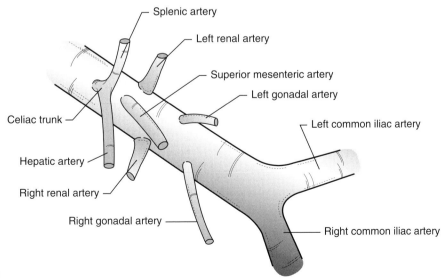

B

Figure 9.10. The abdominal aorta. The relationship of the vasculature of the retroperitoneum are demonstrated in (**A**). The main branches of the abdominal aorta are seen in (**B**).

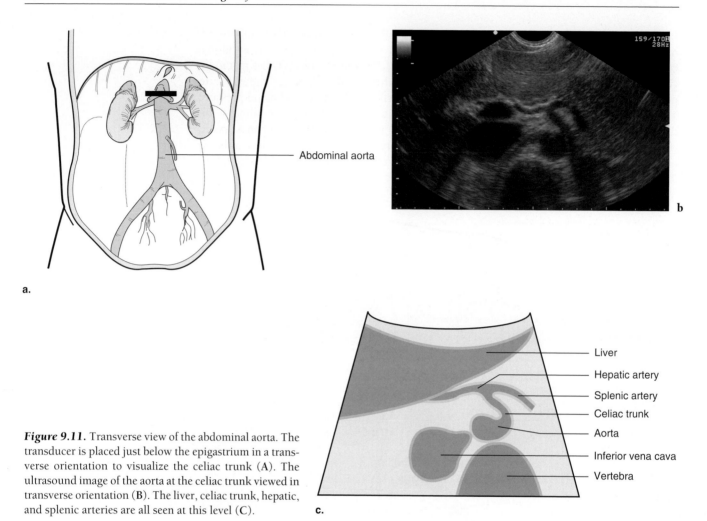

Figure 9.11. Transverse view of the abdominal aorta. The transducer is placed just below the epigastrium in a transverse orientation to visualize the celiac trunk (**A**). The ultrasound image of the aorta at the celiac trunk viewed in transverse orientation (**B**). The liver, celiac trunk, hepatic, and splenic arteries are all seen at this level (**C**).

When the aorta is visualized in transverse orientation at the epigastrium the celiac trunk can be seen to take off nearly perpendicular to the aorta, quickly giving rise to the splenic, hepatic, and left gastric arteries. The ultrasound appearance of the celiac trunk has been described as the "seagull sign;" indeed as the celiac trunk projects off the main body of the aorta, it appears to have the shape of a seagull, with the hepatic and splenic arteries each forming one wing (Fig 9.11). The superior mesenteric artery (SMA) is the largest branch of the aorta and is easily imaged in the epigastrium approximately 2 cm below the celiac trunk (Fig. 9.12). Once the celiac trunk has been identified, the SMA can often be visualized by gently projecting the transducer slightly caudad, without actually moving its position on the body. The SMA is surrounded by fibrofatty tissue that gives it a distinctly echogenic appearance. In cross section it appears to be surrounded by a bright halo. This characteristic aids in identifying it and makes it a valuable ultrasound landmark. The renal arteries arise just below the SMA (Fig. 9.13) followed by the inferior mesenteric artery. The renal and inferior mesenteric arteries may be difficult to image on ultrasound, and views of these individual branches are typically not a necessary aspect of the limited exam. On the other hand, the renal arteries originate from the aorta at a similar point as the SMA, so visualization of the SMA roughly estimates the takeoff of the renal arteries. The aorta bifurcates into the common iliac arteries at the level of the umbilicus or fourth lumbar vertebrae (Fig. 9.6).

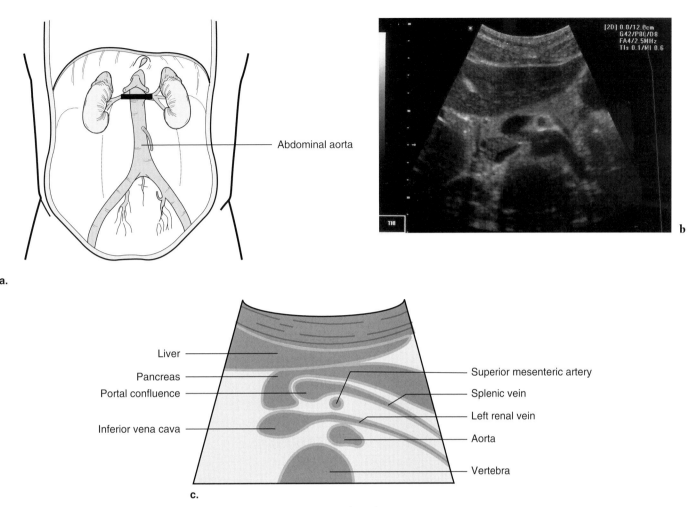

a.

b

Liver

Pancreas

Portal confluence

Inferior vena cava

Superior mesenteric artery

Splenic vein

Left renal vein

Aorta

Vertebra

c.

Abdominal aorta

Figure 9.12. The aorta at the level of the superior mesenteric artery (SMA) in transverse orientation. The transducer is placed approximately 2 cm inferior to the take-off of the celiac trunk in a transverse orientation (**A**). Ultrasound image at the level of the superior mesenteric artery (**B**). The portal confluence, superior mesenteric artery, aorta, and inferior vena cava are all visible at this level (**C**).

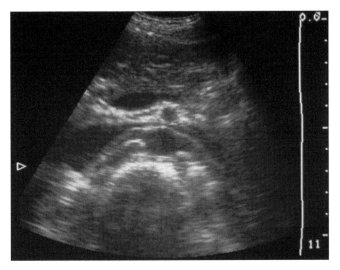

Figure 9.13. Transverse ultrasound image of the aorta at the level of the renal arteries.

PATHOLOGY

The diameter of the aorta is approximately 2 cm in the abdomen and tapers distally. The upper limits of normal are 2.5 cm at the diaphragm and 1.8 cm at the bifurcation. An aneurysm is defined as an abnormal focal dilation of the vessel wall that measures greater than 3 cm (Fig. 9.14). Calcification in the wall of the plaque produces bright linear echoes that are easily visualized on ultrasound. Atherosclerosis is the most common cause of an aneurysm. Cystic medial necrosis, syphilis, and Marfan's syndrome are other causes of aneurysms. The majority of aneurysms are fusiform with uniform circumferential dilation of the vessel wall (Fig. 9.15). A saccular aneurysm, or focal outpouching of a segment of the wall is more rare, and suggests a mycotic aneurysm or pseudoaneurysm (Fig. 9.16). Circumferential thrombus commonly develops in the wall of an aneurysm. This thrombus is easily visualized on ultrasound as increased echoes (Fig. 9.17). The gain on the ultrasound machine should be set to minimize reverberation artifact while still visualizing the clot (17).

The diameter of the aneurysm should be measured in both the longitudinal and transverse planes (Fig. 9.18). The most accurate measurement is the anterior-posterior diameter, outer wall to outer wall in the transverse plane (18). The risk of rupture is directly related to the diameter of the aneurysm with the overwhelming majority of catastrophic ruptures occurring when an aneurysm is greater than 5 cm (19). However, any

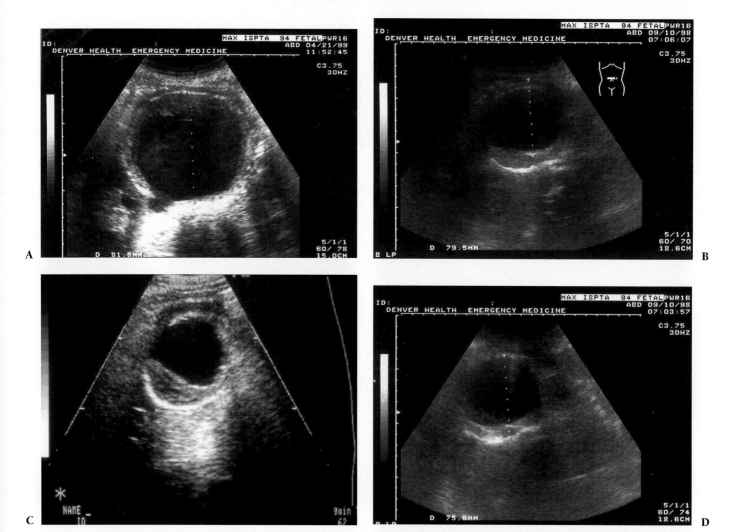

Figure 9.14. Ultrasound images of a variety of abdominal aortic aneurysms (**A, B, C,** and **D**). (Reused with permission from *Ultrasound in Emergency Medicine and Trauma* © 2005, Challenger Corporation.)

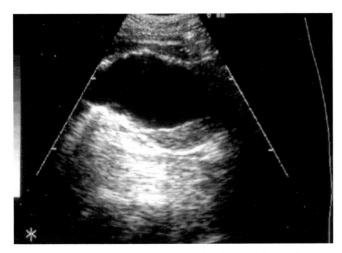

Figure 9.15. Ultrasound image of a fusiform abdominal aortic aneurysm. (Reused with permission from *Ultrasound in Emergency Medicine and Trauma* © 2005, Challenger Corporation.)

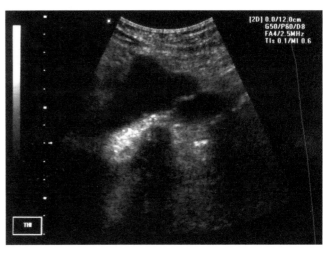

Figure 9.16. Ultrasound image of a saccular aneurysm.

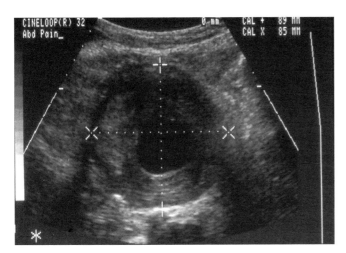

Figure 9.17. Abdominal aortic aneurysm with a large thrombus. (Reused with permission from *Ultrasound in Emergency Medicine and Trauma* © 2005, Challenger Corporation.)

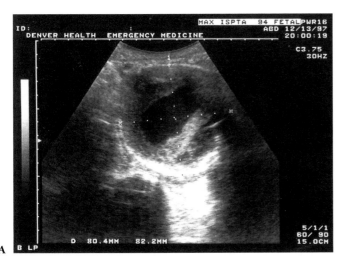

A

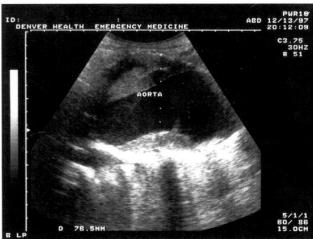

B

Figure 9.18. Measurement of an abdominal aortic aneurysm. Three measurements should be taken to accurately describe the dimensions of an aneurysm. In a transverse view, two measurements are taken of the cross-section of the aneurysm (**A**). An anterior-posterior measurement should be taken in the longitudinal view of the aorta (**B**). The measurements should include any thrombus in the wall of the aneurysm (**A**, **B**).

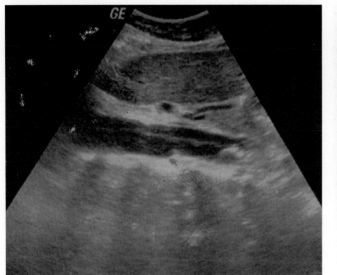

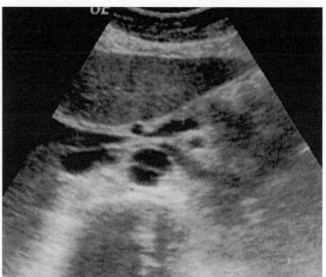

A   B

Figure 9.19. Ultrasound image of an abdominal aorta demonstrating dissection in longitudinal (**A**) and transverse (**B**) orientations.

symptomatic aneurysm, regardless of size, is suspicious for rupture or leak. Up to 40% of aneurysms extend into the iliac arteries.

    Ultrasound may also detect complications of an AAA. For example, compression of the ureter by an expanding aneurysm or retroperitoneal hematoma can lead to hydronephrosis. Hemoperitoneum from intraperitoneal rupture may be seen as fluid in Morison's pouch. As well, 2% to 4% of aortic dissections involve the abdominal aorta. Ultrasound is not a primary modality for evaluating aortic dissections; however an intimal flap, false lumen, or other signs of a dissection may be seen on ultrasound examination of the aorta (Fig. 9.19) (20).

Artifacts and Pitfalls

1. Far and away the greatest pitfall in the sonographic evaluation of the abdominal aorta is failing to fully visualize the entirety of its course from the takeoff of the SMA to the iliac

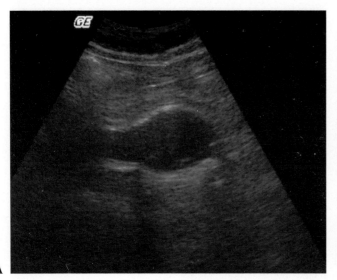

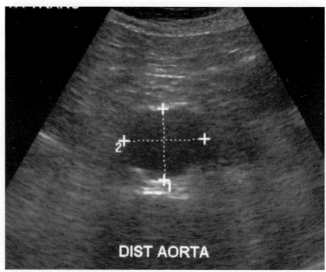

A   B

Figure 9.20. A small distal aortic aneurysm is seen near the bifurcation in an otherwise normal-appearing aorta. This aneurysm would be missed if the scan did not include the distal aorta. (**A**) Longitudinal view. (**B**) Transverse view.

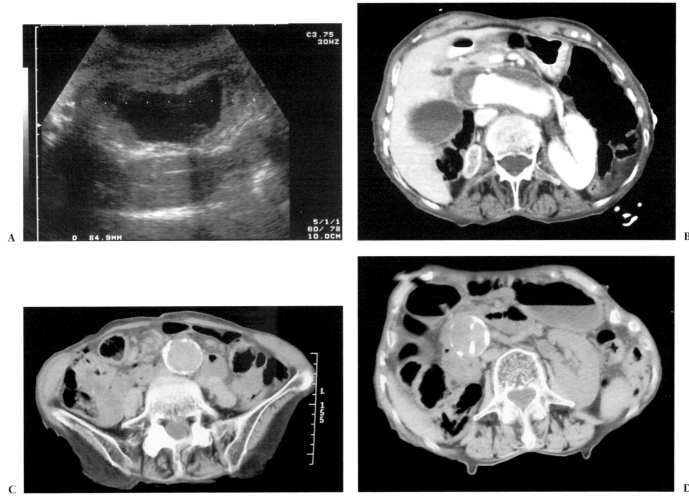

Figure 9.21. Ultrasound image taken with transducer in a transverse orientation demonstrating a tortuous aorta. (**A**). Computer tomography of the same patient (**B, C, D**). Noncontrast computed tomography scan showing the abdominal aortic aneurysm on either side of the vertebral body in two different axial planes (**C–D**).

bifurcation. Failure to visualize the entire aorta may miss an infrarenal aneurysm (Fig. 9.20). The most common obstacle to obtaining an adequate picture of the aorta is overlying bowel gas. Gentle pressure with the transducer may displace the bowel gas and improve the image. As a person ages the aorta may become more tortuous, making it harder to visualize and measure (Fig. 9.21). The aorta is a cylinder, and obtaining an oblique measurement may result in underestimating or even overestimating the diameter (Fig. 9.22). This can be avoided by orienting the transducer directly perpendicular to the aorta.

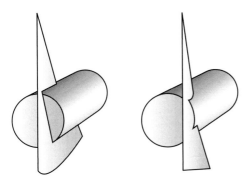

Figure 9.22. The cylinder tangential effect. An oblique view of a cylinder will underestimate the diameter.

Table 9.1: Ultrasound Characteristics of the Aorta versus the Inferior Vena Cava

Inferior Vena Cava	Aorta
Almond shaped	Round
Thin walled, easily compressible	Thicker wall
Varies with respiration	Does not vary with respiration
Located to the right of the vertebral body	Located above the vertebral body

2. The inferior cava is located just to the right of the aorta. Because it has a similar appearance on ultrasound, it is possible to mistake the inferior vena cava for the aorta. The inferior vena cava is almond or tear shaped on cross section, easily compressible, has a thinner wall than the aorta, and varies in size with respiration (Fig. 9.4). Table 9.1 lists the key differences between the inferior vena cava and the aorta that help the examiner differentiate between these two structures.

3. Ruptured AAAs often have retroperitoneal fluid, but not necessarily free intraperitoneal fluid. The absence of free fluid by the FAST exam should not be used to exclude rupture. As well, the site of rupture is rarely visualized by ultrasound (Fig. 9.23).

COMPARISON WITH OTHER IMAGING MODALITIES

There are other imaging modalities available to the physician evaluating for an AAA. Radiographs, especially of the lateral lumbar spine, may increase suspicion for an AAA, but they should never be used to rule out this condition. Abnormalities may include calcification of the aortic wall or a paravertebral soft tissue mass (Fig. 9.24). Less common findings include erosion of vertebral bodies or an obscured renal shadow. Occasionally these findings may be noted incidentally on films and early recognition may clue physicians in to an unsuspected diagnosis (21).

Computed tomography (CT) is highly sensitive for the detection of AAA (Figs. 9.25, 9.26). It is superior to ultrasound for the detection of retroperitoneal hemorrhage or other signs of rupture and it can demonstrate the extent of aneurysmal involvement. Specifically, it can determine whether the aneurysm is above or below the renal arteries, information that is helpful to the surgeon planning a surgical repair. Because an abdominal CT visualizes the entire abdomen, it also has the advantage of revealing alternative diagnoses, such

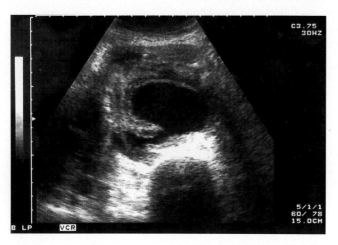

Figure 9.23. Ultrasound image demonstrating the site of rupture of an abdominal aortic aneurysm. (Reused with permission from *Ultrasound in Emergency Medicine and Trauma* @ 2005, Challenger Corporation.)

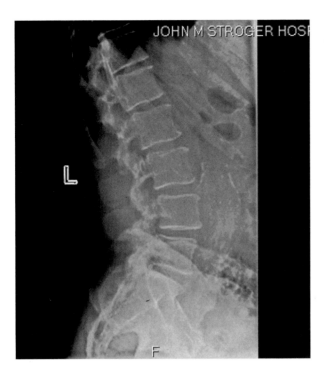

Figure 9.24. Lateral radiograph demonstrating the outline of a calcified aneurysm.

as renal stones or bowel pathology (22). On the other hand, CT scanning takes time to complete and requires moving the patient from the ED—neither of which can be afforded in an unstable patient.

The role of arteriography in the evaluation of AAA has diminished in recent years. Arteriography is useful in defining the extent of involvement of the branch vessels, and gives an accurate assessment of the lumen diameter. However arteriography may underestimate the diameter of the aneurysm because of thrombus in the vessel wall (17). Arteriography is also time intensive, invasive, requires intravenous contrast, and necessitates moving the patient from the ED.

Magnetic resonance imaging (MRI) is very sensitive for the detection of AAA and signs of rupture. Because of the time and effort required to obtain the images, MRI is usually not practical in the acute setting, especially in the unstable patient.

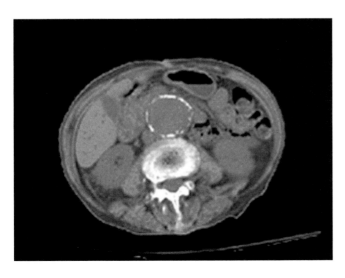

Figure 9.25. Computed tomography scan of the abdomen demonstrating an abdominal aortic aneurysm.

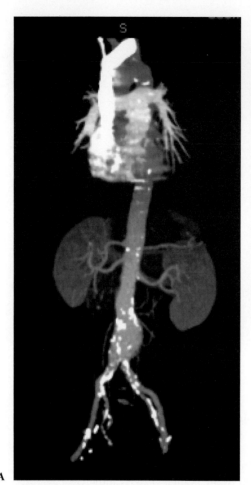

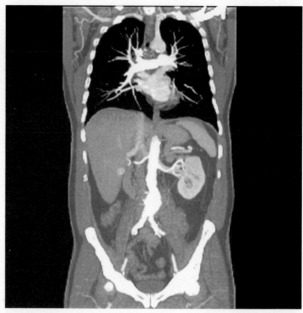

Figure 9.26. Reformatted images from a computed tomography scan of an infrarenal aortic aneurysm (A, B).

USE OF THE IMAGE IN CLINICAL DECISION MAKING

There are two factors that influence the decisions of an emergency physician who detects an AAA: the amount of dilatation of the aorta and the stability of the patient.

Regardless of whether an AAA is detected secondary to an exam done for symptoms or incidentally, if the aorta is greater than 3.0 cm in diameter, the patient should be referred for vascular surgery follow-up with repeat ultrasound exams. Studies that have tracked AAAs longitudinally have found that the natural history of an aneurysm is to expand at an average rate of 0.4 cm per year. More importantly, the risk of rupture is directly related to the diameter of the aneurysm (18). Once an aneurysm reaches 5.0 cm the risk of rupture is 22% in two years (19). Therefore, most surgeons recommend elective repair of the aneurysm once it reaches 5.0 cm and that a vascular surgeon be contacted to arrange close follow-up for the patient. The patient should receive careful instructions to return to the ED immediately if he or she develops any symptoms suggestive of an expanding or leaking aneurysm.

In the hemodynamically unstable patient, the rapid detection of an AAA facilitates immediate vascular surgery consultation. Plummer et al demonstrated that the time to the operating room was decreased from an average of 90 minutes to 12 minutes when an ED ultrasound was performed to detect the aneurysm (23).

INCIDENTAL FINDINGS

The presentation of patients with an AAA may be very nonspecific. For instance, patients may present with pain in the flank, back, abdomen, buttock, leg, groin, scrotum, or chest. Historically, studies have focused on presentations that have led to the misdiagnosis of AAA, but this data was collected in an era lacking significant influence of bedside ultrasound (13). The opposite end of the spectrum is that emergency physicians using broad indications for performing ultrasounds looking for an AAA will encounter patients having a normal caliber aorta, but with other findings such as hydronephrosis, gallstones, or urinary retention that are the actual etiology of the patient's symptoms. To date, the incidence of detecting alternative diagnoses during routine scanning of the abdominal aorta has not been determined.

CLINICAL CASE

A 74-year-old man presents to the ED with a chief complaint of light-headedness. He has a history of hypertension and hypercholesterolemia. He currently takes metoprolol and lisinopril. He has no known drug allergies and quit smoking over 10 years ago. Along with a sensation of light-headedness on standing for the last 2 to 3 days, he also notes a dull abdominal pain most severe in the right lower quadrant, as well as occasional right back pain. He is afebrile, has a heart rate of 78 beats per minute, blood pressure of 88/52 mm Hg and 18 breaths per minute. The physical examination of his head, lungs and heart is unremarkable. His abdomen is slightly distended with normoactive bowel sounds. He is moderately tender in the right lower quadrant and periumbilical region without rebound or guarding. There are no palpable masses. He is guaiac negative on rectal exam. His vascular exam reveals a 2+ left femoral pulse and a 1+ right femoral pulse. The rest of his physical exam is normal.

After adequate intravenous access is established, the patient is started on crystalloid fluids and his blood pressure improves to 104/64. A rapid bedside ultrasound in the ED reveals a 6-cm abdominal aortic aneurysm starting approximately 1 cm below the renal arteries (Fig. 9.27). He remains hemodynamically stable during his ED stay. His hematocrit returns at 22 and a blood transfusion is initiated. An emergent vascular surgery consult is obtained. He is taken immediately to the operating room and has successful repair of his 6.4-cm AAA and is discharged to home on hospital day 7.

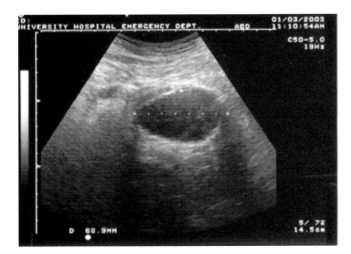

Figure 9.27. An abdominal aortic aneurysm. (Courtesy of Kristen Nordenholz, MD, University of Colorado.)

REFERENCES

1. Minino AM, Arias E, Kochanek KD, et al. Deaths: final data for 2000. *Natl Vital Stat Rep* 2002;50:1–119.
2. Johansson G, Swedenborg J. Ruptured abdominal aortic aneurysms: a study of incidence and mortality. *Br J Surg.* 1986;73:101–103.
3. Ernst CB. Abdominal aortic aneurysm. *N Engl J Med.* 1993;328:1167–1172.
4. Rose WM 3rd, Ernst CB. Abdominal aortic aneurysm. *Compr Ther.* 1995;21:339–343.
5. Fink HA, Lederle FA, Roth CS, et al. The accuracy of physical examination to detect abdominal aortic aneurysm. *Arch Intern Med.* 2000;160:833–836.
6. Kiell CS, Ernst CB. Advances in management of abdominal aortic aneurysm. *Adv Surg.* 1993;26:73–98.
7. Lederle FA, Simel DL. The rational clinical examination. Does this patient have abdominal aortic aneurysm? *JAMA.* 1999;281:77–82.
8. Tayal VS, Graf CD, Gibbs MA. Prospective study of accuracy and outcome of emergency ultrasound for abdominal aortic aneurysm over two years. *Acad Emerg Med.* 2003;10:867–871.
9. Schlager D, Lazzareschi G, Whitten D, et al. A prospective study of ultrasonography in the ED by emergency physicians. *Am J Emerg Med.* 1994;12:185–189.
10. Kuhn M, Bonnin RL, Davey MJ, et al. Emergency department ultrasound scanning for abdominal aortic aneurysm: accessible, accurate and advantageous. *Ann Emerg Med.* 2000;36:219–223.
11. Jehle D, Davis E, Evans T, et al. Emergency department sonography by emergency physicians. *Am J Emerg Med.* 1989;7:605–611.
12. Hendrickson RG, Dean AJ, Costantino TG. A novel use of ultrasound in pulseless electrical activity: the diagnosis of an acute abdominal aortic aneurysm rupture. *J Emerg Med.* 2001;21:141–144.
13. Marston WA, Ahlquist R, Johnson G, Jr., et al. Misdiagnosis of ruptured abdominal aortic aneurysms. *J Vasc Surg.* 1992;16:17–22.
14. Ashton HA, Buxton MJ, Day NE, et al. The Multicentre Aneurysm Screening Study (MASS) into the effect of abdominal aortic aneurysm screening on mortality in men: a randomised control trial. *Lancet.* 2002;360:1531–1539.
15. Mortality results for randomized controlled trial of early elective surgery or ultrasonographic surveillance for small abdominal aortic aneurysms. The UK Small Aneurysm Trial Participants. *Lancet.* 1998;352:1649–1655.
16. Salen P, Melanson S, Buro D. ED screening to identify abdominal aortic aneurysms in asymptomatic geriatric patients. *Am J Emerg Med.* 2003;21:133–135.
17. Plummer D. Abdominal Aortic Aneurysm. In: Ma OJ, Mateer JR, eds. *Emergency Ultrasound.* New York: McGraw-Hill, 2003:129–142.
18. Barkin AZ, Rosen CL. Ultrasound detection of abdominal aortic aneurysm. *Emerg Med Clin North Am.* 2004;22:675–682.
19. Ouriel K, Green RM, Donayre C, et al. An evaluation of new methods of expressing aortic aneurysm size: relationship to rupture. *J Vasc Surg.* 1992:15:12–20.
20. Sherman SC, Cosby K. Emergency physician ultrasonography-aortic dissection. *J Emerg Med.* 2004;26:217–218.
21. LaRoy LL, Cormier PJ, Matalon TA, et al. Imaging of abdominal aortic aneurysms. *AJR Am J Roentgenol.* 1989;152:785–792.
22. Loughran CF. A review of the plain abdominal radiograph in acute rupture of abdominal aortic aneurysms. *Clin Radiol.* 1986;37:383–387.
23. Plummer D, Clinton J, Matthew B. Emergency department ultrasound improves time to diagnosis and survival in ruptured abdominal aortic aneurysm. *Acad Emerg Med.* 1998;5:417 (abstract).

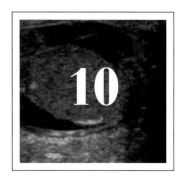

RENAL ULTRASOUND

Michael Blaivas
Matthew L. Lyon

INTRODUCTION

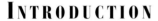

Frequently viewed by emergency physicians as part of other ultrasound examinations, ultrasound of the kidneys is often overlooked as a valuable diagnostic tool. With computed tomography (CT) readily available in many institutions, renal ultrasound is often thought of as a second-line modality (1). However, a focused renal ultrasound can give valuable and rapid information at the bedside about renal obstruction. Consequently, once proficient at this exam, the emergency physician has a powerful tool in the evaluation of flank, abdominal, and pelvic pain.

CLINICAL APPLICATIONS

The primary clinical application of renal ultrasound in the emergency setting is for evaluation of acute flank or abdominal pain and/or hematuria (2). After appropriate training, emergency physicians can learn to identify hydronephrosis and intrarenal stones (3). The detection of hydronephrosis supports a clinical diagnosis of renal colic and possibly ureteral obstruction (4). The presence of bilateral hydronephrosis, in contrast, may be an important clue to a pelvic mass or bladder outlet obstruction such as occurs with benign prostatic hypertrophy, prostate cancer, and bladder cancer (5). The absence of hydronephrosis in the face of acute abdominal pain may, in some cases, lead the clinician to an alternative diagnosis.

In addition, renal ultrasound may aid the clinician in the initial assessment of acute renal failure to rapidly detect bilateral obstruction, which could lead to salvage of renal function (6). This is especially true in patients who may not be able to provide their own histories or make complaints. The clinical presentation of renal colic, pyelonephritis, biliary colic, and aortic aneurysm may overlap. Renal ultrasound examinations often flow into evaluation of other structures such as the gallbladder, liver, common bile duct, and aorta to detect other possible etiologies of acute pain. Once proficiency has been achieved, this simple bedside assessment for hydronephrosis can expedite the evaluation and treatment for many patients with complaints of flank and abdominal pain.

IMAGE ACQUISITION

The ability to obtain quality renal images is one of the easier skills to master in emergency sonography (2). Both kidneys are relatively superficial; both are located adjacent to solid viscera (liver, spleen) that provide favorable acoustic windows. In addition, the kidneys are often used as reference structures for other abdominal ultrasound examinations, particularly the Focused Assessment with Sonography for Trauma (FAST) scan. It is important, nonetheless, to follow the same basic principles of all ultrasound examinations: scan slowly, scan methodically, and image in at least two planes in order to conceptually convert two-dimensional information into three-dimensional mental images.

Patients requiring emergency renal ultrasounds are often in considerable pain, especially those with renal colic. In order to obtain an adequate examination, it is essential that the patient's pain be controlled. It is necessary for patients to cooperate with instructions on how to position themselves and control their respiratory rate and pattern upon request by the sonologist.

The kidneys are best visualized in a fasted and hydrated patient (7). However, this is not always possible in the emergency setting. Bowel gas, ideally absent in the fasted patient, can present considerable interference during a renal ultrasound examination. Hydration status also affects the sonographic appearance of the kidney and bladder. Indeed, the state of hydration can mislead the examiner when attempting to determine the presence or absence of hydronephrosis. A well-hydrated patient may have a dilated renal pelvis that appears similar to mild hydronephrosis (8). A markedly dehydrated patient with obstruction may not demonstrate a dilated renal collecting system (9).

Most sonologists begin with the patient in a supine position similar to that used for general abdominal scans and scan from the anterior or midaxillary line (Figs.10.1 **A–D**, 10.2). This position provides the most intuitive location for anatomical structures when imaged with ultrasound. In order to build a three-dimensional mental image of the kidney from two-dimensional frames, all of the anterior, posterior, superior, inferior, medial, and lateral relationships of the kidney must be understood. Relationships between the liver and right kidney and between the spleen and left kidney are easy to conceptualize (Fig. 10.3).

It is important when using the supine view to have the patient lie as flat as possible. When the head or the trunk is elevated, the kidney tends to tuck under the rib margin, making renal imaging more difficult. In some circumstances, however, adequate visualization is not obtainable from the supine position. In these instances the patient can be moved to alternative positions, such as the right and left lateral decubitus or prone positions (Figs. 10.1**B** and **D**). In the decubitus position the kidney of interest is elevated, i.e., the left lateral decubitus position is used to visualize the right kidney. This allows for better use of both the liver and spleen as acoustic windows for kidney visualization. The prone position is rarely utilized but may be necessary occasionally. In this position, a pillow is placed under the abdomen to use the paraspinal muscles as an acoustic window. Often these positions are utilized in a stepwise fashion to obtain the best view of the kidney.

During the renal ultrasound examination, it may be necessary for patients to hold their breath or vary their respirations. When the patient takes a large breath, the expanding lungs push down the diaphragm and kidney toward the pelvis. This allows more of the kidney to be visualized from an anterior or midaxillary approach. Furthermore, rapid breathing can create so much motion that image quality degrades and interpretation is made more difficult. Therefore, it is often necessary for patients to hold their breath, usually at maximal inspiration, especially if motion-sensitive Doppler ultrasound is utilized during the examination.

A 3- to 5-MHz curvilinear array transducer commonly used for general abdominal scanning is appropriate for most renal scans as well (Fig. 10.4). This frequency provides a good compromise between adequate penetration and good resolution of renal structures. However, the sonologist should recognize small stones that may be encountered in the renal parenchyma might not be visualized at this resolution. Higher-frequency transducers, up to 7.5 MHz, may be used if the person is thin or if a small child is being scanned. If a curvilinear array transducer is used, it is important to recognize that only structures

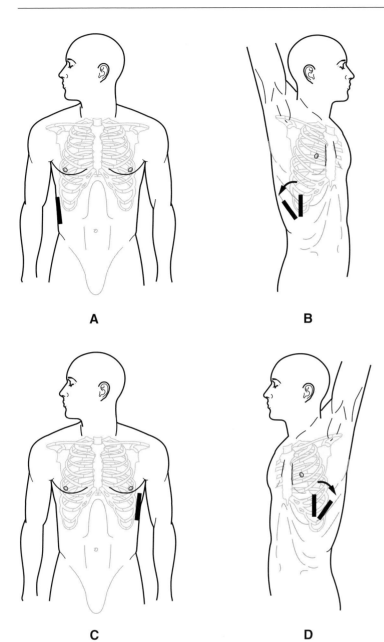

A   B

C   D

Figure 10.1. Guide to Image Acquisition. The kidneys can be imaged with the patient in a supine or lateral decubitus position. Place the transducer in the right flank and first image in the long axis of the kidney (**A**). Rotate the transducer 90° to view the short axis. Alternatively, the kidney may be viewed through an intercostal approach (**B**). The left kidney can be imaged through the spleen from a left flank (**C**) or intercostal (**D**) approach.

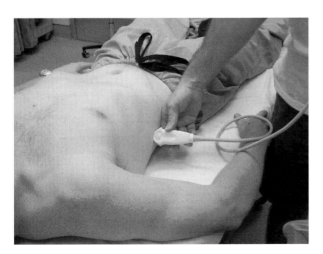

Figure 10.2. A patient is seen in the supine position. This is the typical starting point for an emergency ultrasound of the kidneys.

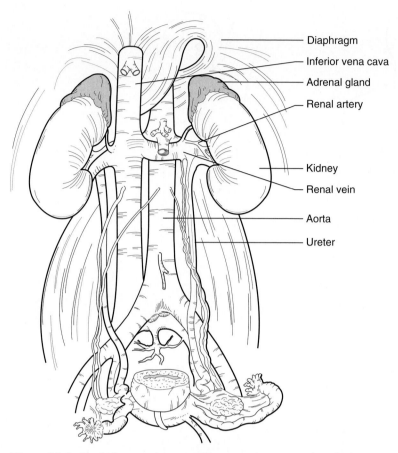

Diaphragm
Inferior vena cava
Adrenal gland
Renal artery
Kidney
Renal vein
Aorta
Ureter

Figure 10.3. The kidneys and surrounding structures. Note the relative positions of the aorta, inferior vena cava, renal vessels, collecting system, and ureters.

directly in line with the footprint of the probe are optimally imaged; thus, structures of interest should be visualized in the central field of the probe.

When the standard axillary approach fails to provide a good image, a transthoracic approach provides an alternative approach (Fig. 10.5). If the sonologist has a choice, a phased array transducer offers some advantages over the curvilinear array transducer; its small footprint facilitates imaging through the narrow rib space, although it offers less definition and a somewhat poorer image quality (Fig. 10.6).

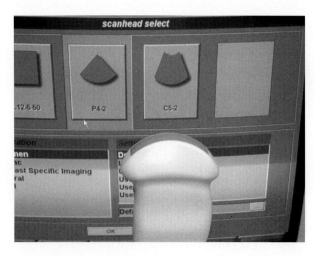

Figure 10.4. An image of a curved linear array transducer typically used for abdominal ultrasound.

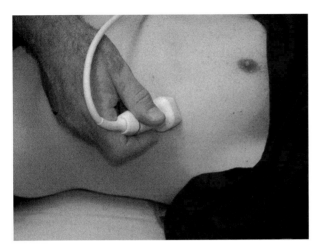

Figure 10.5. The ultrasound transducer is positioned abnormally high over the patient's ribs to attempt visualization of the kidney through the intercostal spaces.

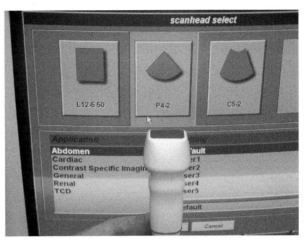

Figure 10.6. An image of a phased array transducer typically used for cardiac ultrasound but one that can be very useful for imaging the kidneys through tight rib spaces.

The images required for a renal ultrasound include both the longitudinal and transverse views through both kidneys (Figs. 10.7, 10.8). Generally the contralateral side is imaged first. This is done in order to have a baseline comparison for evaluating the potentially abnormal kidney. Again, each kidney needs to be imaged in at least two planes in entirety, and "spot checks" scanning only through portions of the kidney, such as the hilar area, are not acceptable.

To image the kidney, place the probe below the ribs in the axillary line with the probe indicator at a 12-o'clock position perpendicular to the costal margin (Figs. 10.1A and B, 10.9). Sweep the probe from an anterior to posterior direction until the kidney is located. It may be necessary in some cases to direct the ultrasound beam cranially, under the costal margin. Once located, rotate the probe until the long axis of the kidney is in full view (Fig. 10.7). In this longitudinal view, the superior pole of the kidney should be on the left side of the ultrasound screen and the inferior pole on the right side of the screen (Fig. 10.10). As the probe is swept in this plane, a three-dimensional construct of the long axis of the kidney can be mentally assembled. In most cases the liver or spleen is used as an acoustic

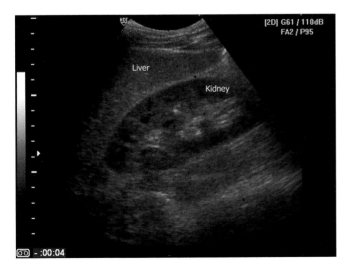

Figure 10.7. A longitudinal image of the right kidney is seen. No hydronephrosis or other pathology is noted. The superior pole of the kidney is on the left side of the image and inferior pole on the right side.

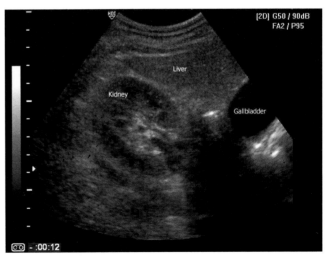

Figure 10.8. The normal right kidney is shown in short axis.

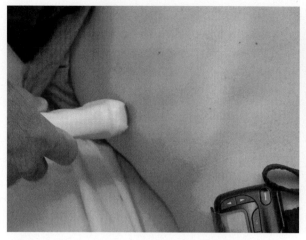

Figure 10.9. An ultrasound transducer is positioned on the patient's right side in preparation for a renal scan.

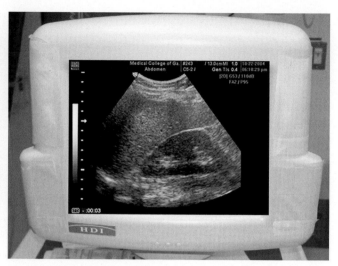

Figure 10.10. Image of the kidney on an ultrasound monitor.

window to provide an optimal image of the kidney. A noticeable difference will be appreciated in most cases when the liver or kidney is no longer under the transducer to provide a favorable window. When the transcostal approach is used, it is important to position the probe in a manner to minimize rib shadowing. It should be noted that the kidneys lie in an oblique orientation relative to the long axis of the body (Fig. 10.3). A true long axis view of the kidney may require that the transducer be rotated slightly away from the long axis of the body. For the right kidney, the probe indicator more commonly comes to rest at a 10-o'clock position to view the long axis; for the left kidney, the indicator may need to be oriented at 2 o'clock (Figs. 10.1B and D). Once the kidney is visualized, the sonologist should obtain the proper images based on internal guidelines and not artificial external landmarks. In other words, the image on the screen is matched to the sonologist's mental image of a standard renal view.

The transverse position view is obtained by rotating 90 degrees counterclockwise from the longitudinal view (Fig. 10.8). Transverse images of the kidney are made from the cranial to the caudal poles by angling the transducer along the length of the kidney. The hilum (located in the midportion of the kidney) should be imaged to assess the renal artery, vein and ureter (Fig. 10.11).

The right kidney is usually best imaged near the anterior to midaxillary line. This kidney is slightly more inferior in location than the left because the right kidney is displaced

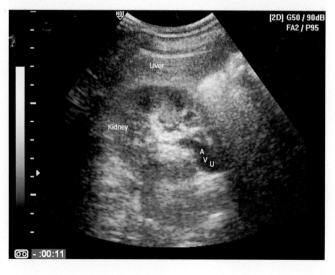

Figure 10.11. Short axis image of the right kidney through the hilum. The artery (*A*), vein (*V*) and ureter (*U*) are seen exiting the kidney.

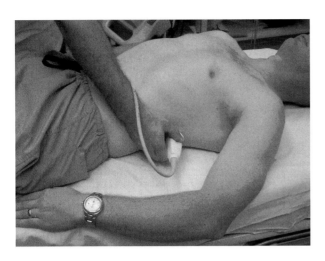

Figure 10.12. The transducer is positioned more posteriorly on the left side. This position may be required in many patients.

by the liver. The left kidney is typically best imaged between the midaxillary line and the posterior axillary line depending upon the size and location of the spleen (Fig. 10.12).

Once both kidneys are imaged in both the longitudinal and transverse views, comparison views are made. The dual function on the ultrasound allows display of both kidney images on one screen (Fig. 10.13). Similar views of each kidney are obtained. This allows for the comparison of the two kidneys. Labeling of each kidney is essential to prevent confusion.

Before concluding the renal scan the bladder should also be imaged. The transducer should be placed in the midline just above the pubis and the bladder imaged in two dimensions (Fig. 10.14). The bladder provides additional information that is often relevant to the renal scan. Occasionally pelvic pathology may be noted that will explain abnormalities detected in the kidneys, such as a dilated (obstructed) bladder.

ULTRASOUND ANATOMY AND LANDMARKS

The kidneys are paired retroperitoneal organs that lie lateral to the aorta and the inferior vena cava, and inferior to the diaphragm (Fig. 10.3). The kidneys are bounded by Gerota's fascia, a tough connective tissue that also surrounds the adrenal glands, renal hila, proximal collecting system, and the perinephric fat. The right kidney is bounded by the liver anteriorly, the liver and diaphragm superiorly, and the psoas and quadratus lumborum

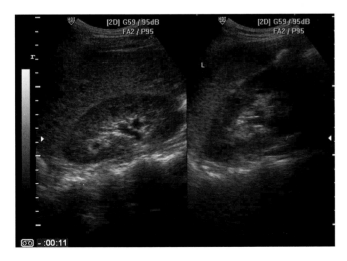

Figure 10.13. Both kidneys are shown side by side to allow direct comparison.

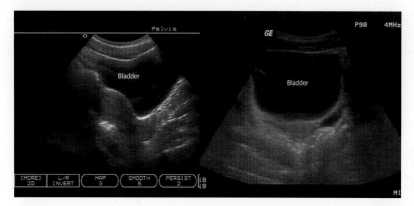

Figure 10.14. The bladder is seen in long and short axis. This should be part of every complete renal ultrasound examination.

muscles posteriorly. The left kidney is bounded by the spleen, large and small bowel, and stomach anteriorly; the diaphragm superiorly; and the psoas and quadratus lumborum muscles posteriorly. Both kidneys lie between the 12th thoracic and the 4th lumbar vertebrae. Usually, the right kidney is located more inferior than the left due to displacement by the liver, but position will vary with changes in posture and respiration.

The kidneys are connected to the body via the renal artery and vein and the ureter (Fig. 10.15). The renal arteries branch directly from the aorta laterally (10). Most of the population has a single renal artery; an accessory artery is present in 30% of the population (11). The renal vein drains directly into the inferior vena cava. The left renal vein crosses the midline of the body and can be seen in a transverse plane crossing between the aorta and the superior mesenteric artery as it crosses the midline toward the inferior vena cava (IVC). The right renal vein lies more proximate to the IVC and has a shorter course. The renal

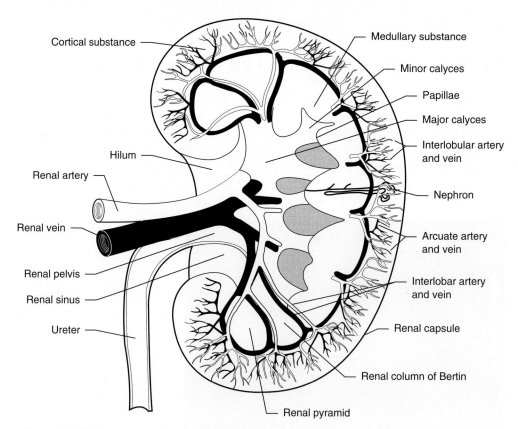

Figure 10.15. A cut section through a normal kidney shows the renal pelvis, the renal vessels, and the parenchyma. (Redrawn from Ma and Mateer, eds. *Emergency Ultrasound*. New York: McGraw-Hill Companies, 2003.)

pelvis drains into the ureter that travels parallel to the psoas muscles en route to the bladder (Fig. 10.3).

The kidneys are bean-shaped structures that average 9 to 13 cm in length, 4 to 6 cm in width, and 2.5 to 3.5 cm in thickness (Fig. 10.15) (12). Each kidney is surrounded by a fibrous capsule, the true capsule; an adipose capsule that contains perirenal fat; and the renal fascia known as Gerota's fascia. The kidney can be divided into two major parts: the parenchyma and the renal sinus.

The central portion of the kidney is referred to as the renal sinus. The sinus is comprised of the major and minor calyces, arteries, veins, lymphatics, and peripelvic fat (Fig. 10.15). The fibrofatty tissue within the renal sinus imparts a characteristic echogenicity. When the sinus is distended by excessive hydration or in the face of obstruction, the central renal sinus will be anechoic. The entrance to the sinus is referred to as the hilum. The minor calyces join to form the major calyces, which in turn join to form the renal pelvis.

The parenchyma surrounds the renal sinus on all sides except at the hilum and is composed of the cortex and the medulla. The cortex outlines the medulla, the functional unit of the kidney that is responsible for the formation of urine. The renal cortex tends to be slightly less echodense than the adjacent liver and spleen (Fig. 10.7). Abnormalities in this echotexture may reflect suboptimal gain control or intrinsic renal disease. The inner medulla consists of 8 to 18 renal pyramids that pass the formed urine to the minor calyces of the renal sinus. The pyramids of the medulla are called such because their structure resembles a pyramid with the base, the broader portion, directed toward the outer surface and the apex, or papillae, toward the sinus. The medulla is less echodense than the renal cortex. These subtle variations in echotexture within the kidney allow the sonologist to appreciate fine anatomical detail.

The renal arteries arise from the aorta. The renal arteries branch into the interlobar arteries and course between the medullary pyramids. The interlobar arteries divide into the arcuate arteries, which are found at the base of the medullary pyramid, and then into the interlobular arteries in the cortex.

PATHOLOGY

HYDRONEPHROSIS

When the ureter is unable to empty properly, the renal pelvis becomes distended with urine as long as urine production continues. The central renal sinus is composed of fibrofatty tissue that has a distinctly echogenic appearance. As fluid fills the collecting system, the usual echogenic (white) renal sinus becomes anechoic (black) surrounded by the thick, hyperechoic rim of the distended sinus (Fig. 10.16). The anechoic space takes the form and

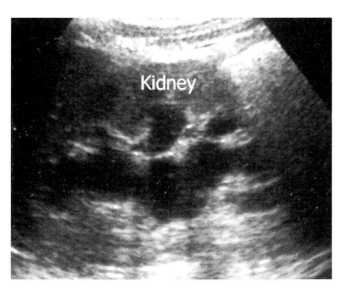

Figure 10.16. Moderate hydronephrosis is shown in a long axis image of the left kidney.

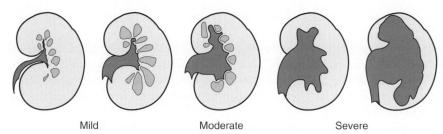

Mild   Moderate   Severe

Figure 10.17. The grading of hydronephrosis. Mild hydronephrosis is noted by distension of the typically echogenic renal pelvis. Moderate hydronephrosis is seen to splay the calyces and distend the medullary pyramids. Marked hydronephrosis extends to the cortex. (Redrawn from Ma and Mateer, eds. *Emergency Ultrasound.* New York: McGraw-Hill, 2003.)

shape of the renal calyces and communicates with the dilated renal pelvis. The appearance of hydronephrosis is visually distinct and easily appreciated by ultrasound in most cases. Hydronephrosis is evidence of pathology within the collecting system, ureter, bladder, or even urethra. Hydronephrosis can be graded in several different ways. Perhaps the most common is mild, moderate, and severe (Fig. 10.17). Other grading systems such as 1, 2, and 3 are also used and are typically based on the appearance of the calyces (13). Mild hydronephrosis is characterized by prominence of the calyces and slight splaying of the renal pelvis (Fig. 10.18). Specifically, the renal pelvis does not appear as white as it does on the affected side and an area of darkness is seen. This grade of hydronephrosis may not be identifiable unless a comparison between the affected and unaffected sides is made (Fig. 10.19). On occasion a comparison to the contralateral side will reveal that no difference exists and

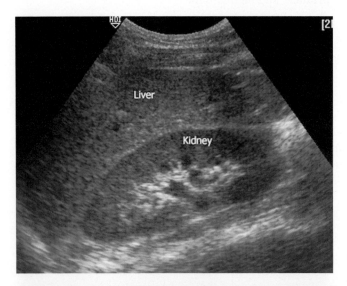

Figure 10.18. Mild hydronephrosis is seen in a long axis image of the right kidney.

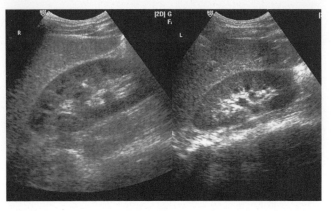

Figure 10.19. A dual view helps compare the mild hydronephrosis of the left kidney (seen on the right) with the normal right kidney (seen on left).

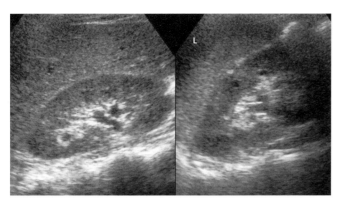

Figure 10.20. Dual view for comparison of mild hydronephrosis of the left kidney (image shown on right) that is identical to the image of the right kidney (shown on the left).

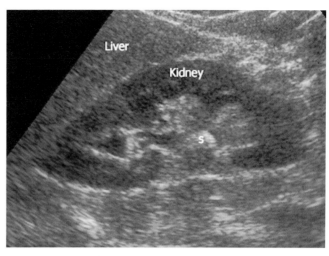

Figure 10.21. Moderate hydronephrosis is seen in the long axis of the right kidney. A large intrarenal stone (*S*) is also present.

the patient may simply be well hydrated (Fig. 10.20). Moderate hydronephrosis is typically obvious without comparison to the contralateral side, a comparison that should still be made for completeness (Fig. 10.21). The typically white renal pelvis is dilated with a large amount of dark space. The cortex is of normal echogenicity. It is of utility to use color Doppler to insure that what appears to be hydroureter is not actually ureter, renal vein, and artery laying side by side and giving the appearance of a dilated ureter (Fig. 10.22). Severe hydronephrosis shows significant dilation of the renal pelvis extending into the medullary pyramids toward the cortex (Fig. 10.23). The cortex is typically more echogenic and when the obstruction has been present for a long time the cortex can become very bright and may signify damage. Again, a comparison of the two sides is warranted.

Hydronephrosis itself is only a sign of pathology and does not identify a particular illness itself. Hydronephrosis occurs as a result of obstruction, either intrinsic or extrinsic to the genitourinary tract. The most common cause of hydronephrosis seen by the emergency physician is ureteral obstruction from nephrolithiasis. Up to 5% of the population will have renal stones identified at some point in their lifetime. Certainly, it seems that rarely a day goes by in many emergency medicine practices where renal colic is not seen or suspected.

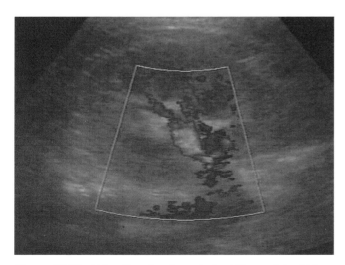

Figure 10.22. Color Doppler through the hilium of the kidney shows that an apparent enlarged ureter is actually vascular structures superimposed on the collecting system. (See color insert.)

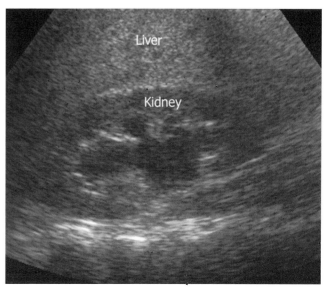

Figure 10.23. A long axis image of severe hydronephrosis.

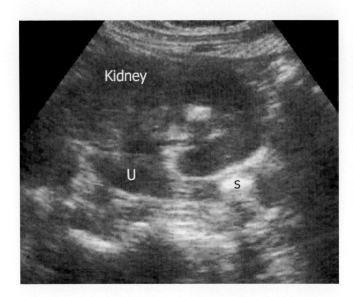

Figure 10.24. A large stone (*S*) is seen in the proximal ureter (*U*).

Hydronephrosis can also be caused by obstruction from other causes. Pelvic masses may cause unilateral or bilateral ureteral obstruction. These include ovarian, uterine, prostatic, and bladder masses, as well as retroperitoneal infiltrative processes. Some of these processes may be neoplastic, others benign.

NEPHROLITHIASIS

Renal calculi may lodge anywhere within the genitourinary tract and can be visualized within the kidney itself, the ureter, and the bladder. Like calculi elsewhere in the body, they appear as echogenic structures with posterior shadowing. Stones that are large and/or proximal are easiest to visualize. Ureteral stones are unfortunately more difficult, often obscured by bowel gas. Occasionally, a stone may be visualized in a hydroureter when scanning conditions are optimal (Fig. 10.24). Whenever possible, it is helpful to locate the obstructing stone and describe its position and size. Stones larger than 7 mm are less likely to pass spontaneously and may require instrumentation. The ability to detect and describe these details can help determine the most appropriate management for individual patients. However, most emergency scans will not detect the stone and even experienced scanners will have to rely on clinical parameters or alternative imaging to make some management decisions.

URINARY RETENTION

Optimal renal scans should include the ureters and bladder. The bladder can be imaged from a suprapubic position. Assuming that the patient has not recently voided, the degree of bladder distention can give clues regarding the patient's volume status and renal function. When a patient presents with signs and symptoms suggesting urinary retention, the diagnosis can be confirmed by a scan at the suprapubic position. A distended urinary bladder is simple to detect by ultrasound. With limited experience, the sonologist may learn to recognize bladder wall thickening, evidence of chronic bladder outlet obstruction. In addition, scans of the bladder may help detect bladder calculi.

ARTIFACTS AND PITFALLS

Like any ultrasound examination, the renal exam comes with several pitfalls and challenges.

1. One of the most frequently overlooked limitations is the time course for hydronephrosis to develop. Patients that present and are seen rapidly after the onset of pain may not

have had enough time to develop hydronephrosis. This is especially true for patients who are not well-hydrated. Patients with significant pain can present with nausea and vomiting and thus have depleted intravascular volume and reduced urine production. In such patients, hydronephrosis is more likely to be seen after receiving intravenous fluid boluses (14).

2. Renal, ureteral, and bladder stones may be difficult to visualize. The ability to image an obstructing stone will depend upon the size of the stone, the location, and the quality of the ultrasound image (15). Small stones, nonobstructing stones, and stones obscured by bowel gas present a challenge. Ultrasound alone is not sufficient to image all stones; the inability to detect a stone does not rule out a stone. A few guidelines may help detect stones. A stone is typically lodged at the cutoff of a hydroureter. When the pain of renal colic seems localized to the pelvis, additional transabdominal views of the bladder and/or endovaginal views in women patients may be productive.

3. Not all stones that can be visualized are responsible for acute pain. Large proximal stones may be easy to visualize, but often serve as a source for smaller stones that themselves create the clinical picture of renal colic.

4. There are multiple causes of hydronephrosis, and clinical correlation is necessary to detect causes other than nephrolithiasis. Urinary catheter obstruction is a common cause of hydronephrosis in immobilized and chronically ill patients. In such cases the hydronephrosis is bilateral, unless one of the kidneys is nonfunctional. Bilateral hydronephrosis can also be seen in bladder tumors and prostate enlargement. Unilateral hydronephrosis can be caused by obstruction from any tumor or abscess constricting one of the ureters and typically arise from the bowel, ovary, or uterus.

5. The grade of hydronephrosis does not necessarily correlate well with either acuity or degree of obstruction (16). A recent but high-grade obstruction may have only mild hydronephrosis. Likewise, severe hydronephrosis may be due to past disease and not related to the acute illness. Patients with protracted hydronephrosis may develop permanent changes in the renal parenchyma. In the face of new symptoms and a complicated history, ultrasound may be difficult to interpret.

6. Of all pitfalls to avoid, the most significant one is fixating on the scan and neglecting sound clinical judgment. The ability to scan should not inhibit the emergency physician from keeping a broad differential and considering diagnoses outside the area scanned. Hydronephrosis has been described in cases of appendicitis and diverticulitis, when inflammatory masses obstruct the ureter. Flank pain can be the only symptom associated with an aortic disaster. The ability to image should enhance the bedside diagnostic skills, not distract or detract.

USE OF THE IMAGE IN CLINICAL DECISION MAKING

How individuals incorporate bedside imaging of the kidneys into their clinical practice may vary significantly depending upon one's practice setting. The addition of fluid boluses to a patient's care who has a suspected renal stone is likely to result in hydronephrosis if a significant obstruction exists. Thus, if a large stone is present, signs of it should be found on ultrasound examination. Obviously mild or moderate hydronephrosis may be expected in most stones, and pain control will be the order of the visit. Follow-up can assure that pain resolves and the stone is passed. Marked hydronephrosis will be more likely to require earlier consultation and intervention. It is important to remember that, unlike intravenous pyelography (IVP) and CT scans, the ultrasound examination does not assess renal function to any degree. If bilateral severe hydronephrosis is identified then suspicion of decreased renal function is raised. Unilateral severe hydronephrosis may damage renal function on the affected side, but a check of the blood urea nitrogen (BUN) and creatinine may not indicate this if the other kidney is working properly.

Hydronephrosis itself does not pose a significant immediate danger to renal function (17). Studies differ on just how long is safe. Most cases of hydronephrosis secondary to renal stones will eventually resolve on their own as the stone traverses the ureter, bladder, and finally, the urethra (18). With relief of short-lived obstruction the hydronephrosis should decrease rapidly. If the hydronephrosis is severe and persists longer than two weeks, permanent renal damage may occur. This timeline is debated, although most physicians are surprised to find that hydronephrosis can be tolerated for so long. The management of obstructing renal stones and hydronephrosis will require consultation with and follow-up by a urologist to optimize outcome.

In all cases of flank pain, the clinician should always harbor some concern of the risk of aortic disease in the appropriate patient population. Whenever indicated, renal scans done to assess flank pain should progress to views of the aorta, particularly in the older patient.

CORRELATION WITH OTHER IMAGING MODALITIES

Intravenous pyelography is the former gold standard for the evaluation of suspected renal stones and is still favored by some urologists (19). However, it has a number of disadvantages compared to newer imaging modalities (20). The use of intravenous contrast poses a risk of allergy and renal toxicity. In the abnormal scan, delayed images that are labor-intensive and time-consuming limit its usefulness clinically (21). IVP has largely been replaced by newer generations of spiral CT scanners that are now available in most hospitals. CT scans can give an indication of renal function (when contrast is used), and are excellent in visualizing renal stones. They provide additional information when the source of pain lies outside the genitourinary tract (22). Ultrasound occupies a unique role in the evaluation of flank pain. The use of bedside ultrasound by clinicians allows a rapid, noninvasive, and essentially risk-free method to rapidly detect hydronephrosis. Because the scan is quick and available at the bedside, serial exams can be performed if desired. Ultrasound is highly sensitive for the detection of hydronephrosis and is the test of choice for hydronephrosis (23). Compared to spiral CT, it is less sensitive for the detection and localization of renal stones (24). The combination of plain abdominal films combined with ultrasound may improve the ability to detect stones (25). The ability to detect other abdominal pathology is determined by the skill level and expertise of the sonologist. However, CT offers excellent detail and is generally cited as better than ultrasound at visualizing other conditions.

In general, ultrasound is unequivocally the best screening test for hydronephrosis available at the bedside at all hours. In patients with very typical renal colic and mild to moderate hydronephrosis, additional imaging may not be necessary. Emphasis for these patients can be focused on hydration and pain control. Patients with equivocal scans, those with marked hydronephrosis, those without hydronephrosis after adequate hydration, or patients in whom alternative diagnoses are under consideration may benefit from CT. Regardless, the use of bedside emergent ultrasound can expedite the evaluation and treatment for most patients.

INCIDENTAL FINDINGS

A variety of masses may be detected incidentally during renal ultrasound examinations (26). Renal masses may present with acute flank pain from rapid expansion, mass effect with obstruction, bleeding, or abscess formation. The most common renal masses are simple cysts; occasionally more complex cysts and solid masses are seen (27). Renal masses can originate from the kidney or from adjacent organs. Differentiating an intrinsic renal mass from one that simply abuts the kidney may be difficult.

Simple cysts have a relatively smooth internal contour and few if any internal echoes (Fig.10.25). They typically occur on the cortical surface of the kidney and are peripheral in location, distinguishing them from an abnormal collecting system in the central kidney. However, perihilar cysts can occur and may be easily mistaken as hydronephrosis (Fig. 10.26). Simple renal cysts are common and rarely of any clinical significance unless they

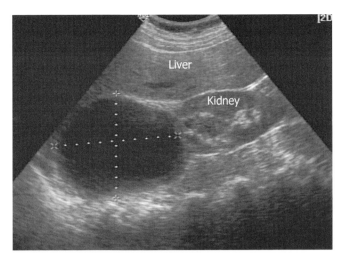

Figure 10.25. A large simple renal cyst is shown.

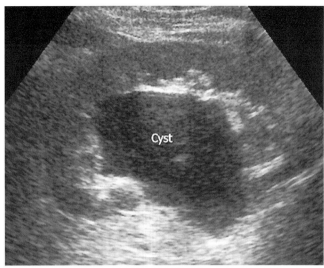

Figure 10.26. A perihilar cyst is shown. Such cysts can be confused for hydronephrosis or a hydroureter.

enlarge to a significant enough size to impair function of the kidney (28). If large enough they can distort the normal renal architecture. Occasionally renal cysts may become infected and present with flank pain and fever. In such cases, the patient may need emergent evaluation for drainage and antibiotics. Multiple simple cysts should raise the suspicion of polycystic renal disease, a diagnosis that will require long-term follow-up to detect and treat potential complications such as pain, hypertension, renal failure and associated liver disease (Fig. 10.27).

Complex cysts have a combination of echopoor and echogenic areas (Fig. 10.28). They differ from solid masses that have no cystic component. Complex cysts are more concerning than simple renal cysts; they may signify abscess, hemorrhage, or cancer. Occasionally solid masses may be identified within the kidney. Ultrasound criteria alone cannot distin-

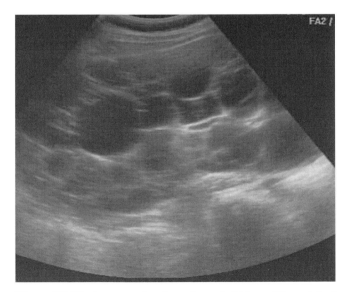

Figure 10.27. An example of a polycystic kidney. The original architecture of kidney is completely obscured by multiple cysts of various sizes.

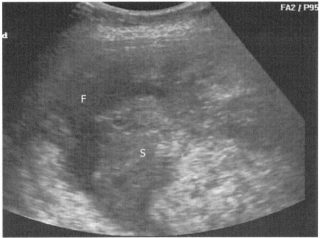

Figure 10.28. A complex renal cyst is shown with a mixture of fluid (*F*) and solid (*S*) components. The rest of the kidney is obscured by the abscess.

guish benign from neoplastic masses. Renal cell carcinoma has a variable appearance by ultrasound and can be hypoechoic, hyperechoic, or complex. All solid masses need definitive follow-up plans.

It is important to note that while some masses are obvious, some isoechoic masses may be difficult to detect by ultrasound. Emergency sonologists should not consider screening for renal masses a goal for emergency sonography. However, in the course of routine scanning of symptomatic patients, emergency sonologists will likely encounter incidental findings and should be prepared to obtain confirmatory imaging studies and appropriate, timely care. Nonetheless, the ability to detect and refer patients with renal masses is valuable and such findings should not be discounted or ignored because of indecision concerning the relevance of such abnormalities.

On some occasions, the sonologist may fail to visualize a kidney. The most likely cause is simply technique when bowel gas obscures the image in an obese or inadequately prepped patient. However, the sonologist should scan down to the pelvis, as occasionally a pelvic kidney may be found. This anatomical variant predisposes to stasis and infection and should have follow-up. Rarely, a patient may have renal agenesis. Again, such a finding deserves recognition and follow-up.

CLINICAL CASE

A 26-year-old female presents to the emergency department with the chief complaint of right-sided abdominal pain. The patient states that the pain began two days ago primarily in her right flank and has moved over the last 24 hours to the right middle abdomen. The pain is constant and throbbing but waxes and wanes throughout the day. There are no modifying factors and she has never had this type of pain before. There is no history of trauma.

She has no past medical history, but is pregnant at 32 weeks gestation. This is her first pregnancy and she has had routine prenatal care and an uncomplicated prenatal course. She has had no past surgery. She takes prenatal vitamins and has no allergies.

Her review of systems is positive for several episodes of nausea and vomiting and mild dysuria. She denies fever, vaginal discharge or bleeding, and hematuria.

On exam, her temperature is 37.8 °C, her blood pressure is 110/70 mm Hg, pulse is 95 beats per minute, and respirations are 18 breaths per minute. She has a gravid uterus consistent with 30 weeks gestation. Her abdomen is nontender except for mild right flank and right costovertebral angle tenderness. She has fetal heart tones at 156 beats per minute. She has no vaginal discharge or bleeding; her cervical os is closed.

Significant laboratory results include 20 to 50 white blood cells (wbc) and 20 to 50 red blood cells (rbc) per high-power field, positive leukocyte esterase, small blood, bacteruria, and negative nitrate.

Her emergency ultrasound is shown in Figure 10.29.

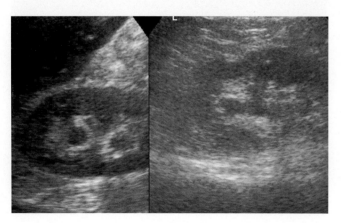

Figure 10.29. Bilateral hydronephrosis is shown.

The differential diagnosis in this patient can be quite varied. Though most consistent with a urinary tract infection or pyelonephritis, other diagnoses include renal colic due to an obstructing stone, biliary colic or cholecystitis, preterm labor, appendicitis, or placental abruption. Though a renal ultrasound may be useful in the evaluation of these other diagnoses, the presence of bilateral hydronephrosis may be confusing to the novice user of ultrasound. In this case, the bilateral hydronephrosis is likely due to ureteral compression due to the growing uterus and fetus.

REFERENCES

1. Kobayashi T, Nishizawa K, Watanabe J, et al. Clinical characteristics of ureteral calculi detected by nonenhanced computerized tomography after unclear results of plain radiography and ultrasonography. *J Urol.* 2003;170:799–802.
2. American College of Emergency Physicians. ACEP emergency ultrasound guidelines—2001. *Ann Emerg Med.* 2001;38:470–481.
3. Noble VE, Brown DF. Renal ultrasound. *Emerg Med Clin North Am.* 2004;22:641–659.
4. Mostbeck GH, Zontsich T, Turetschek K. Ultrasound of the kidney: obstruction and medical diseases. *Eur Radiol.* 2001;11:1878–1889.
5. Tan YH, Foo KT. Intravesical prostatic protrusion predicts the outcome of a trial without catheter following acute urine retention. *J Urol.* 2003;170:2339–2341.
6. Knobel B, Rosman P, Gewurtz G. Bilateral hydronephrosis due to fecaloma in an elderly woman. *J Clin Gastroenterol.* 2000;30:311–313.
7. Nicolau C, Vilana R, Del Amo M, et al. Accuracy of sonography with a hydration test in differentiating between excretory renal obstruction and renal sinus cysts. *J Clin Ultrasound.* 2002; 30:532–536.
8. Morse JW, Hill R, Greissinger WP, et al. Rapid oral hydration results in hydronephrosis as demonstrated by bedside ultrasound. *Ann Emerg Med.* 1999;34:134–140.
9. Morin ME, Baker DA. The influence of hydration and bladder distension on the sonographic diagnosis of hydronephrosis. *J Clin Ultrasound.* 1979;7:192–194.
10. Rha SE, Byun JY, Jung SE, et al. The renal sinus: pathologic spectrum and multimodality imaging approach. *Radiographics* 2004;24:S117–S131.
11. Kapoor A, Kapoor A, Mahajan G, et al. Multispiral computed tomographic angiography of renal arteries of live potential renal donors: a review of 118 cases. *Transplantation.* 2004;77:1535–1539.
12. Lewis E, Ritchie WG. A simple ultrasonic method for assessing renal size. *J Clin Ultrasound.* 1980;8:417–420.
13. Hagen-Ansert S. (ed). *Textbook of Diagnostic Ultrasonography*, 4th ed. St. Louis: Mosby; 1995: 219–230.
14. Chau WK, Chan SC. Improved sonographic visualization by fluid challenge method of renal lithiasis in the nondilated collecting system. Experience in seven cases. *Clin Imaging.* 1997; 21:276–283.
15. Fowler KA, Locken JA, Duchesne JH, et al. US for detecting renal calculi with nonenhanced CT as a reference standard. *Radiology.* 2002;222:109–113.
16. Coll DM, Varanelli MJ, Smith RC. Relationship of spontaneous passage of ureteral calculi to stone size and location as revealed by unenhanced helical CT. *AJR Am J Roentgenol.* 2002;178:101–103.
17. Sibai H, Salle JL, Houle AM, et al. Hydronephrosis with diffuse or segmental cortical thinning: impact on renal function. *J Urol.* 2001;165:2293–2295.
18. Irving SO, Calleja R, Lee F, et al. Is the conservative management of ureteric calculi of > 4 mm safe? *BJU Int.* 2000;85:637–640.
19. Juul N, Brons J, Torp-Pedersen S, et al. Ultrasound versus intravenous urography in the initial evaluation of patients with suspected obstructing urinary calculi. *Scand J Urol Nephrol Suppl.* 1991;137:45–47.
20. Stewart C. Nephrolithiasis. *Emerg Med Clin North Am.* 1988;6:617–630.
21. Pfister SA, Deckart A, Laschke S, et al. Unenhanced helical computed tomography vs intravenous urography in patients with acute flank pain: accuracy and economic impact in a randomized prospective trial. *Eur Radiol.* 2003;13:2513–2520.
22. Colistro R, Torreggiani WC, Lyburn ID, et al. Unenhanced helical CT in the investigation of acute flank pain. *Clin Radiol.* 2002;57:435–441.
23. Webb JA. Ultrasonography in the diagnosis of renal obstruction. *BMJ.* 1990;301:944–946.

24. Smith RC, Coll DM. Helical computed tomography in the diagnosis of ureteric colic. *BJU Int.* 2000;86(Suppl):33–41.

25. Henderson SO, Hoffner RJ, Aragona JL, et al. Bedside emergency department ultrasonography plus radiography of the kidneys, ureters, and bladder vs intravenous pyelography in the evaluation of suspected ureteral colic. *Acad Emerg Med.* 1998;5:666–671.

26. Mandavia DP, Pregerson B, Henderson SO. Ultrasonography of flank pain in the emergency department: renal cell carcinoma as a diagnostic concern. *J Emerg Med.* 2000;18:83–86.

27. Terada N, Arai Y, Kinukawa N, et al. Risk factors for renal cysts. *BJU Int.* 2004; 93:1300–1302.

28. Holmberg G. Diagnostic aspects, functional significance and therapy of simple renal cysts. A clinical, radiologic and experimental study. *Scand J Urol Nephrol Suppl.* 1992;145:1–48.

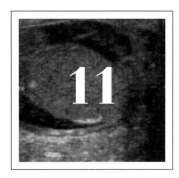

LOWER EXTREMITY VENOUS STUDIES

J. Christian Fox
JoAnne McDonough

INTRODUCTION

The possibility of a lower extremity deep venous thrombosis (DVT) is a frequent clinical concern in emergency medicine, arising in patients with varied presentations, from painless leg swelling to impending cardiopulmonary arrest. DVT and pulmonary embolus (PE) can be difficult to diagnose and carry significant morbidity and mortality. Physical exam findings have a low sensitivity for the detection of DVT (1). Historical factors can aid in risk stratification, but not ultimate diagnosis (2). Although there are numerous diagnostic possibilities for patients in whom a DVT is suspected, venous compression ultrasonography is the most practical test for the emergency department (ED) setting.

In many institutions, consultative vascular studies are not available outside of regular business hours (3). Given this lack of availability, many clinical decision rules combining risk factor assessment and the use of a quantitative D-dimer assay have been proposed (4). These protocols decrease the need for vascular studies in low-risk patients, but still leave many patients requiring a service that is often not available. When a DVT is suspected, emergency physicians are often faced with three options: admit the patient, hold the patient in the ED awaiting the availability of venous studies, or discharge the patient after anticoagulation in the ED with arrangement for an outpatient study as soon as possible. This is especially troublesome for patients without primary care physicians, patients presenting early in the weekend, or patients without reliable follow-up. In response to these many concerns, emergency physicians began performing their own bedside examinations of the lower extremity venous system to evaluate for the presence of DVT. Although traditional venous compression ultrasonography is thorough and time-consuming, a limited approach that is more practical for emergency medicine practice can be applied. Poppiti et al. demonstrated that limited venous ultrasound can be done with a dramatic reduction in the usual time required for a complete consultative exam, taking 5.5 minutes for a targeted emergency ultrasound compared with 37 minutes for the complete vascular exam of the lower extremity (5,6). It has been shown that emergency physicians can accurately detect DVT on focused ultrasound (3,7–10). Limited emergency ultrasound is thus both accurate and fast enough to be practical for typical emergency medicine practice (3,8).

CLINICAL APPLICATIONS

Lower extremity venous compression ultrasonography is indicated any time there is a suspicion of a lower extremity DVT. In terms of clinical presentation, leg pain, leg swelling, or symptoms concerning for PE may prompt a clinician to proceed with the exam. There are no absolute contraindications to this noninvasive exam.

IMAGE ACQUISITION

The bedside exam has primary and secondary components. The primary component visualizes the venous structures and detects gray-scale compressibility. The literature suggests that only the primary component can be adequately relied upon for confirming the presence or absence of a DVT (11,12). Lack of compressibility defines a DVT. The secondary component involves the use of Doppler to evaluate for abnormalities in flow. The Doppler exam is an adjunct measure of lesser importance. Note that the diagnosis of DVT does not rest with direct visualization of thrombus within the lumen.

PRIMARY COMPONENT

Lower extremity studies are best performed with a high-resolution linear transducer with a frequency of 5.0 to 7.0 MHz. Use of higher frequency will give images with better resolution, but lower frequency may be needed in larger patients. Depth should be adjusted based on the physical characteristics of the patient. There are several options for patient positioning, the choice of which will vary with the patient's clinical condition, body habitus, and physician choice. Generally, the patient is supine. If the patient's hemodynamic status will allow it, placing the patient in 35° to 40° of reverse Trendelenburg (head up) will increase venous distention and aid in visualization. Also, the patient's leg can be slightly flexed at the knee and hip and the hip externally rotated to ease visualization of the vessels (Figs. 11.1, 11.2).

Begin the exam in the region of the common femoral vein, in the transverse plane just distal to the inguinal ligament (Fig. 11.3). Gel should be applied to the transducer or along the course of the vessel. The transverse view is first used to locate the vessel and to evaluate for compression. Once a good transverse view of both the common femoral vein and artery is obtained (Fig. 11.4), apply direct pressure. In a normal exam, complete coaptation of the vein occurs with pressure (Figs. 11.5, 11.6). In cases in which the vein does not appear to completely compress, there are two main possibilities: 1) presence of a clot, or 2) inadequate pressure on the transducer. Adequate pressure has been applied to the vein when one can observe the artery being deformed by the pressure (Fig. 11.7). Next, proceed distally and medially, following the course of the vessel (Fig. 11.2). In general, visualization of the common femoral vein should continue in 1-centimeter increments until the vein descends into the adductor canal, generally about two thirds down the thigh.

Now begin evaluation of the popliteal region. If possible, have the patient dangle his/her leg off the bed to improve access to the region (Figs. 11.1b, 11.8). Apply gel to the transducer or the skin surface at the popliteal fossa (Fig. 11.9). Visualize the popliteal artery and vein in the transverse view, noting that the vein is more superficial than the artery (Fig. 11.10). The rhyme "the vein comes to the top in the pop" may be helpful to remember this. Then proceed with compression in 1-centimeter increments throughout the popliteal fossa. The popliteal vein requires significantly less pressure than the common femoral vein, and in some patients even the pressure from the transducer on the skin may be enough to collapse the vessel.

SECONDARY COMPONENT

The use of Doppler, while confusing at first, can provide additional useful information. Doppler measures the frequency shift from approaching and/or receding red blood cells. This can aid the emergency physician by identifying which structures have flow (blood

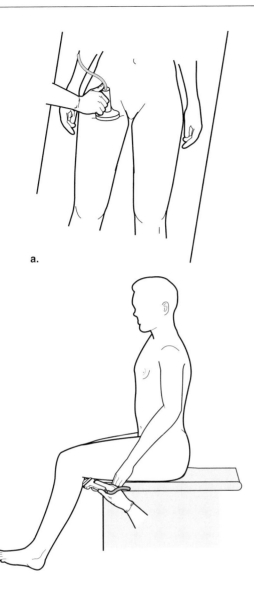

a.

b.

Figure 11.1. Guide to Image Acquisition. Begin with the patient semi-recumbent, with hip externally rotated and leg slightly flexed (**A**). Scan in a transverse orientation, beginning just distal to the inguinal ligament. Identify the common femoral vein, then scan distally to view the junction of the common femoral, deep femoral, and superficial femoral vessels. To view the popliteal vein, begin with the patient sitting with leg dangling (**B**). Scan in the popliteal fossa and identify the popliteal vein in transverse view.

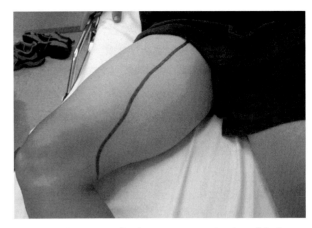

Figure 11.2. Position for the venous examination of the lower extremity. The leg is externally rotated and flexed at the knee. The line represents the surface landmark of the femoral vein.

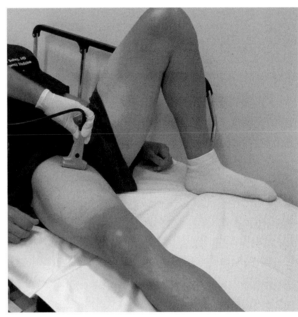

Figure 11.3. The venous study of the lower extremity begins with the femoral vessels.

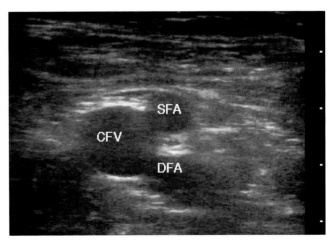

Figure 11.4. Transverse view of the left femoral region showing the common femoral vein (*CFV*), superficial femoral artery (*SFA*), and the deep femoral artery (*DFA*).

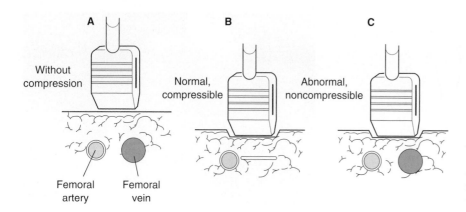

Figure 11.5. The venous exam. Visualize the relevant vein (**A**). A normal vein will compress with pressure (**B**). Noncompressibility indicates an abnormal vein, consistent with a deep venous thrombosis (**C**).

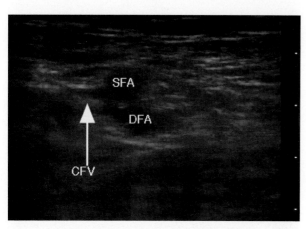

Figure 11.6. Ultrasound showing normal compression of the left common femoral vein (CFV). (Superficial femoral artery: SFA; Deep Femoral Antery: DFA.)

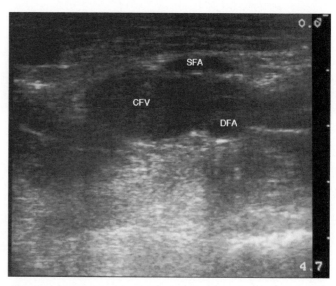

Figure 11.7. Ultrasound showing the common femoral vein (*CFV*) with thrombosis, with lack of compressibility despite adequate pressure, as evidenced by deformity of the superficial femoral artery (*SFA*) and deep femoral artery (*DFA*).

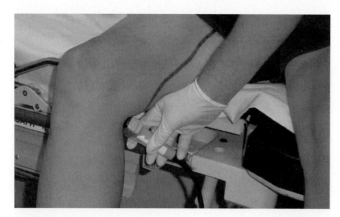

Figure 11.8. The leg is dangled off the bed for the venous study of the popliteal vessels.

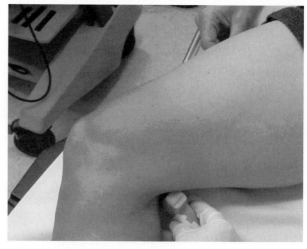

Figure 11.9. Probe placement for the examination of the popliteal vessels.

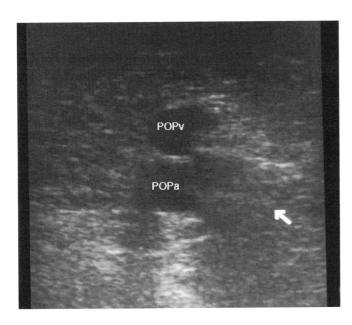

Figure 11.10. Ultrasound of the popliteal area in transverse orientation. (POPa, popliteal artery; POPv, popliteal vein).

vessels) and which do not (cysts or fluid-filled organs). Veins have a characteristic color flow pattern in a normal individual. Loss of this pattern may suggest occlusion at a site directly beneath the transducer, or more proximally. There are three aspects to the Doppler exam for DVT: augmentation, spontaneity, and phasic variation. Augmentation occurs when the examiner or an assistant uses their hand to squeeze the calf while the Doppler signal is being taken. In the normal individual a blush of color fills the vein (augments); a filling defect is observed in patients with DVT (Fig. 11.11). Spontaneity is the detection of flow in the larger vessels that should occur without squeezing the calf. Variation of the venous flow that occurs during the respiratory cycle is termed phasic variation. In the normal study, the Doppler signal of the lower extremity veins increases during expiration and decreases during inspiration. The mechanism of this seemingly counterintuitive Doppler signal is as follows: on inspiration the diaphragm descends causing intra-abdominal pressure to rise, compressing the vena cava and impeding venous outflow from the legs. Loss of phasic variation and loss of spontaneity of flow in the face of a negative compressibility study can be a result of a clot in the inferior vena cava (IVC).

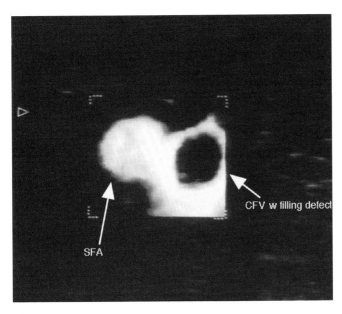

Figure 11.11. A filling defect is seen during augmentation. (CFV, common femoral vein; SFA, superficial femoral artery.) (See color insert.)

CONSULTATIVE TECHNIQUE CONTRASTED WITH LIMITED EMERGENCY ULTRASOUND

Traditionally, lower extremity venous Doppler studies performed by the department of radiology or vascular laboratories visualize the entire deep venous system in the affected extremity, a process that can be very time-consuming. This comprehensive method involves compressing the deep venous system of the leg in 1-centimeter increments starting proximally at the level of the common femoral vein and proceeding down through the superficial femoral canal. This is followed by an evaluation of the popliteal system, extending distally to the level of the trifurcation in the upper calf. In contrast, emergency physicians perform a limited examination involving evaluation of vein compressibility at the common femoral and popliteal veins (Fig. 11.1). This limited evaluation of the deep venous system has been shown to be adequate because of the rarity with which clots are isolated to the superficial femoral canal. Pezzullo reviewed 146 scans that were positive for DVT and concluded that only 1% of clots were isolated to the superficial femoral canal (6,11,13).

NORMAL ULTRASOUND ANATOMY AND LANDMARKS

The deep veins of the lower extremity include the popliteal, deep femoral, superficial femoral, and common femoral veins. It is worth noting that despite its name, the superficial femoral vein is in fact part of the deep system, not the superficial system. To avoid confusion, it is sometimes simply referred to as the femoral vein. (Fig. 11.12). The popliteal vein is formed by the merger of the anterior and posterior tibial veins with the peroneal

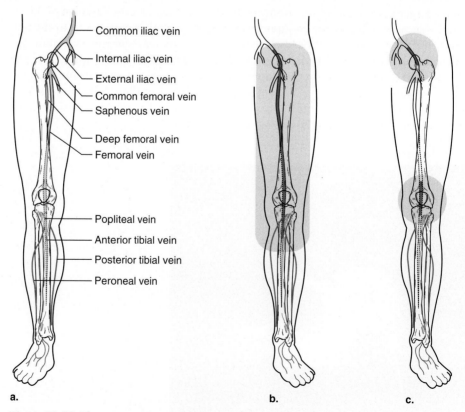

Common iliac vein
Internal iliac vein
External iliac vein
Common femoral vein
Saphenous vein
Deep femoral vein
Femoral vein
Popliteal vein
Anterior tibial vein
Posterior tibial vein
Peroneal vein

a.   b.   c.

Figure 11.12. The venous system of the lower extremity (**A**). The entire system is visualized by traditional studies (**B**). The more focused exam for emergency ultrasound targets the inguinal and popliteal regions (**C**).

vein. Continuing proximally, the popliteal vein becomes the superficial femoral vein in the distal thigh. The superficial femoral vein joins the deep femoral vein to form the common femoral vein, which becomes the external iliac vein at the level of the inguinal ligament. At the level of the inguinal ligament, the great saphenous vein (a superficial vein) merges with the common femoral vein. In relation to the companion arteries, the popliteal vein is superficial to the artery. The common femoral vein lies medial to the artery only in the region immediately surrounding the inguinal ligament. The vein abruptly runs posterior to the artery distal to the inguinal region.

There is limited anatomic variation in this area. Approximately one third of the population will have a duplicated popliteal vein. Additionally, although the common femoral vein is classically taught to be medial to the artery, there is some variability in its position relative to the artery. In some situations it may be necessary to confirm a venous structure. This is done by placing spectral flow Doppler onto the vein to observe for venous waveforms.

PATHOLOGY

The most common pathological finding in lower extremity venous studies is noncompression of the vessel. Noncompression is the inability to completely compress the vessel with proper pressure (enough to slightly deform the artery) after ensuring good position (Fig. 11.7). It is important to remember that only complete compression of the vessel rules out DVT, and only the lack of total compression is a hard finding for DVT. Although findings such as direct visualization of clot or the absence of flow may suggest a DVT, only compression findings stand alone as rule-out/rule-in criteria.

ARTIFACTS AND PITFALLS

1. In general, clot echogenicity increases with the age of the clot. However, this is highly variable and therefore not clinically reliable. The direct visualization of clot in the lumen of the vessel is potentially misleading for three reasons. First, the flow of blood can occasionally be echogenic and therefore mimic the presence of a clot. Second, artifact can often appear as echogenic material in the vessel lumen and be mistaken for a clot (Fig. 11.13). This is especially true in larger patients. Finally, the nonvisualization of a clot does not rule out DVT because clots themselves may lack echogenicity altogether.

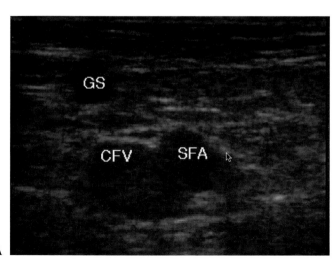 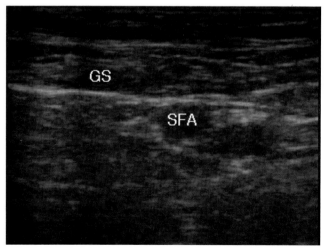

A
B

Figure 11.13. The common femoral vein (*CFV*) demonstrates artifact resembling thrombus. GS, great saphenous vein (**A**). Same CFV demonstrating full compression (**B**).

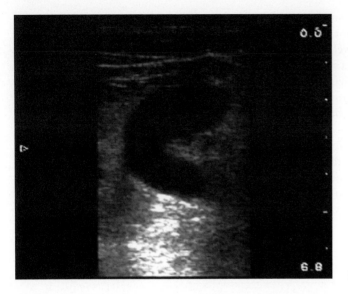

Figure 11.14. Image of Baker's cyst in the popliteal fossa.

2. Cysts will sometimes be encountered in the popliteal region. The most common cyst seen during lower extremity scanning is a Baker's cyst in the popliteal fossa (Fig. 11.14). Following the Baker's cyst in a longitudinal plane will typically reveal its confluency with the joint space. It may be helpful in equivocal cases to help differentiate a cyst from a vessel by using Doppler.

3. In addition to misinterpretation of images, pitfalls in bedside venous ultrasonography include challenging subjects and lack of understanding of the limits of bedside ultrasonography. Subjects who are obese or have significant edema are more difficult to image. In these patients, it is often necessary to use lower frequencies (3.5- to 5.0-MHz range) for tissue penetration, which decreases the image quality.

4. It is important to understand the limits of bedside ultrasonography. The focused exam is not a complete vascular study in which every vessel is interrogated along its entire course. Focused venous ultrasound is not a good choice to evaluate for isolated calf DVT. Several studies suggest that calf vein DVTs can propagate to more proximal locations. Hollerweger et al. showed that the embolic frequency for isolated calf vein thrombosis and muscular calf vein thrombosis was 48% and 50%, respectively (14). In a patient for whom there exists a moderate to high clinical suspicion for DVT with a negative focused ultrasound exam, it is advisable to obtain confirmatory studies in a timeframe in keeping with the level of clinical suspicion, in three to five days.

5. A few common technical problems may be encountered. If the vein is not visualized, pressure from the transducer may be collapsing the vein. Consider lessening the transducer pressure. If that does not help, reposition the patient and check landmarks. If the vein doesn't compress but no clot is seen, consider repositioning the patient and/or the transducer to apply pressure from a different angle.

USE OF THE IMAGE IN CLINICAL DECISION MAKING

A focused lower extremity ultrasound exam will generate two data points for each vein: the ability to compress the vein, and Doppler findings. A normal exam will have complete compression of the vessel and a phasic Doppler signal that augments with distal compression. In an abnormal exam the vessel will either be able to be compressed partially, or not at all. The Doppler signal may be normal or abnormal. It is important to stress that the most important finding is the presence or absence of complete compression.

Table 11.1: Wells criteria

Wells explicit assessment
■ Active cancer ■ Paralysis, paresis or recent plaster, or immobilization of lower limb ■ Recently bedridden for more than 3 days or major surgery in the past 4 weeks or more ■ Localized tenderness ■ Entire leg swollen ■ Calf swelling >3 cm compared with asymptomatic leg ■ Pitting edema ■ Collateral superficial veins ■ Alternative diagnosis as likely or greater than deep venous thrombosis
Each positive response is 1 point, except if an alternative diagnosis is as likely or greater than **deep vein thrombosis** DVT, where 2 points are deducted. Low probability: 0 or fewer points Moderate probability: 1 to 2 points High probability: 3 or more points

The question of whether or not a lower extremity DVT can be excluded by normal findings on a venous ultrasound was reviewed by the American College of Emergency Physicians Clinical Policies Subcommittee on Suspected Lower-Extremity Deep Venous Thrombosis (15). Its conclusion was that in patients with a low clinical probability for DVT, negative findings on a single venous ultrasound scan in symptomatic patients exclude proximal DVT and clinically significant distal DVT. However in patients with moderate to high pretest probability of DVT, serial ultrasound exams are needed. Furthermore, patients with a high suspicion of pelvic or IVC thrombosis may require additional imaging techniques such as contrast venography, computed tomography (CT), or magnetic resonance imaging (MRI). Pretest probability is assessed using the Wells criteria that take into account both historical features and physical exam findings to risk-stratify patients (Table 11.1) (16). Patients in whom there is a clinical suspicion of PE but who are either too unstable to leave the department for diagnostic testing, or in whom testing is not available in a timely fashion, can be evaluated at the bedside for DVT. In the appropriate clinical setting, a positive lower extremity study can strongly support the diagnosis of pulmonary embolism.

In many cases an emergency ultrasound can guide disposition and treatment decisions. When the vascular structures are adequately visualized but lack compressibility, the diagnosis of DVT is established and treatment is indicated. If the ultrasound examination is normal (vessels are visualized and compressible), disposition depends upon the pretest probability guided by Wells criteria. Low-risk patients with normal ultrasounds can be discharged home with no need for a repeat study. If patients have moderate to high probability, two options are available. Either an alternative test can be done (CT, MRI, or venogram), or arrangements made for a follow-up ultrasound in three to five days, assuming that the patient has access to care and is reliable. If any ultrasound is indeterminant, alternative testing will be necessary.

CORRELATION WITH OTHER IMAGING MODALITIES

Compression sonography remains the primary diagnostic modality in the evaluation of the lower extremity venous system. Additional modalities include contrast venography, CT, and MRI. Contrast venography is the gold standard for the diagnosis of DVT, especially for calf veins and upper extremity vessels. It is particularly helpful in differentiating between acute and chronic DVT. However, venography is invasive; painful; expensive; time-consuming; cannot be performed at the bedside; and places the patient at risk for phlebitis, hypersensitivity reactions, and even DVTs (17). For these reasons, it is typically used only when other tests are nondiagnostic or unavailable.

CT has been well studied in the literature and compared to ultrasonography and contrast venography (18,19). CT provides the ability to simultaneously evaluate for both PE and DVT. It is accurate; less operator-dependent; and not limited by casts, burns, open wounds, obesity, or severe pain. Also, CT enables one to visualize the opposite limb, IVC, superior vena cava, and heart. CT has the disadvantage of exposing the patient to radiation and risk of contrast reaction. In addition, it requires potentially unstable patients to be moved from the emergency department.

MRI is an alternative seldom used by EDs. It has the ability to directly image the thrombi and visualize nonocclusive clots (17). MRI is also effective for imaging pelvic, IVC, and upper extremity vessels. It can help differentiate acute from chronic DVT's. As opposed to CT, there is no radiation, and the scan can be performed without contrast, making it useful for pregnant patients. However, an accurate study requires the active involvement of an experienced radiologist and resources that are often not available at all hours.

Venous ultrasound can aid in the evaluation of PE as well as DVT. In patients who are being evaluated for PE but are unable to undergo CT or ventilation perfusion scans, the presence of a DVT on ultrasound greatly simplifies the evaluation. This can be especially helpful in an unstable, hypotensive patient in whom the rapid diagnosis of a DVT may significantly alter management. Combining the use of bedside ultrasound for DVT and bedside cardiac ultrasound for right ventricular strain in patients unstable for CT or angiography may, in some cases, prove lifesaving (see Chapter 5) (20).

INCIDENTAL FINDINGS

Many patients in whom we consider the diagnosis of DVT actually have cellulitis causing their legs to be swollen. Lymph nodes, especially in the femoral region, can be mistaken for a vessel with intraluminal clot (Fig. 11.15). Lymph nodes can be differentiated from DVT's in two ways. First, lymph nodes are superficial structures located 2 to 3 cm from the skin surface, while the deep venous system is significantly more posterior, in the range of 4 to 5 cm from the skin surface. Second, enlarged lymph nodes are highly vascularized structures and therefore exhibit high Doppler signals in contrast to a venous clot.

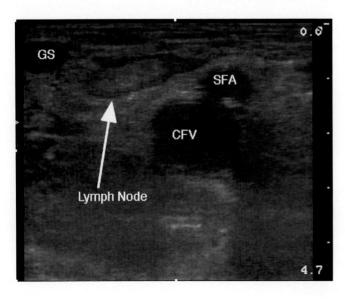

Figure 11.15. A lymph node (arrow) can be mistaken for a vessel with intraluminal clot. (GS, greater saphenous vein; SFA, superficial femoral artery; CFV, common femoral vein)

CLINICAL CASE

A 65-year-old male presents at 7 PM on a Friday complaining of right leg swelling and pain, worst behind the knee, for 1 day. His past medical history includes congestive heart failure and significant osteoarthritis, and a recent hospitalization for subdural hematoma. His vital signs include a heart rate of 94 beats per minute, blood pressure of 147/82 mm Hg, respiratory rate 14 breaths per minute, oxygen saturation 95% on room air, and temperature 99.2 °F. On exam, his right knee is swollen and tender to palpation in the popliteal region. The swelling appears to extend distally, however he has 2+ edema bilaterally, making it difficult to compare. On direct measurement, the right calf measures 2.5 cm larger than the left. A focused bedside ultrasound showed a femoral and popliteal vein that compressed easily, with no visible echogenicity visible in the lumen. Doppler evaluation was normal. The patient was discharged home from the ED on an anti-inflammatory for presumed arthritis, and followed up for complete vascular evaluation on Thursday, to be followed by his primary physician.

The application of focused bedside ultrasound of the lower extremity saved this gentleman three to four days of unnecessary anticoagulation or Greenfield filter, and possibly unnecessary hospitalization.

REFERENCES

1. Kennedy D, Setnik G, Li J. Physical examination findings in deep venous thrombosis. *Emerg Med Clin North Am.* 2001;19:869–876.
2. Kahn SR, Joseph L, Abenhaim L, et al. Clinical prediction of deep vein thrombosis in patients with leg symptoms. *Thromb Haemost.* 1999;81:353–357.
3. Blaivas M, Lambert MJ, Harwood RA, et al. Lower-extremity Doppler for deep venous thrombosis—can emergency physicians be accurate and fast? *Acad Emerg Med.* 2000;7:120–126.
4. Anderson DR, Wells PS, Stiell I, et al. Management of patients with suspected deep vein thrombosis in the emergency department: combining use of a clinical diagnosis model with D-dimer testing. *J Emerg Med.* 2000;19:225–230.
5. Poppiti R, Papanicolaou G, Perese S, et al. Limited B-mode venous imaging versus complete color-flow duplex venous scanning for detection of proximal deep venous thrombosis. *J Vasc Surg.* 1995;22:553–557.
6. Pezzullo JA, Perkins AB, Cronan JJ. Symptomatic deep vein thrombosis: diagnosis with limited compression US. *Radiology.* 1996;198:67–70.
7. Theodoro D, Blaivas M, Duggal S, et al. Real-time B-mode ultrasound in the ED saves time in the diagnosis of deep vein thrombosis (DVT). *Am J Emerg Med.* 2004;22:197–200.
8. Jang T, Docherty M, Aubin C, et al. Resident-performed compression ultrasonography for the detection of proximal deep vein thrombosis: fast and accurate. *Acad Emerg Med.* 2004;11:319–322.
9. Frazee BW, Snoey ER, Levitt A. Emergency department compression ultrasound to diagnose proximal deep vein thrombosis. *J Emerg Med.* 2001;20:107–112.
10. Frazee BW, Snoey ER. Diagnostic role of ED ultrasound in deep venous thrombosis and pulmonary embolism. *Am J Emerg Med.* 1999;17:271–278.
11. Lensing AW, Prandoni P, Brandjes D, et al. Detection of deep-vein thrombosis by real-time B-mode ultrasonography. *N Engl J Med.* 1989;320:342–345.
12. Birdwell BG, Raskob GE, Whitsett TL, et al. The clinical validity of normal compression ultrasonography in outpatients suspected of having deep venous thrombosis. *Ann Intern Med.* 1998; 128:1–7.
13. Frederick MG, Hertzberg BS, Kliewer MA, et al. Can the US examination for lower extremity deep venous thrombosis be abbreviated? A prospective study of 755 examinations. *Radiology.* 1996;199:45–47.
14. Hollerweger A, Macheiner P, Rettenbacher T, Gritzmann N. [Sonographic diagnosis of thrombosis of the calf muscle veins and the risk of pulmonary embolism]. *Ultraschall Med.* 2000;21:66–2.
15. American College of Emergency Physicians (ACEP) Clinical Policies Committee; ACEP Clinical Policies Subcommittee on Suspected Lower-Extremity Deep Venous Thrombosis. Clinical policy: critical issues in the evaluation and management of adult patients presenting with suspected lower-extremity deep venous thrombosis. *Ann Emerg Med.* 2003;42:124–135.

16. Wells PS, Anderson DR, Bormanis J, et al. Value of assessment of pretest probability of deep venous thrombosis in clinical management. *Lancet*. 1997;350:1795–1798.
17. Kelly J, Hunt BJ, Moody A. Magnetic resonance direct thrombus imaging: a novel technique for imaging venous thromboemboli. *Thromb Haemost*. 2003;89:773–782.
18. Lim KE, Hsu WC, Hsu YY, et al. Deep venous thrombosis; Comparison of indirect multidetector CT venography and sonography of lower extremities in 26 patients. *Clin Imaging*. 2004;28:439–444.
19. Baldt MM, Zontsich T, Stumpflen A, et al. Deep venous thrombosis of the lower extremity: efficacy of spiral CT venography compared with conventional venography in diagnosis. *Radiology*. 1996;200:423–428.
20. Lim KE, Hsu YY, Hsu WC, et al. Combined computed tomography venography and pulmonary angiography for the diagnosis PE and DVT in the ED. *Am J Emerg Med*. 2004;22:301–306.

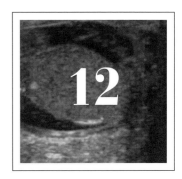

TESTICULAR ULTRASOUND

Paul R. Sierzenski

Stephen J. Leech

INTRODUCTION

The patient presenting to the emergency department (ED) with acute scrotal pain represents a high-risk, time-urgent complaint. The differential diagnosis includes testicular torsion with potential organ loss and loss of fertility. In addition the clinician must also consider epididymitis, orchitis, trauma, hemorrhage, and tumor as a potential diagnosis. Many signs, symptoms, and physical findings of these diagnoses overlap and do not discriminate between disease states. One series demonstrated that up to 50% of cases of acute scrotal pain could not be discriminated on the basis of patient symptom history, physical exam, and lab work (1). Patients with equivocal findings on history and exam often receive diagnostic imaging because many urologists are hesitant to operate on such cases. Testicular ultrasound with power and spectral Doppler has become the imaging modality of choice in patients with acute scrotal pain or swelling (2–9). Emergency physicians can utilize the increased availability of bedside ultrasound in the ED to expedite patient care and prompt referral to specialists. Studies have shown that emergency physicians with expertise in ultrasound can accurately identify and discriminate causes of the acute scrotum when compared to radiology-based studies and surgical findings (10–12).

CLINICAL APPLICATIONS

Any patient with acute scrotal pain, trauma, or a scrotal mass is a candidate for bedside testicular ultrasound. Ultrasound is sensitive and specific for diagnosing and differentiating the causes of acute scrotal pain, with characteristic findings dependent upon the underlying cause.

TESTICULAR TORSION

Testicular torsion represents a true surgical emergency, and any patient with acute scrotal pain or swelling should be suspected to have torsion until proven otherwise. Patients with a "bell-clapper" deformity lack the normal posterior fixation of the testicle to the scrotal wall. Testicular torsion results from the twisting of redundant spermatic cord on its pedunculated blood supply, causing testicular ischemia. Venous thrombosis then occurs, followed by arterial thrombosis. The degree of twisting of the testicle about its axis affects how rapidly testicular infarction can occur. In an animal model, 90 degrees of torsion caused no testicular necrosis at 7 days, 360 degrees of torsion resulted in necrosis in 12 to 24 hours, and 1440 degrees of torsion caused necrosis in 2 hours (13). It is generally thought that rotation of at least 450 degrees is needed to cause complete testicular torsion (14). In addition, spontaneous torsion-detorsion and incomplete torsion can occur. Torsion occurs at two age peaks, the first during infancy, and the second during puberty. However the emergency physician must still consider the diagnosis of torsion after puberty, as up to 20% of cases occur postpubescently (15).

Prompt diagnosis and treatment lead to higher salvage rates. Reported salvage rates range from 80% to 100% for patients treated within 6 hours of symptom onset, 70% to 83% between 6 and 12 hours, and 20% to 80% after 12 hours (16–19). No successful testicular salvage has been reported after 48 hours of torsion (19).

EPIDIDYMITIS AND ORCHITIS

Epididymitis is the most common cause of acute scrotal pain in adults and also represents the most common misdiagnosis in cases of missed testicular torsion (20). This mistake is usually made in men under age 35, in whom testicular torsion and epididymitis are both common. Epididymitis occurs in patients of all ages, from infants to the elderly. It can result from either viral or bacterial infection with inflammation.

In most cases, epididymitis is caused by extension of infection from the lower urinary tract. In men under 35 years old, epididymitis is most often a sexually transmitted disease, with *Chlamydia trachomatis* or *Neisseria gonorrhoeae* as common etiologic agents. In older males, epididymitis is usually caused by gram-negative pathogens as a result of a urinary tract infection or recent urinary instrumentation (20). Occasionally, epididymitis results from trauma, and some cases are idiopathic with no definite cause. Severe cases of epididymitis can result in abscess formation.

Orchitis is an acute infection of the testis and usually results following an initial episode of epididymitis. The infectious agents implicated in orchitis are similar to those that cause epididymitis. In some cases, an isolated orchitis occurs in the setting of viral infection. Several etiologic agents have been implicated, with mumps being the most common cause.

SCROTAL TRAUMA

Direct trauma to the scrotum can result in contusion, hematoma formation, and testicular fracture. Ultrasound is helpful in defining the location and extent of injury and can help guide management. When the tunica albuginea is ruptured, surgical intervention is required to prevent an autoimmune reaction against the testicle and resultant sterility (21).

SCROTAL MASSES

Ultrasound is very sensitive for the identification of scrotal masses, and can help differentiate intratesticular masses from extratesticular masses. The majority of extratesticular masses are benign, while intratesticular masses must be presumed to be neoplastic until proven otherwise. Testicular cancer accounts for 1% to 2% of all malignant tumors in men and is the fifth leading cause of death in men aged 15 to 34 years (22). The majority of testicular tumors are of germ cell origin; seminoma is the most common cell type. If ultrasound demonstrates an intratesticular mass, urgent urologic consultation is required. Common extratesticular scrotal masses include hydroceles, spermatoceles, varicoceles, and inguinal hernias.

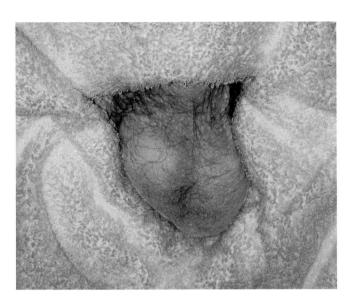

Figure 12.1. Patient preparation for testicular ultrasound. Note the scrotum is supported for patient comfort and to facilitate testicular scanning.

GUIDE TO IMAGE ACQUISITION

ULTRASOUND TECHNIQUE

The patient should be placed in a supine position and made as comfortable as possible. The scrotum is elevated and immobilized by a towel rolled and placed between the patient's thighs behind the scrotum (Fig. 12.1). The penis should be folded back onto the patient's abdomen and covered with a towel. Ample amounts of warm gel should be used. A high frequency linear array transducer provides the greatest detail and resolution (Fig. 12.2). Frequencies used range from 5 to 10 MHz, with lower frequencies being reserved for settings where increased tissue penetration is needed.

SCANNING PROTOCOL

When scanning the scrotum it is important to start with the unaffected testicle. This will allow for comparison of size, texture, and echogenicity between the testicles, as well as allowing for the Doppler settings to be oriented toward the unaffected side. A standard protocol should be followed in order to allow for complete visualization of the scrotal con-

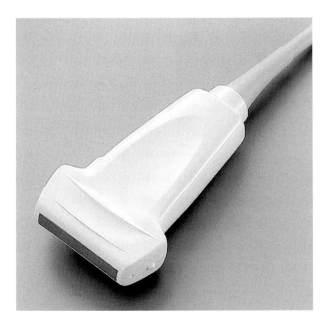

Figure 12.2. A linear high-frequency transducer. (Courtesy of Sono Site, Inc. Bothell, WA).

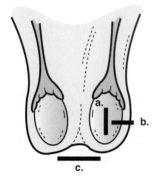

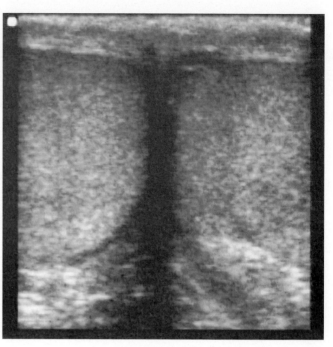

Figure 12.3. Transducer placement for ultrasound of the testicle. (*A*) Sagittal orientation. (*B*) Transverse view. (*C*) Transverse comparative view of both testicles.

Figure 12.4. Transverse comparative view. Transverse bilateral view of normal testes in B-Mode. Allows comparison of testicular echotexture as well as a side-by-side comparison of color Doppler imaging.

tents. Both testicles should be scanned in their entirety in the sagittal and transverse planes. In addition, a transverse view across the median raphe should be included in order to compare the gray scale anatomy, as well as blood flow patterns between testicles (Fig. 12.3).

The normal sonographic appearance of the testicle has been described as similar to the liver, with a homogenous, uniform echogenic pattern (Fig. 12.4). The mediastinum testis appears as a bright echogenic band running in the long axis of the testicle (Fig. 12.5). Attention should also be focused in the epididymis as it courses superiorly and posterior to

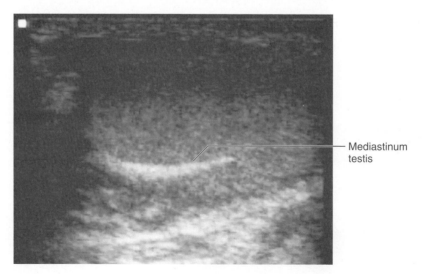

Mediastinum testis

Figure 12.5. Sagittal image of normal testis showing mediastinum testis as an echogenic band (*arrows*).

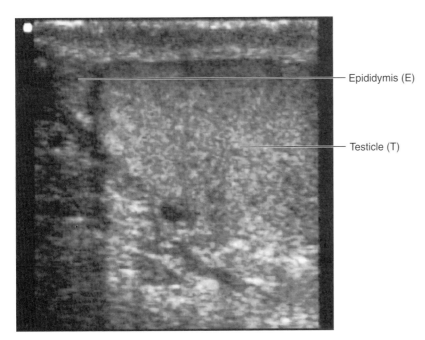

Figure 12.6. Normal testis. Sagittal B-Mode image of a normal testis showing testicle (*T*) and epididymis (*E*).

the testicle (Fig. 12.6). Sonographically, the epididymis is usually isoechoic when compared to the testicle. The head is the most prominent portion, and the body and tail may be difficult to clearly visualize in its normal state.

After a thorough survey of the testicle in B-mode imaging, color or power Doppler should be used to identify intratesticular vessels (Fig. 12.7). This is best achieved in the transverse plane near the mediastinum testis. Spectral Doppler interrogation should then be used to identify both arterial and venous waveforms. It is important to demonstrate both arterial and venous flow to exclude testicular torsion with a high degree of certainty. Side-by-side comparisons should be performed to assess for symmetric flow, and any difference noted should raise the clinician's suspicion for an incomplete torsion or torsion-detorsion.

The spermatic cord is located superior to the testicle. Arterial waveforms obtained in this area will have a high resistive pattern consistent with peripheral vessels. The sper-

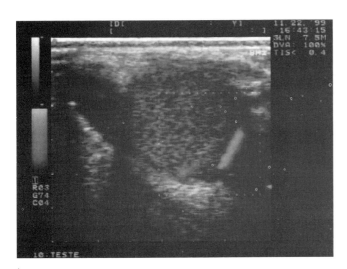

Figure 12.7. Color Doppler imaging (CDI). Power Doppler showing testicular blood flow. Power Doppler displays color-coding in one color that can vary with the velocity of flow but is not directionally dependent. (See color insert.)

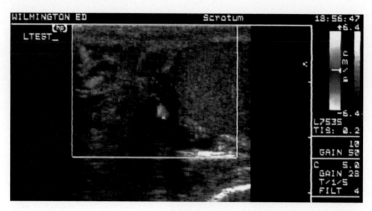

Figure 12.8. Spermatic cord. Doppler of the spermatic cord as well as the upper pole of the testicle. (See color insert.)

matic cord should be surveyed for evidence of a varicocele if clinical suspicion exists (Fig. 12.8).

DOPPLER

An understanding of Doppler ultrasound is crucial to evaluating the patient with suspected testicular torsion or scrotal pain. The ultrasound transducer emits and receives ultrasound frequencies; the central processing unit in turn converts the signal into ultrasound images. When an ultrasound wave strikes a moving object, such as a blood cell inside a vessel, shifting of the original ultrasound frequency occurs. The difference between the original and returned frequency is known as "Doppler shift." The magnitude of the frequency shift is dependent on the angle at which sound strikes the moving object, as well as the direction and speed of the object. The usual frequency range of Doppler frequency shifts that occurs in normal circumstances in situations involving blood flow is measured in kilohertz. These shifts can provide important diagnostic information regarding flow in the testicle.

Two main types of Doppler are used in scanning the testicles, color Doppler imaging (CDI) and spectral Doppler. CDI displays Doppler shift overlaid on a gray scale B-mode image, which provides information regarding flow velocity and flow direction. Colors are assigned to velocities either toward or away from the transducer, with the intensity of color increasing with increased velocity. Shift toward the transducer is color coded in one color, and shift away from the transducer is coded in another. Power color Doppler displays only the intensity of the Doppler shift, without information regarding the direction of shift (Fig. 12.7). In testicular ultrasound, the detection of flow is the most important use of Doppler, and the increased sensitivity in detecting lower-flow states makes power Doppler imaging preferable to color Doppler for the evaluation of the testicles and scrotum.

Color and power Doppler are both helpful in identifying flow and excluding complete testicular torsion from arterial compromise. It is important to note that partial torsion, or early torsion where venous occlusion is the principle finding, is best excluded using spectral Doppler with the identification of venous flow by the presence of a spectral venous waveform. Spectral Doppler allows quantification of velocities and differentiates between arterial and venous blood flow (Fig. 12.9). The centripetal testicular arteries have a characteristic low-resistive pattern, with a low systolic peak, and a wide diastolic peak. The testicular veins display a low-flow, phasic pattern (Fig. 12.10). It is important to document both arterial and venous waveforms during an exam for possible torsion. During torsion, the venous flow pattern is lost first, followed by dampening of the arterial waveform, and then all flow to the testicle is lost. By seeing both arterial and venous spectral waveforms, torsion and incomplete torsion can be essentially ruled out.

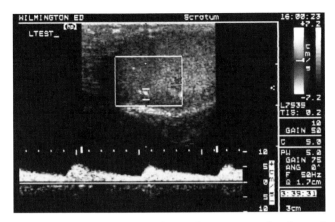

Figure 12.9. Arterial spectral Doppler. Directional color and spectral Doppler waveform is displayed. A normal arterial spectral waveform is demonstrated. (See color insert.)

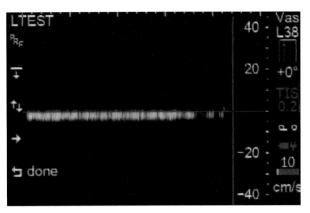

Figure 12.10. Venous spectral Doppler. A venous spectral Doppler waveform from a normal testicle is displayed. A continuous waveform is visualized.

Doppler settings should be adjusted to allow for maximum sensitivity. Physicians should review the adjustable Doppler parameters with the applications specialist for their ultrasound equipment. Briefly, the wall filter eliminates or diminishes unwanted echoes that occur from vessel wall motion. The pulse repetition frequency (PRF) helps to determine the measurable velocity by Doppler ultrasound. The PRF (sometimes called scale) and wall filter should initially be programmed or adjusted to their lowest settings, then adjusted to eliminate background noise and false signals. This will allow for visualization of the lower-flow velocities commonly found in testicular ultrasound scanning. The Doppler gain should also be decreased to its lowest setting and then slowly increased as needed. This should ensure that any color flow seen inside the testicle represents true flow versus artifact from improper gain settings.

NORMAL ULTRASOUND ANATOMY AND LANDMARKS

The scrotum is a cutaneous pouch divided into two lateral compartments by the median raphe, and each side contains a testicle, epididymis, vas deferens, and spermatic cord. The normal testes are oval in shape and measure approximately 5 by 3 by 3 cm (Figs. 12.6, 12.11). The normal lie of the testicles is within a vertical axis, with a slightly anterior tilt. The scrotal sac is lined by the tunica vaginalis, which is reflected over the exterior surface of each testicle. The tunica albuginea forms the exterior capsule of the testicle and gives rise to multiple septations that run through the testicle and separate the testicle into lobules. The mediastinum testis is a dense band of connective tissue that provides structural support for the testicular vessels and ducts (Fig. 12.5).

The epididymis is the ductal system through which the sperm travel and is located posterior to the testicle. The epididymis is divided into the head, body, and tail. The head is located adjacent to the superior pole of the testis, and measures 1 to 1.2 cm in diameter (Fig. 12.6). The epididymis eventually becomes the vas deferens as it courses superiorly into the spermatic cord. The spermatic cord contains the testicular artery, cremasteric artery, pampiniform plexus, lymphatic structures, and genitofemoral nerve (Fig. 12.11).

The testicular artery is the primary arterial blood supply of the testicles and is a direct branch of the abdominal aorta. After entering the scrotum, the testicular artery runs posteriorly to the testicle and forms capsular arteries that run just beneath the tunica albuginea. The capsular arteries give off centripetal branches that run toward the mediastinum testis. Additional blood supply to the scrotum is provided by the cremasteric and deferential arteries that supply the epididymis, vas deferens, and peritesticular tissues.

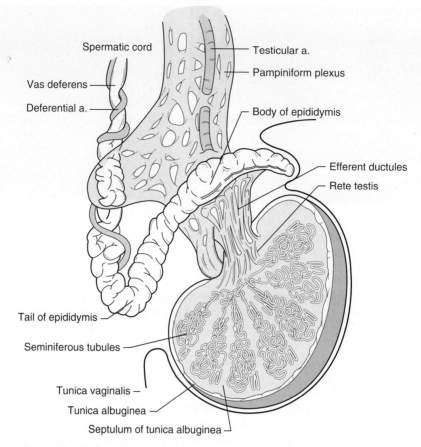

Figure 12.11. Normal testicular anatomy.

Both of these arteries anastomose with the testicular artery but their contribution to testicular blood flow is minimal. Testicular veins flow from the mediastinum testis outward to the pampiniform plexus in the spermatic cord. The right testicular vein empties directly into the inferior vena cava, while the left testicular vein empties into the left renal vein before draining into the inferior vena cava. As with other solid organs, the testicle has a low-resistive arterial waveform on spectral Doppler.

PATHOLOGY

EPIDIDYMITIS AND ORCHITIS

Epididymitis with or without orchitis represents a spectrum of testicular inflammation that is the most common diagnosis in patients presenting to the ED with testicular pain, swelling, or mass (20). Though epididymitis is the most common diagnosis for those with testicular complaints, it is not the most time-critical, as testicular torsion represents the clinical diagnosis that must be excluded. Since testicular torsion and epididymitis/orchitis are difficult to differentiate based on history, symptoms, and physical exam, diagnostic testing is often required. Today CDI has become the accepted modality of choice for the diagnostic evaluation of the patient with acute testicular complaints (2–9).

Sonographic findings of epididymitis include thickening and enlargement of the epididymis (Fig. 12.12A). This occurs most frequently in the epididymal head, followed by the body, and least frequently the epididymal tail. However, in up to 50% of cases, the epididymis is inflamed from the body through the tail (23). Decreased echogenicity is common on 2-D B-mode ultrasound with a coarse and heterogenous appearance, the result of

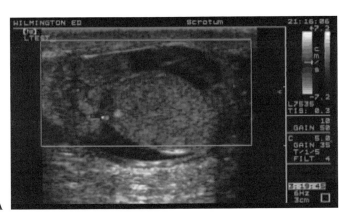
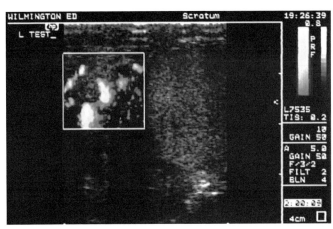

A B

Figure 12.12. (**A**) Epididymitis with orchitis. Sagittal image from a 13-year-old who presented with a painful swollen testicle. Note the enlarged epididymis superior to the testicle. (**B**) Epididymitis. Power Doppler showing increased flow within and around the epididymis. (See color insert.)

edematous inflammation. A "reactive hydrocele" is common in epididymitis and orchitis, as well as nearly all acute testicular pathology including testicular torsion (24). The key diagnostic sonographic finding for epididymitis is increased color or power Doppler flow when compared to the asymptomatic testicle (Fig. 12.12B). If spectral Doppler ultrasound is performed, then a decreased resistive index (RI) less than 0.5 can often be identified, further supporting the diagnosis of orchitis (25).

TESTICULAR TORSION, TESTICULAR ISCHEMIA, AND TESTICULAR INFARCTION

Testicular torsion occurs when the blood supply to the testicle is partially or completely obstructed as a result of first venous, and then arterial compression during coiling of the testicles' pedunculated blood supply. Since torsion may be complete or partial, the sonographic diagnosis of this entity can be difficult, even for the experienced sonographer. Previous studies have consistently shown that the most accurate means to diagnose torsion, regardless of sonographic or radiographic findings, is via surgical exploration (26). Therefore, a high suspicion of testicular torsion should trigger one to obtain immediate urologic consultation. Since an observed difference in flow between the affected and unaffected testicle is key to the diagnosis of torsion, a working and fundamental understanding and performance of CDI and spectral Doppler ultrasound is essential.

The sonographic appearance of the torsed testicle is dependent upon the degree of testicular torsion, as well as the time from symptom onset (24). If the ultrasound is performed within the first 4 hours of torsion, the testicle will likely appear enlarged with a decreased echogenicity resulting from venous congestion (Fig. 12.13). CDI will reveal diminished or absent central testicular blood flow when compared to the asymptomatic testicle. However, CDI alone may not be sufficient in the evaluation of patients with testicular pain with demonstrated flow in both testicles. The identification of intratesticular arterial and venous spectral Doppler waveforms has a greater negative predictive value than the presence of color or power Doppler flow (7). This is believed to be the result of the physiology of early torsion described earlier in this chapter.

TESTICULAR TRAUMA

Testicular fracture and testicular infarction are the principal concerns in patients presenting with either blunt or penetrating testicular trauma. A testicular fracture occurs when the integrity of the tunica albuginea is disrupted. The pathophysiology of testicular rupture is similar to that of a ruptured globe. If struck with sufficient force, the internal pressure

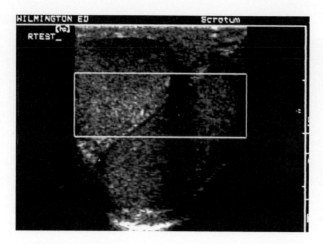

Figure 12.13. Acute left testicular torsion. Note absence of color power Doppler flow compared to right testicle. An edge artifact obscures a portion of the left testicle. (See color insert.)

within the testicle exceeds that of the structural resistance integrity of the tunica albuginea, with leakage of its internal contents. Sonographically the perimeter of the testicle is often noncontiguous and irregular, with a hemorrhagic region at the area of the fracture (Fig. 12.14). A hematocele may be present and can be difficult to distinguish from testicular tissue. A hematocele in the patient with acute scrotal trauma may be an indirect indicator of a testicular fracture, much like free fluid in the trauma exam may represent a solid organ injury. Furthermore, recognition of increased antiplatelets and anticoagulation use for patients who are of childrearing age should raise the emergency physician's concern of hematocele progression. Several case reports describe testicular ischemia and infarction re-

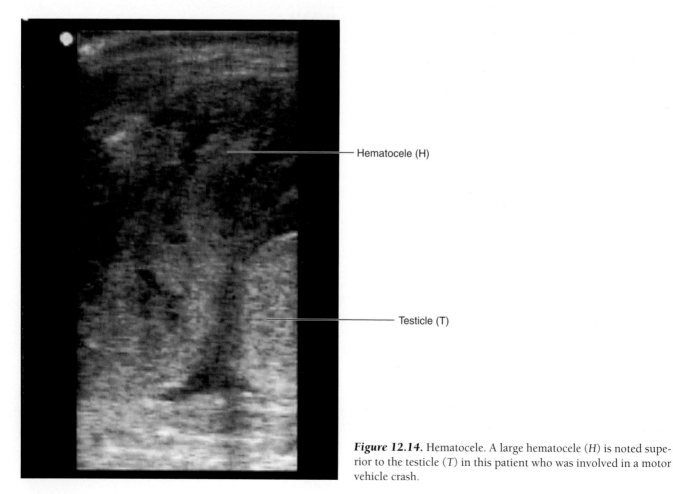

Figure 12.14. Hematocele. A large hematocele (*H*) is noted superior to the testicle (*T*) in this patient who was involved in a motor vehicle crash.

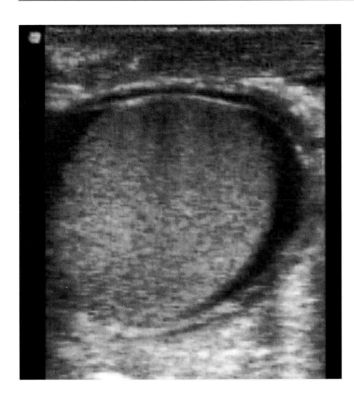

Figure 12.15. Hydrocele. An anechoic circumferential hydrocele is noted to surround the testicle.

sulting from vascular compromise following development of large hydroceles or hematoceles, requiring scrotal decompression (25). Testicular fracture and its associated findings represent a surgical emergency, as testicular function and fertility may be lost if the testicle is not repaired. The suspicion of a testicular fracture should prompt immediate urologic, and potentially further radiologic evaluation.

EXTRATESTICULAR CAUSES OF SCROTAL SWELLING OR MASSES: HYDROCELE, HEMATOCELE, AND PYOCELE

A hydrocele is defined as a fluid collection that is located between the visceral and parietal layers of the tunica vaginalis. These can be congenital or acquired in nature and are often asymptomatic. However, acquired hydroceles or their associated scrotal swelling can represent the initial presenting symptom and finding associated with several clinical entities relevant to the emergency physician. Causes of acquired hydroceles include testicular torsion, epididymitis, trauma, orchitis, and tumors (24). Sonographically, most hydroceles are anechoic in nature, with low attenuating fluid that results in posterior acoustic enhancement (Fig. 12.15). If the fluid collection in the hydrocele is blood, this is termed a "hematocele" and internal echoes from blood cells can be noted. When associated with inflammatory states, internal echoes from white blood cells and debris may be identified on ultrasound and this is then termed a "pyocele."

A varicocele is an extratesticular dilatation and elongation of the veins of the pampiniform plexus. Varicoceles generally occur in the left scrotum, a result of the anatomic venous connection of the left gonadal vein as it drains into the left renal vein. Anatomically the left renal vein traverses between the aorta and superior mesenteric artery, placing it at risk for compression by the "nutcracker syndrome," resulting in higher venous pressures throughout its distal venous system. This can result in the formation of varicoceles. Patients will present with either an asymptomatic or mildly painful mass. The classically defined "bag of worms" on physical exam is often only noted in patients with advanced large varicoceles. Sonographically, enlarged veins greater than 2 to 3 mm in diameter are located superior to the testis but may also be noted posterior and lateral to the testis (Fig. 12.16). When a patient stands or performs a Valsalva maneuver these veins dilate with a classic increased flow on

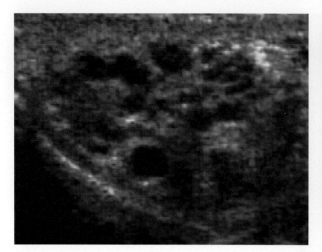

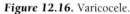

Figure 12.16. Varicocele.

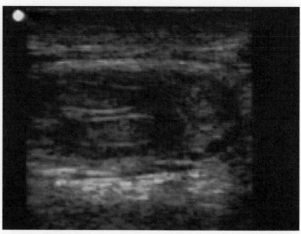

Figure 12.17. Inguinal hernia. An inguinal hernia is noted as intestine loops back upon itself in the inguinal canal.

CDI or a reversal of venous flow noted on spectral Doppler analysis. Though varicoceles rarely represent an immediate testicular emergency (unless venous thrombosis is suspected), they have been implicated and are felt to be a significant cause of decreased fertility or infertility in men. Therefore, the finding of a varicocele does require appropriate urology consultation and follow-up. Finally, the presence of an isolated right-sided varicocele should raise the possibility of potential right-sided venous obstruction such as a right renal mass.

SCROTAL HERNIA

A scrotal hernia is a protrusion of intra-abdominal contents, which is often bowel, through the processes vaginalis into the scrotal sac. Patients often present with either acute onset of pain and swelling, or with complications that may occur with chronic herniation such as bowel strangulation or even obstruction. Sonographically one can usually distinguish the testicle from this extratesticular mass if they are clearly distinct from each other, or if the mass has evidence of peristalsis, fluid, air artifact, or a reactive hydrocele (Fig. 12.17) (27,28).

ARTIFACTS IN TESTICULAR ULTRASOUND IMAGING

Several artifacts can be encountered during testicular ultrasound.

1. Posterior Acoustic Enhancement. The far field beyond an anechoic or hypoechoic area will have increased echogenicity. This is commonly observed in the far field beyond cysts (such as epididymal cysts), hydroceles, and varicoceles (Fig. 12.18).
2. Color Doppler Flash Artifact. Color or power Doppler artifact results from movement of the transducer or the testicle in the area of the Doppler box. This may be confused for blood flow. This commonly occurs when the Doppler gain is set too high, the color filter set too low, or when the patient or transducer is moved during evaluation (Fig. 12.19).
3. Refraction (Edge Artifact, Lateral Cystic Shadowing). The ultrasound image displayed may be lost from the curved border of a structure. This is commonly seen at the head of the epididymis, and in some intratesticular masses (Fig. 12.18).
4. Shadowing. This is the loss of a displayed ultrasound image immediately beyond a structure with a high acoustic impedance such as a dense calcium-containing structure. This occurs with tissue calcifications and in some tumors with calcifications.

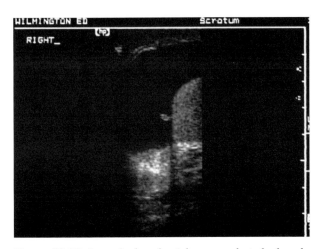

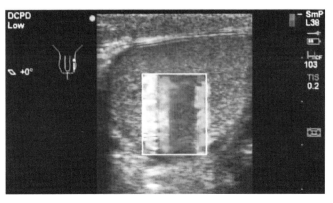

Figure 12.18. Large hydrocele. A large anechoic hydrocele is noted to display posterior acoustic enhancement. Edge artifact/ lateral cystic shadowing is also evident extending into the far field from the superior testicle edge. The appendix testis is seen.

Figure 12.19. Color Doppler "flash" artifact. This image shows color filling within the sample volume that results from the Doppler shift caused by either the patient or the transducer moving. Though this is an extreme example, it is critical that Doppler signals be clearly identified resulting from true venous and arterial flow rather than from either patient movement or transducer movement artifacts. (See color insert.)

PITFALLS IN THE USE OF TESTICULAR ULTRASOUND

Pitfalls in testicular ultrasound may be divided into several categories. It is essential that the emergency sonographer be familiar with these in order to avoid misdiagnosis or a delay in care.

1. The most significant pitfall for performance and optimization of the image and diagnostic information relates to understanding and the skill with using color, power, or spectral Doppler. The emergency sonographer should have an understanding of Doppler physics and its interplay in the performance of testicular ultrasound. Minimizing the effect of Doppler filters and using lower Doppler scales and pulse repetition frequencies should be emphasized and practiced. Our training in emergency medicine often has us focus on the patient's area of complaint, and although we do this with testicular ultrasound, it is critical to first optimize Doppler settings on the asymptomatic side (if one exists) prior to evaluating the symptomatic testicle.

2. Diagnostically, testicular torsion, late torsion, intermittent torsion, and focal infarcts can present a sonographic color and spectral evaluation that is confusing. In all of these states there can exist the presence of peripheral testicular blood flow, with a relative deficiency or absence of central testicular blood flow.

3. It is essential to realize that the diagnosis of testicular torsion does not mandate an "absence of any blood flow" on ultrasound, but rather a "critical deficiency" in testicular blood flow that can result in infarction. To avoid this potential pitfall it is critical that the emergency sonographer scan the asymptomatic testicle initially to obtain baseline Doppler settings, adjust the Doppler filter, pulse repetition frequency (PRF), and the Doppler gain. If perimeter blood vessels appear hyperemic with increased flow, yet clear central testis color and spectral arterial and venous Doppler signals are difficult to identify, then one of two scenarios exists. The system may not be optimized, or the patient has a central flow deficiency that may represent torsion, an intermittent torsion, or a focal infarct, all of which require immediate urology consultation and potentially further diagnostic evaluation; time is critical for the viability of the testis.

USE OF THE IMAGE IN CLINICAL DECISION MAKING (FIG. 12.20)

It is important to recognize that the history, physical exam, and urinalysis are not 100% specific for the diagnosis of epididymitis or testicular torsion. Even pyuria is unreliable in distinguishing between infection and inflammation. The simplest use of emergency testicular ultrasound is to use the positive predictive value for the inclusion of inflammatory states. It is often easier to rule in a specific diagnosis with a positive result than it is to rule out a diagnosis such as torsion that relies on the absence of findings (i.e., blood flow). This is not an unusual concept in medicine. For example, an electrocardiogram (EKG) showing an inferior wall myocardial infarction can aid in rapid disposition and management of patients, while the nondiagnostic EKG in the patient with chest pain requires further evaluation. Using this same mentality, consider a real life example. A 16-year-old male presents with three days of intermittent testicular pain and swelling and admits to sexual activity and dysuria. He is afebrile. His exam shows a swollen left testis that is tender but has a normal cremasteric reflex. At this point, let's presume two different potential emergency ultrasound scan results. The patient's ultrasound scan reveals an enlarged testis with decreased echogenicity and hyperemic flow throughout the testicle and epididymis as compared to the asymptomatic side.

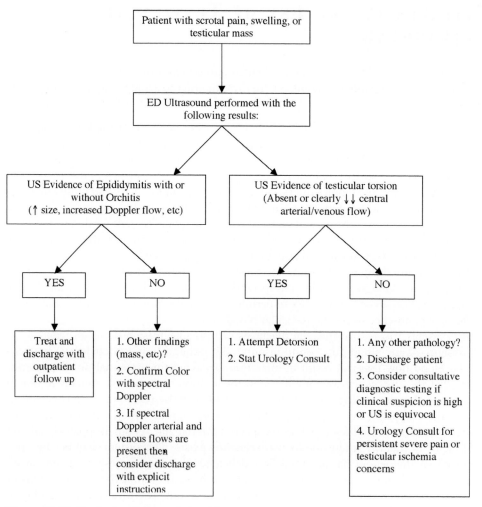

Figure 12.20. Testicular ultrasound algorithm.

Centrally both arterial and venous spectral Doppler waveforms are identified. The patient is diagnosed as epididymo-orchitis and appropriately discharged on analgesics and antibiotics with urology follow-up. If the ultrasound had instead shown peripheral hyperemia with the absence of central flow, torsion could not be ruled out. Urology should be consulted and the diagnosis confirmed. This example illustrates a conservative approach to emergency testicular ultrasound that is likely to fit within the practice patterns of most emergency physicians, that is to say, when conditions other than torsion are evident and the testicular ultrasound supports a specific diagnosis, then disposition can be made. In the case of torsion when complete torsion without central flow is evident on ultrasound, operative disposition and consultation is immediate. However when partial flow is noted on testicular ultrasound and inflammatory states (epididymitis/orchitis) cannot be confirmed, further immediate consultative evaluation or diagnostic testing is reasonable and suggested.

The sonographic evidence for torsion or testicular emergencies may not be as clear as the presence or absence of an abdominal aortic aneurysm or a pericardial effusion. When doubt or clinical concern remains high, further testing beyond the emergency ultrasound and immediate consultation with urology is essential, as a delay in diagnosis can result in a poor outcome.

CORRELATION WITH OTHER IMAGING MODALITIES

Prior to the widespread use of color duplex ultrasound, nuclear imaging was the diagnostic test of choice for the assessment of the acute scrotum. In nuclear imaging, a radioactive isotope, generally technetium-99 with a chemical vector, is intravenously injected into the patient. Serial time-dependent images using a gamma radiation detection scanner are obtained usually at 1-minute intervals, with delayed images at 10 to15 minutes as needed. This allows a radioisotope tagged assessment of perfusion of the testicle and the surrounding tissues. Several key differences exist between nuclear imaging and ultrasound. First, ultrasound does not employ ionizing radiation, and this is a clear benefit if diagnostic information can be obtained without radiation exposure. The second key difference is based on the time to obtain the diagnostic information. The diagnostic information by ultrasound is immediate; in contrast, nuclear imaging requires up to 60 minutes following isotope injection. Although both modalities offer information about blood flow to the scrotum and testicles, ultrasound provides sonographic anatomic information that nuclear imaging cannot. While both modalities have a high sensitivity for detecting scrotal pathology, these advantages have made color Doppler ultrasound the principal modality for evaluating scrotal and testicular pathology.

INCIDENTAL FINDINGS

TESTICULAR MASS

The majority of intratesticular masses are malignant germ cell tumors. For this reason it is essential that patients identified with a testicular mass on ultrasound receive definitive and rapid consultative follow-up. Sonographic differentiation of testicular germ cell tumors is generally beyond the scope of practice for emergency physicians, and will not be discussed in this chapter.

Patients with testicular masses can present with complaints including testicular or groin pain, testicular enlargement, a palpable mass, hematuria, or scrotal swelling. Sonographically, intratesticular masses are usually "hypoechoic" when compared to the surrounding testicular tissue (Fig. 12.21). They can further display *heterogenicity*, focal areas of necrosis, echogenic calcified foci, and necrotic or cystic regions (Fig. 12.22). A "reactive hydrocele" is frequently present, and CDI may reveal increased flow within the mass, unless infarction or hemorrhage occurs within the mass.

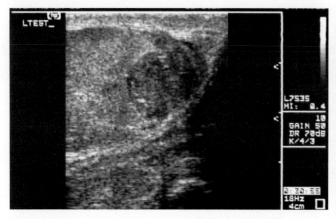

Figure 12.21. Left testicular mass. Hypoechoic mass at the inferior pole of the left testicle in a patient who presented with a painless, firm mass noted on self-exam.

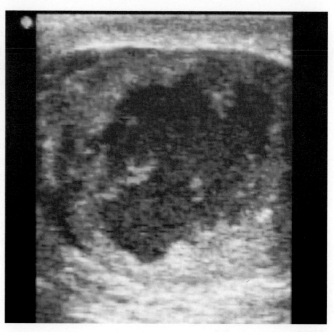

Figure 12.22. Intratesticular mass. Longitudinal, sagittal view of a hypoechoic mass within the center of the testicle with irregular borders.

Epididymal cysts and spermatoceles represent a common finding in patients presenting with either a painful or painless palpable scrotal mass. They can be located anywhere along the length of the epididymis but are frequently found at the head of the epididymis. Sonographically these cysts usually are anechoic, display posterior acoustic enhancement and lateral cystic shadowing (edge artifact), and have no internal CDI flow (Fig. 12.23). It is important to recognize that if the transmit frequency for the transducer can be increased, this may aid in the recognition of posterior acoustic enhancement and help with the sonographic diagnosis of cysts and fluid collections.

MICROLITHIASIS

Microlithiasis is noted on ultrasound as diffuse punctate echogenic calcifications throughout the testicles. The image pattern is described sonographically as a "starry night." The clinical significance of this is debatable. Concern exists that intratesticular calcifications may represent a precancerous state. Any patient with this incidental finding should have appropriate specialist follow-up.

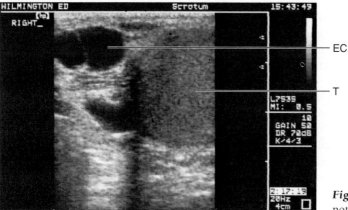

Figure 12.23. Epididymal cyst (EC). Two epididymal cysts are noted in the head of the epididymis superior to the testis (T).

CLINICAL CASES

CASE ONE

A 34-year-old male presents with complaints of 3 days of increasing persistent testicular pain and right testicular swelling. He complains of dysuria and states that the symptoms became worse today. His vitals include a temperature of 38.7 °C, pulse of 105 beats per minute, and a blood pressure of 135/65 mmHg. A urinalysis shows moderate bacteria with 30 to 40 white blood cell count (WBC) and 5 to 10 red blood cell count (RBC) per high-power field. On exam he has a swollen right testicle that is warm and tender to the touch. He has a cremasteric reflex present. An emergency ultrasound reveals an enlarged epididymal head and testicle with a significant increase color flow on Doppler as compared to the left testicle (Figs 12.12A and B). He is diagnosed with acute epididymitis with orchitis and placed on antibiotic therapy with an outpatient follow-up with a urologist.

CASE TWO

A 16-year-old male presents with 3 days of intermittent testicular pain that completely resolved during each episode. He states that while working out on an exercise bike he noted the sudden onset of severe left testicular and groin pain with nausea and vomiting. He presents in obvious distress 3 hours after the onset of pain today. His vitals include a temperature of 37.8 °C, pulse of 115 beats per minute, and a blood pressure of 145/84 mmHg. A urinalysis shows trace bacteria with 0 to 10 WBC and 5 to 10 RBC per high-power field. On exam he has a swollen left testicle that is tender to the touch. No cremasteric reflex is present, and the testicle rests in an oblique position. An emergency ultrasound reveals a slightly enlarged testicle with some peripheral testicular flow but a significant decrease in color flow on Doppler as compared to the right testicle. (Figs.12.24A and B). A small hydrocele is also noted on the left. He is given intravenous analgesia with procedural sedation and manual detorsion is attempted without success. He is diagnosed with acute left

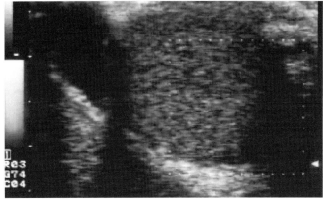

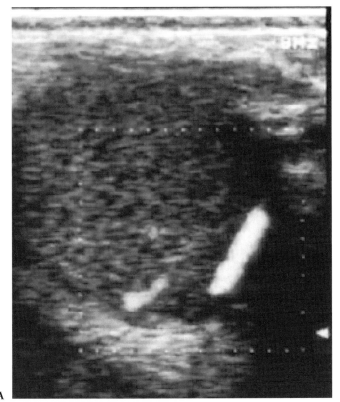

Figures 12.24. Acute left testicle torsion. Sagittal images of patient's testicles 3 hours after onset of acute left testicular pain. Note power color Doppler flow in the unaffected right testicle (**A**) compared to the absence of flow in the color gate for the left testicle with superior reactive hydrocele (**B**). (See color insert.)

testicular torsion with a stat urology consult for operative detorsion. Operative findings confirmed a testicular torsion with bell-clapper deformity requiring bilateral surgical repair.

REFERENCES

1. Mueller DL, Amundson GM, Rubin SZ, et al. Acute scrotal abnormalities in children: diagnosis by combined sonography and scintigraphy. *AJR Am J Roentgenol.* 1988;150:643–646.
2. Nussbaum Blask AR, Bulas D, Shalaby-Rana E, et al. Color Doppler sonography and scintigraphy of the testis: a prospective, comparative analysis in children with acute scrotal pain. *Pediatr Emerg Care.* 2002;18:67–71.
3. Kravchick S, Cytron S, Leibovici O, et al. Color Doppler sonography: its real role in the evaluation of children with highly suspected testicular torsion. *Eur Radiol.* 2001;11:1000–1005.
4. Weber DM, Rosslein R, Fliegel C. Color Doppler sonography in the diagnosis of acute scrotum in boys. *Eur J Pediatr Surg.* 2000;10:235–241.
5. Cook JL, Dewbury K. The changes seen on high-resolution ultrasound in orchitis. *Clin Radiol.* 2000;55:13–18.
6. Lerner RM, Mevorach RA, Hulbert WC, et al. Color Doppler US in the evaluation of acute scrotal disease. *Radiology.* 1990;176:355–358.
7. Sanelli PC, Burke BJ, Lee L. Color and spectral Doppler sonography of partial torsion of the spermatic cord. *AJR Am J Roentgenol.*1999;172:49–51.
8. Dogra VS, Sessions A, Mevorach RA, et al. Reversal of diastolic plateau in partial testicular torsion. *J Clin Ultrasound.* 2001;29:105–108.
9. Middleton WD, Middleton MA, Dierks M, et al. Sonographic prediction of viability in testicular torsion: preliminary observations. *J Ultrasound Med.* 1997;16:23–27.
10. Blaivas M, Sierzenski P. Emergency ultrasonography in the evaluation of the acute scrotum. *Acad Emerg Med.* 2001;8:85–89.
11. Blaivas M, Batts M, Lambert M. Ultrasonographic diagnosis of testicular torsion by emergency physicians. *Am J Emerg Med.* 2000;18:198–200.
12. Blaivas M, Sierzenski P, Lambert M. Emergency evaluation of patients presenting with acute scrotum using bedside ultrasonography. *Acad Emerg Med.* 2001;8:90–93.
13. Williamson, RC. Torsion of the testis and allied conditions. *Br J Surg.*1976;63:465–476.
14. Janetschek G, Schreckenberg F, Grimm W, et al. Hemodynamic effects of experimental testicular torsion. *Urol Res.* 1987;15:303–306.
15. Krone KD, Carroll BA. Scrotal Ultrasound. *Radiol Clin North Am.* 1985;23:121–139.
16. Hricak H, Lue T, Filly RA, et al. Experimental study of the the sonographic diagnosis of testicular torsion. *J Ultrasound Med.* 1983;2:349–356.
17. Knight PJ, Vassy LE. The diagnosis and treatment of the acute scrotum in children and adolescents. *Ann Surg.* 1984;200:664–673.
18. Rampaul MS, Hosking SW. Testicular torsion: most delays occur outside the hospital. *Ann R Coll Surg Engl.* 1998;80:169–172.
19. Witherington R. The 'acute' scrotum. Lesions that require immediate attention. *Postgrad Med.* 1987;82:207–216.
20. Selected Urologic Problems In: Rosen P, et al., eds. *Emergency Medicine Concepts and Clinical Practice.* 5th edition. St. Louis (MO): Mosby; 2002. 94:1422–1426.
21. Jeffrey RB, Laing FC, Hricak H, et al. Sonography of testicular trauma. *AJR Am J Roentgenol.* 1983;141:993–995.
22. Grantham JG, Charboneau JW, James EM, et al. Testicular neoplasms: 29 tumors studied by high-resolution ultrasound. *Radiology.* 1985;157:77–780.
23. Benson CB, Doubilet PM, Richie JP. Sonography of the male genital tract. *AJR Am J Roentgenol.* 1989;153:705–713.
24. Stewart R, Carroll B. The Scrotum. In: Rumack CM, Wilson SR, Charboneau JW, eds. *Diagnostic Ultrasound.* 2nd ed. St. Louis (MO): Mosby; 1998:791–821.
25. Dogra VS, Rubens DJ, Gottlieb RH, et al. Torsion and beyond: new twists in spectral Doppler evaluation of the scrotum. *J. Ultrasound Med.* 2004; 23:1077–1085.
26. Rivers KK, Rivers EP, Stricker HJ, et al. The clinical utility of serologic markers in the evaluation of the acute scrotum. *Acad Emerg Med.* 2000;7:1069–1072.
27. Korenkov M, Paul A, Troidl H. Color duplex sonography: diagnostic tool in the differentiation of inguinal hernias. *J Ultrasound Med.* 1999;18:565–568.
28. Ogata M, Imai S, Hosotani R, et al. Abdominal ultrasonography for the diagnosis of strangulation in small bowel obstruction. *Br J Surg.* 1994;81:421–424.

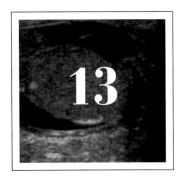

13

EMERGENT PROCEDURES

Robert S. Park
Jeffrey C. Metzger
Susan B. Promes

INTRODUCTION

Emergency ultrasound has been adapted for use in guiding a variety of diagnostic and therapeutic procedures. Traditionally many of these procedures have relied on external anatomical landmarks. The ability to visualize internal landmarks offers potential for improving the ease, efficiency, and safety of many procedures. This chapter describes techniques for the use of ultrasound guidance for a number of common procedures.

ADULT CENTRAL VENOUS ACCESS

CLINICAL APPLICATIONS

In the emergency department (ED), central venous catheter (CVC) insertion may be performed daily and is often a lifesaving procedure. Once established, CVCs can be used for fluid resuscitation, to administer inotropic and vasoactive medications, and to monitor central venous pressures. CVC insertion can aid the placement of a transvenous pacemaker. At times a CVC can serve simply as an alternative for venous access when peripheral venous access is limited. Blind central venous punctures guided only by external landmarks are associated with significant morbidity and rarely mortality. Failure rates for placement of CVCs have been reported to be 10% to 19% (1,2). Mechanical complication rates are reported to occur in 5% to 19% of patients (1–5). These complications are dependent upon the site chosen for insertion, nature of underlying disease (emphysema, bleeding dyscrasia, mechanical ventilation), patient anatomy, prior CVC insertion, and physician experience (1–3,6). The most common complications include arterial puncture, hematoma, and pneumothorax (1). Other reported complications include catheter malposition, adjacent nerve injury, artery or vein wall laceration, cardiac arrhythmias, hemothorax, chylothorax, pericardial tamponade, hemomediastinum, pneumomediastinum, air embolism, guidewire embolism, and death (6–12).

Traditionally CVCs have been inserted using "blind techniques" that rely on anatomical landmarks and their relationship to the underlying target vessel. More recently, real-time two-dimensional (2-D) ultrasound machines have been used to aid CVC insertion.

Advantages of 2-D ultrasound include exact localization of the target vein, visualization of the relationship of the target vein to the adjacent artery (13,14), detection of anatomic variations (15–17), avoidance of veins with preexisting thrombosis, and real-time guidance of the needle into the target vein. There have been numerous prospective, randomized, controlled trials revealing that real-time ultrasound guidance is superior to traditional landmark techniques (18–28). This literature has been critically evaluated with several meta-analyses (29–33). Real-time 2-D ultrasound improves catheter insertion success rates, reduces the number of venipuncture attempts prior to successful placement, and reduces the number of complications associated with catheter insertion (31). The strength of evidence has prompted the Agency for Healthcare Research and Quality (AHRQ) to publish a report stating that ultrasound-guided insertion of CVCs is a top 10 patient safety practice to prevent hospital iatrogenesis and is specifically among the practices " . . . most highly rated in terms of strength of evidence supporting more widespread implementation" (32). The National Institute of Clinical Excellence performed a technology appraisal for the United Kingdom's National Health Service that stated, " . . . the use of 2-D imaging ultrasound guidance should be considered in most clinical circumstances where CVC insertion is necessary either electively or in an emergency situation" (33).

IMAGE ACQUISITION

A 7.5- to 10-MHz linear array transducer is typically used for real-time ultrasound-guided CVC insertion. Other necessary components include a sterile ultrasound transducer sleeve, gel, and rubber bands (Fig. 13.1). Smaller and more portable ultrasound machines have been designed specifically for vascular access, but traditional cart-based ultrasound machines may be used for this purpose as well (Fig. 13.2). Ultrasound transducer needle guide attachments designed to ensure accurate insertion are available but not required (Fig. 13.3). These needle guides may be particularly helpful for novice ultrasound users until the freehand ultrasound technique has become completely familiar. Ultrasound images of central vessels may be obtained in either short or long axis depending on the orientation of the ultrasound transducer (Figs. 13.4–13.7). Ultrasound-guided needle insertion has been described using both approaches. In general, visualizing and subsequently accessing the target vessel in short axis has been shown in one study to be easier to learn for novice users, but either approach may be employed, depending on the site of access and the experience of the person performing the procedure (34).

Position the patient in usual fashion according to the desired anatomic approach. Position the ultrasound screen directly in front of the operator while performing the procedure. This allows smooth transitions between viewing the CVC insertion site and the ultrasound screen. Perform a brief nonsterile ultrasound scan of the CVC insertion site. Regardless of anatomic approach, there is typically a pair of nonechogenic blood vessels running side by side (Fig. 13.5A). The artery is usually rounder, smaller in diameter, and more

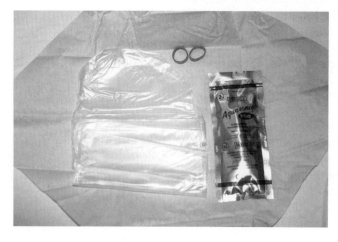

Figure 13.1. Sterile ultrasound transducer packet. Includes non-latex sleeve, rubber bands, and gel.

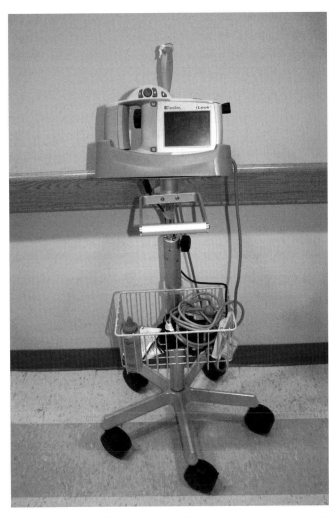

Figure 13.2. Handheld vascular ultrasound machine on a roll stand.

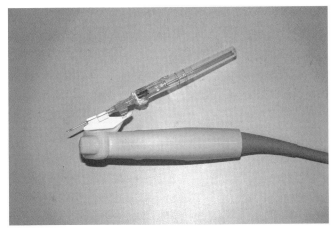

Figure 13.3. Ultrasound transducer needle guide attachment to ensure accurate placement.

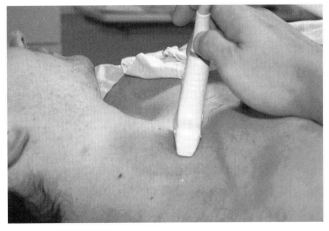

Figure 13.4. Transverse ultrasound transducer orientation of the right internal jugular vein and carotid artery.

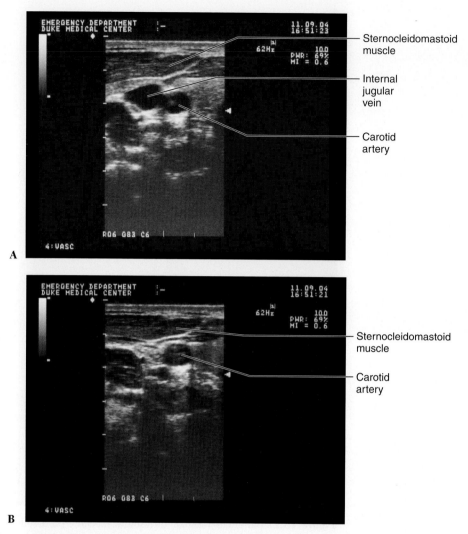

Sternocleidomastoid muscle

Internal jugular vein

Carotid artery

Sternocleidomastoid muscle

Carotid artery

Figure 13.5. **(A)** Corresponding ultrasound short axis view of the internal jugular vein and carotid artery. **(B)** Ultrasound short axis view of the internal jugular vein compressed with gentle transducer pressure. The carotid artery is patent.

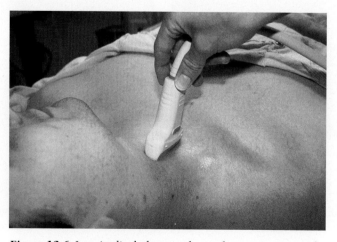

Figure 13.6. Longitudinal ultrasound transducer orientation of the right internal jugular vein.

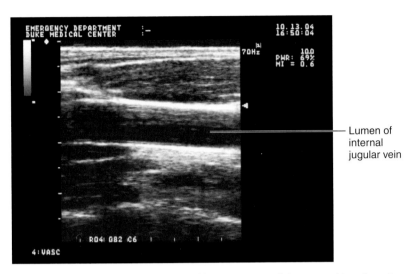

Figure 13.7. Corresponding ultrasound long axis view of the internal jugular vein.

prominently pulsatile. The central vein is larger, more irregular in shape, and has a subtle undulating pulsatile quality. Localize the vein definitively by applying gentle pressure with the ultrasound transducer. The vein should compress easily and completely, while the artery will stay patent (Fig. 13.5B). Prepare the ultrasound transducer for sterile use as shown in Figures 13.8–13.11. Apply a copious amount of ultrasound gel (sterile or nonsterile) directly to the transducer footprint. Slip the sterile sleeve over the transducer. Smooth all air bubbles away from the scanning surface to prevent imaging artifact. Secure the sleeve with rubber bands. Place sterile gel on the sleeved ultrasound transducer. An alternative sterile barrier can be made using a sterile glove. Nonsterile gel can be put inside the glove, followed by placing the glove over the transducer. The fingers of the glove can be folded over and held next to the base of the transducer so that the palmar surface of the glove becomes the scanning surface. Sterile gel is then placed on the outer surface of the glove to complete this rudimentary sterile cover.

ANATOMY AND LANDMARKS

Internal jugular vein approach
Place the patient in the Trendelenburg position with head turned contralaterally 30 degrees. Place the ultrasound transducer just superior to the clavicle between the two heads of the

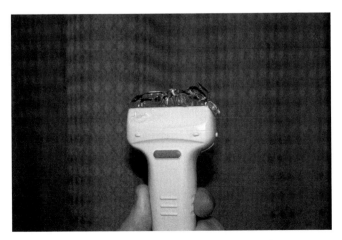

Figure 13.8. Ultrasound transducer with copious gel.

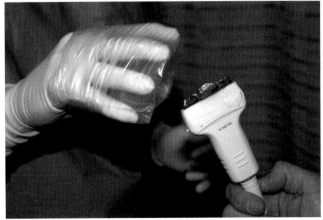

Figure 13.9. Rolled ultrasound transducer sleeve used to grab the transducer and maintain sterility.

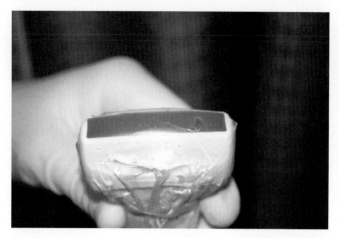

Figure 13.10. Transducer with air bubbles on the footprint that need smoothing away. Air bubbles cause significant imaging artifact.

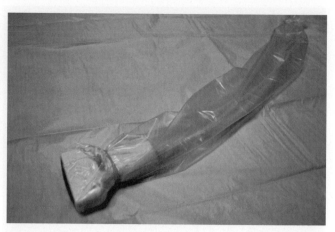

Figure 13.11. Ultrasound transducer with sterile sleeve in place.

sternocleidomastoid muscle (Fig. 13.12). The right internal jugular vein anatomy and corresponding normal ultrasound findings are shown in Figures 13.13–13.14. The internal jugular vein is anterior and lateral to the carotid artery with the widest diameter just superior to the clavicle. Scan the length of the vein from the clavicle to the thyroid cartilage taking into account the widest diameter, relationship to the carotid artery, and any variations of normal anatomy.

Subclavian vein approach (Axillary vein)

Place the patient in the Trendelenburg position with a small rolled towel between the shoulder blades. The patient's arm is abducted 90 degrees to straighten the axillary vessels. The axillary vein travels from the axillary fold to the lateral border of the first rib where it becomes the subclavian vein. The subclavian vein runs obliquely and posterior to the clavicle making ultrasound imaging of this vessel nearly impossible. The more distal axillary vein, on the other hand, is exposed for ultrasound examination. Place the ultrasound transducer just inferior to the most lateral aspect of the clavicle as in Figure 13.15. Right axillary vessel anatomy and corresponding ultrasound findings are depicted in Figures 13.16 and 13.17. With the transducer indicator directed toward the patient's head, the axillary vein is typically inferior to the axillary artery. Note that transducer pressure may not collapse the vein completely due to its slightly deeper location beneath the skin. The axillary vein will completely collapse when the patient inhales against a closed glottis; this technique should

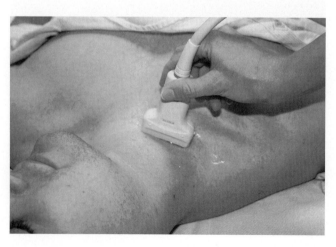

Figure 13.12. Internal jugular vein transducer placement. Transducer is placed just above the clavicle in between the two heads of the sternocleidomastoid.

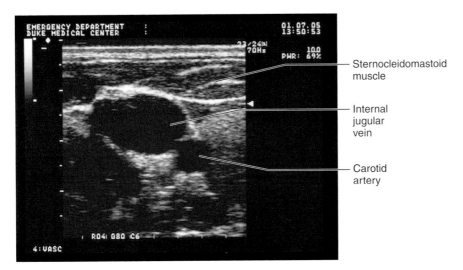

Figure 13.13. Corresponding ultrasound short axis views of the right internal jugular vein and carotid artery.

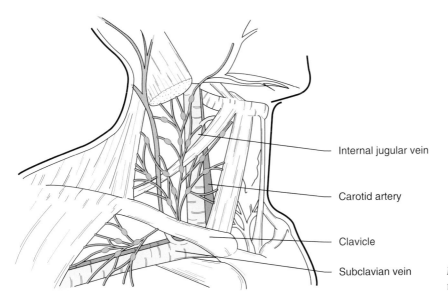

Figure 13.14. Corresponding anatomy of the right internal jugular vein and carotid artery.

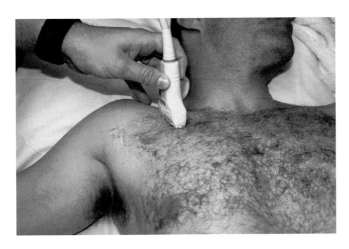

Figure 13.15. Axillary vein transducer placement for subclavian vein catheter insertion. Transducer is placed inferior to the most lateral aspect of the clavicle.

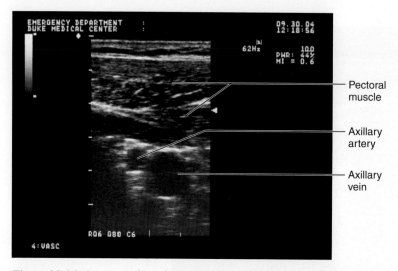

Figure 13.16. Corresponding ultrasound short axis views of the right axillary artery and vein. Note the increased depth of the vessels (3.5cm) with the pectoral muscle in the near field.

be used to identify the vein and ensure absence of thrombus (Fig. 13.18). As the axillary vein travels medially, it runs adjacent to the pleura of the lung (Fig. 13.19). To avoid pneumothorax, care must be taken to place the transducer several centimeters lateral to the thoracic cage. Alternatively, approaching the cannulation of the axillary vein in the long axis will allow for the tip of the needle to be identified through the entirety of its course, thereby avoiding puncturing the posterior vessel wall and entering the pleural space.

Femoral vein approach

The patient should be in the supine position. Place the ultrasound transducer transversely just inferior to the inguinal ligament (Fig. 13.20). The anatomy of the right femoral vessels and corresponding ultrasound images are shown in Figures 13.21 and 13.22. The femoral vein is just medial to the femoral artery at this level. As the femoral vessels course more

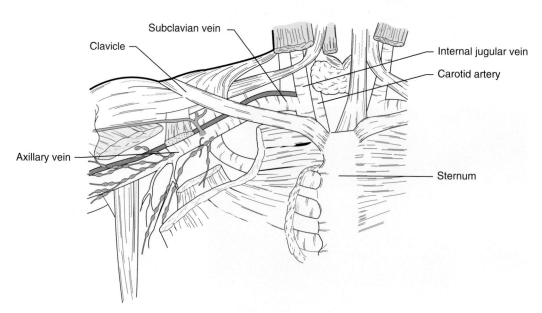

Figure 13.17. Corresponding anatomy of the axillary and subclavian vessels.

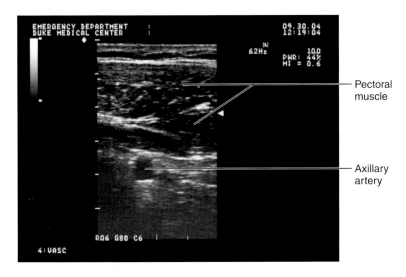

Pectoral
muscle

Axillary
artery

Figure 13.18. Complete collapse of the axillary vein. This is achieved by asking the patient to place a thumb in his/her mouth. Request the patient to breathe in through the imaginary straw. The negative inspiratory force achieved by inhaling against a closed glottis collapses the axillary vein.

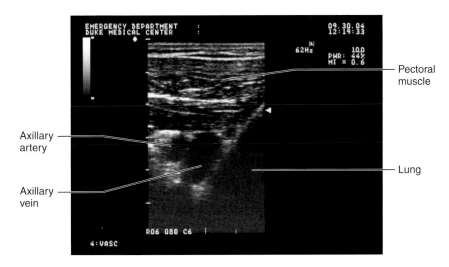

Pectoral
muscle

Axillary
artery

Axillary
vein

Lung

Figure 13.19. Ultrasound short axis views of the right axillary artery, vein, and lung. This is seen when the ultrasound transducer is placed several centimeters medial to the proper position. Note that the axillary vein is adjacent to lung and CVC insertion at this site is at risk for pneumothorax.

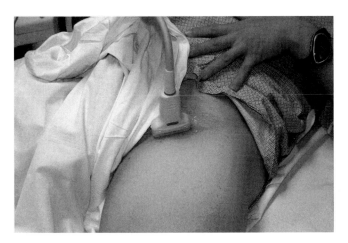

Figure 13.20. Femoral vein transducer placement. The transducer is placed just inferior to the inguinal ligament.

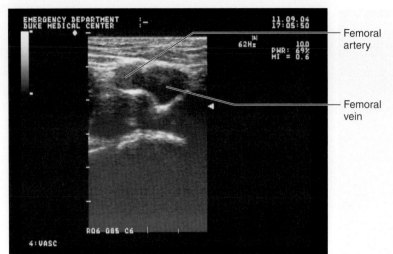

***Figure* 13.21.** Corresponding ultrasound short axis views of the femoral artery and vein.

distally in the leg, they migrate toward each other with the femoral artery usually anterior to the femoral vein. To avoid arterial puncture care must be taken to avoid an insertion site that is too distal from the inguinal ligament.

PROCEDURE

After completion of the brief nonsterile ultrasound scan, proper ultrasound and patient positioning, and sterile preparation of the ultrasound transducer and patient, the operator is ready to perform the procedure. Note that the procedure can be done with one or two operators. The following is a description of a one-operator procedure using the short axis approach. The ultrasound transducer should be held in the nondominant hand while the needle and syringe are in the other. Depending on the anatomic approach, use the

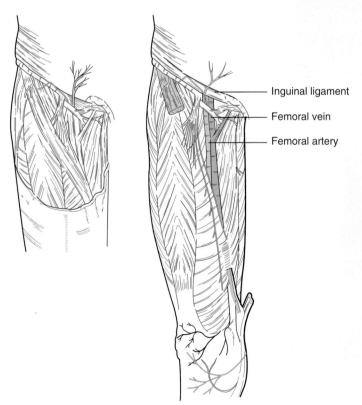

***Figure* 13.22.** Corresponding anatomy of the femoral vessels.

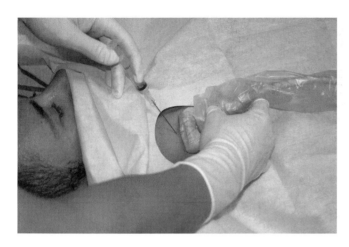

Figure 13.23. Internal jugular vein CVC insertion using real-time ultrasound guidance. Single operator procedure is depicted. Note the steeper needle trajectory than traditional landmark technique due to the more distal insertion site and closer proximity to lung.

landmarks described above and locate the vessels and optimal site of insertion. Once the target vessel is identified, center it on the ultrasound screen. The target vein is now beneath the center of the ultrasound transducer and its depth below the skin can be determined by using the measurement markers on the side of the ultrasound image. Using the center of the transducer as a reference, apply local anesthetic to the skin and proposed needle path, then insert the needle at a 45- to 60-degree angle (Fig. 13.23). The goal is to insert the needle at the correct angle and depth so that the tip of the needle intersects the segment of the vein that is directly under the transducer. This will allow visualization of needle entry into the vessel. Once the needle enters subcutaneous tissue, gently aspirate. As the needle is slowly advanced, look at the ultrasound screen, being careful not to slide the hand holding the ultrasound transducer. The needle may appear as a small brightly echogenic dot; however, the needle is not typically visualized on the ultrasound screen. Instead secondary markers of needle location are used. These include ring down artifact, acoustic shadowing, and buckling of the vein contour correlating with the needle entering the vessel (Fig. 13.24–13.26). If the acoustic shadow or ring down artifact is off-center of the vessel, slowly withdraw the needle and redirect appropriately. Free return of venous blood confirms vessel entry. Frequently the needle tip will traverse both the anterior and posterior walls of the vessel as the needle hits and buckles the vein. When this happens little or no flash of blood

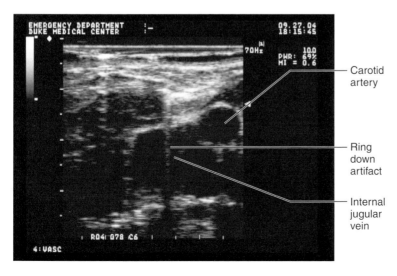

Carotid artery

Ring down artifact

Internal jugular vein

Figure 13.24. Ring down artifact. This artifact is created by the needle and can be used as a marker for where the needle is located relative to the target vessel. Here the artifact is directly centered over the internal jugular vein.

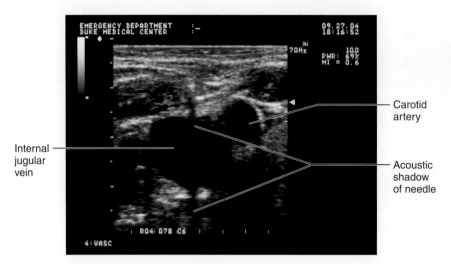

Figure 13.25. Acoustic shadow. This artifact is created by the needle, and can be used as a marker for where the needle is located relative to the target vessel. Here the artifact is directly centered over the internal jugular vein.

will occur. Using continued gentle aspiration, slowly withdraw the needle until the tip is pulled back into the lumen of the vessel, resulting in venous blood return. With free return of blood, the ultrasound transducer can be placed aside onto the sterile drape. Continue central line placement with the usual standard Seldinger technique.

PITFALLS

For the internal jugular vein approach, the transducer is located just a few centimeters away from the lung. Typically the widest diameter of the internal jugular vein is just superior to the clavicle. This location of needle insertion is much closer to the lung than the traditional landmark "central approach," which inserts the needle at the apex of the triangle formed by

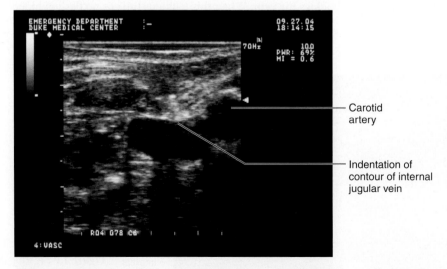

Figure 13.26. Buckling of the vein contour. This is created when the needle tip is entering the vessel. To actually visualize this, the needle tip has to enter the segment of blood vessel directly underneath the ultrasound transducer. Otherwise, the needle tip will enter a portion of the vein not "visualized" by the ultrasound.

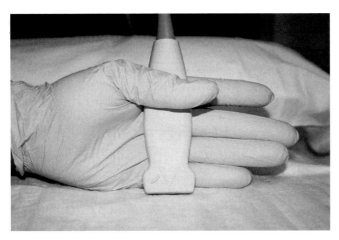 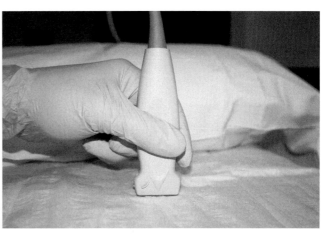

Figure 13.27. Proper technique to brace the ultrasound transducer during CVC insertion. By bracing the hand as well as the probe onto the patient's skin, subtle transducer drift is prevented.

Figure 13.28. Improper technique. Slippery ultrasound gel will cause transducer movement that will interfere with proper alignment of the target vessel.

the joining of the two heads of the sternocleidomastoid muscle. Hence, at the skin surface, the needle must be inserted steeply at a 45- to 60-degree angle in order to safely avoid the lung. Similarly, the axillary vein approach requires a lateral transducer placement to avoid puncture of the lung. Once the transducer is placed several centimeters lateral to the thoracic cage, introduction of the needle should be 45 to 60 degrees to avoid pneumothorax.

Real-time ultrasound allows the operator to visualize the needle advancing towards a target; however, when the initial insertion is off line the needle must be withdrawn and redirected. Ensure proper transducer orientation so that if redirection is necessary, adjustments are done in the proper direction.

Finally, a steady ultrasound transducer position is necessary throughout the entire procedure. Slippery ultrasound gel causes subtle drifts in transducer position that are detrimental to proper needle insertion. Rest both the hand and transducer onto the patient's body so that there is no drift of the transducer during the procedure; however, be careful not to place undue pressure that will collapse the target vessel during the procedure (Figs. 13.27, 13.28).

USE IN DECISION MAKING

Performing a brief nonsterile ultrasound scan of the proposed CVC insertion site before preparing a sterile field is extremely useful. This allows the operator to affirm normal anatomic relationships, ensure absence of thrombosis, and determine the optimal segment of the target vein for catheterization. This optimal segment, regardless of anatomic approach, is one where the vein has the largest diameter, least overlap of the adjacent artery, and no evidence of thrombosis. Any abnormality will often preclude insertion at the initial site and an alternate location should be chosen.

PERIPHERAL VENOUS ACCESS

CLINICAL APPLICATIONS

In the ED, establishing peripheral intravenous access can be challenging. Patients with peripheral edema, obesity, severe dehydration, intravenous drug abuse, and nonvisible, nonpalpable veins are all predisposed for this difficulty. Ultrasound guidance can be used to obtain peripheral venous catheter (PVC) insertion. This has best been shown in adult and pediatric studies describing ultrasound-guided placement of peripherally inserted central venous catheters (PICCs) in the vessels of the upper extremity (35–38). Ultrasound-guided PICCs are successfully placed by both physicians and nurses (39–41). PICCs are long small-caliber catheters inserted through a peripheral extremity vein and then positioned in the central circulation for long-term therapy with antibiotics, chemotherapy, or total parenteral nutrition. These same vessels of the upper extremity can be used for short-term vascular access in the ED with smaller catheters. One study using ultrasound guidance to cannulate the deep brachial or basilic vein showed a 91% success rate with 73% of these achieved on the first attempt. Complications included brachial artery puncture (2%), brachial nerve irritation (1%), and catheter dislodgement or intravenous fluid infiltration (8%) (42). This ultrasound-guided technique is a safe, rapid, and successful method of gaining peripheral intravenous access when traditional methods fail.

Image Acquisition

A 7.5-to 10-MHz linear array transducer is used to perform the procedure. Because this is peripheral intravenous access, a sterile sleeve, gel, and povidone-iodine are not required for this procedure. Ultrasound transducer needle guide attachments designed to ensure accurate insertion are available but not required (Fig. 13.3). Ultrasound images of the vessels may be obtained in either short or long axis depending on the orientation of the ultrasound transducer. Position the ultrasound screen directly in front of the operator while performing the procedure. This allows smooth transitions between viewing the PVC insertion site and the ultrasound screen.

Anatomy and Landmarks

The patient is placed supine with the upper extremity abducted exposing the anteromedial aspect of the upper arm. Place a tourniquet on the upper extremity as close to the axilla as possible. The ultrasound transducer is placed transversely and the vessels from the antecubital fossa to the proximal humerus are scanned. A reliable image pattern seen at the midhumerus is depicted in Figure 13.29A. In the far field is the hyperechoic cortical rim of the humerus. Anterior to the humerus are several round anechoic vessels in short axis cross section. These are the deep brachial veins on either side of the brachial artery and the more superficial basilic vein. The corresponding anatomy is depicted in Figure 13.30. Veins can be identified by applying gentle pressure on the transducer, which causes complete collapse of these vessels, compared to the noncollapsible artery

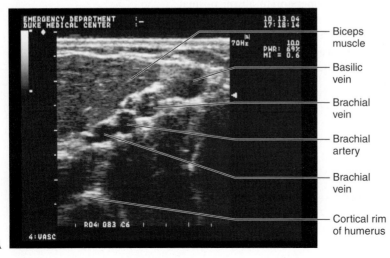

Figure 13.29. (A) Ultrasound image of the short axis views of the two brachial veins, brachial artery, and basilic vein. Note that the basilic is typically larger in diameter, closer to the skin, and has no corresponding artery.

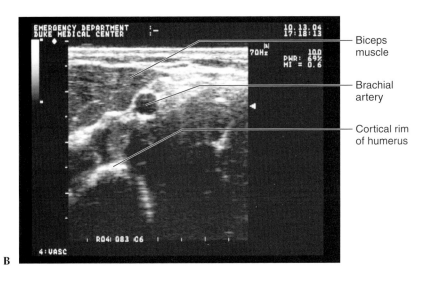

Biceps
muscle

Brachial
artery

Cortical rim
of humerus

B

Figure **13.29.** *(continued)* (B) Ultrasound image showing complete collapse of the two brachial veins and basilic vein. Only the brachial artery remains patent when gentle transducer pressure is used to compress the vessels. Note the hyperechoic cortical rim of the humerus in the far field. This is a useful reference to find the blood vessels which typically course several centimeters superficial to it.

(Fig. 13.29B). By scanning the entire length of the upper arm, one can find the ideal insertion site. This is the segment of vein that has the largest diameter, is away from an adjacent artery, is closest to the skin surface, and travels a straight course. Sometimes the cephalic vein, located anterolaterally, is also a suitable option. Like the basilic, the cephalic vein has no adjacent nerve or artery (43).

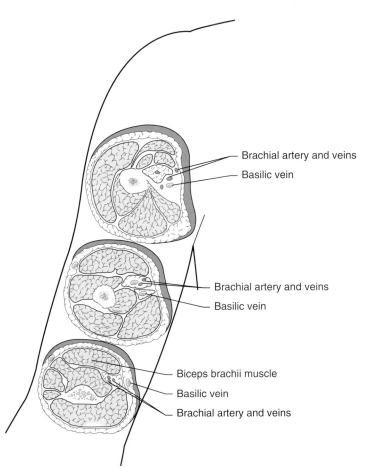

Brachial artery and veins
Basilic vein

Brachial artery and veins
Basilic vein

Biceps brachii muscle
Basilic vein
Brachial artery and veins

Figure **13.30.** Corresponding anatomy of the vessels located at the midhumerus. Redrawn from Netter, F.H., *Atlas of Human Anatomy,* 2d ed. (East Hanover, NJ: Novartis Medical Education, 1997, plate 410.)

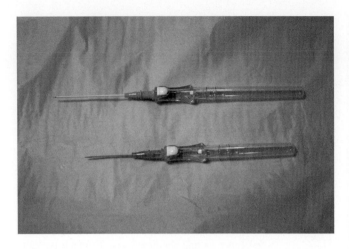

Figure 13.31. Longer 1.88-inch angiocatheter used for brachial or basilic vein cannulation adjacent to usual peripheral IV angio-catheter.

Procedure

It is important to note that regular PVCs are too short for this ultrasound-guided technique. At least a 1.88-inch angiocath, shown in Figure 13.31, is required due to the increased depth of the vein. Shorter catheters used for most peripheral lines are unable to reach or stay within the lumen of the vein. This procedure can be done with one or two operators. The following is a description of a one-operator procedure using the short axis approach. Once the target vein and ideal insertion site have been identified, the operator holds the ultrasound transducer in the nondominant hand and the needle in the other. Center the vessel on the ultrasound screen. The target vein is now beneath the center of the ultrasound transducer and its depth below the skin can be determined by using the measurement markers on the side of the ultrasound image. Local anesthetic can be applied to the skin and proposed needle path using the center of the transducer as a reference. Again using the center of the ultrasound transducer as a reference, insert the needle at a 30- to 45-degree angle (Fig. 13.32). The goal is to insert the needle at the correct angle and depth so that the tip of the needle intersects the segment of the vein that is directly under the transducer. This will allow visualization of needle entry into the vessel. As the needle is slowly advanced, look at the ultrasound screen, being careful not to slide the hand holding the ultrasound transducer. The needle may appear as a small brightly echogenic dot (Fig. 13.33); however, the needle is not typically visualized on the ultrasound screen. Instead, secondary markers of needle location are used. These include ring down artifact, acoustic shadowing, and buckling of the vein

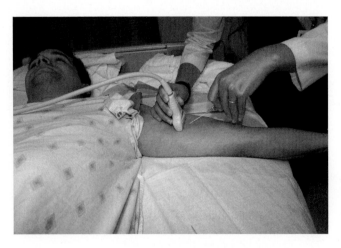

Figure 13.32. Peripheral venous catheter placement using real-time ultrasound guidance. Note that the arm is supinated providing access to the medial aspect of the upper arm. Note that this is not a sterile procedure given that this is a peripheral IV placement.

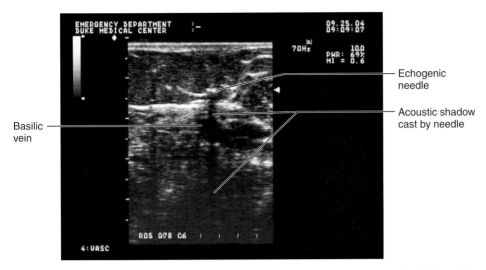

Figure 13.33. Ultrasound of basilic vein in short axis view. Note the echogenic dot of the needle with acoustic shadow cast down the center of the vein.

contour correlating with needle entering the vessel (Fig. 13.34). If the acoustic shadow or ring down artifact is off-center of the vessel, slowly withdraw the needle and redirect appropriately. When free returning blood flash confirms vessel entry, the ultrasound transducer can be placed to the side. Slide the plastic angiocatheter sheath over the needle. After withdrawal of the needle, ensure proper catheter placement with obvious free flow of blood and infusion of saline without infiltration.

PITFALLS

Sometimes as the angiocatheter hits and buckles the vein the needle tip will traverse both the anterior and posterior walls of the vessel. When this happens blood flash might occur but, after advancing the plastic sheath, there will be no free return of blood because the catheter is not in the lumen. In this case do not remove the indwelling catheter. Instead attach a saline-filled syringe to the catheter. Using continued gentle aspiration, slowly

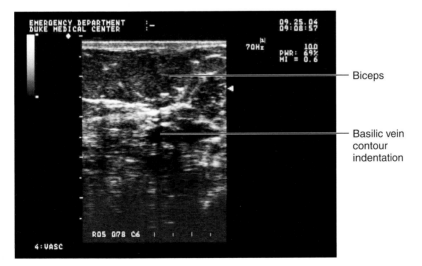

Figure 13.34. Ultrasound of basilic vein contour buckling. This corresponds to the needle tip entering vein.

withdraw the catheter until the tip is pulled back into the lumen of the vessel, resulting in venous blood return. As soon as there is free return of blood, stop withdrawal and carefully advance the catheter in the direction of proper vein placement.

A second pitfall to avoid involves intravenous line infiltration. Make sure to take down the tourniquet prior to flushing the peripheral line just placed. This simple mistake will frequently result in a ruptured vessel and a nonworking line. Alternatively, this approach can be attempted without using a tourniquet, but the veins are much more likely to collapse with either transducer pressure or the advancing catheter.

USE IN DECISION MAKING

All physicians and nurses in the ED have encountered patients who have difficult peripheral intravenous access. Often, these patients are not critically ill and simply need intravenous fluid, medication, or possibly an imaging study that requires intravenous contrast. Each of these situations requires venous access. When venous access is challenging clinicians may use CVCs or venous cutdowns, both relatively invasive procedures for short-term access needs. Ultrasound-guided PVC insertion is an extremely useful safe alternative that, in many instances, obviates the need for more invasive procedures and their associated risks.

ARTHROCENTESIS

CLINICAL APPLICATIONS

Arthrocentesis can be a useful diagnostic and therapeutic procedure in the emergency setting. Unfortunately, it is often done on a joint that is swollen and tender, making the use of bony landmarks difficult. Ultrasound guidance helps locate the bony landmarks and may indicate the part of the joint that has the most fluid, increasing the success rate while decreasing the chance of complications and injury from misplaced needles. There are several locations amenable to ultrasound-guided arthrocentesis. Large joints such as the hip, shoulder, knee, or ankle and smaller joints like the elbow or interphalangeal joint may all be aspirated under ultrasound guidance.

IMAGE ACQUISITION

When performing arthrocentesis, a linear array, high-frequency (5 to 10 MHz) transducer is usually preferred, although deep joints such as the hips may require a lower frequency (3 to 5 MHz) for greater tissue penetration. It is important to point out that small or superficial effusions may be masked by applying too much pressure to the transducer, therefore gentle pressure may allow better image acquisition and more precise localization of the largest fluid collection.

HIP ARTHROCENTESIS

ANATOMY AND LANDMARKS

The most common approach to the hip is the anterior approach (44–50). The attempted view is an oblique sagittal plane parallel to the long axis of the femoral neck. With the patient supine, slightly flex and internally rotate the hip. This relaxes the anterior portion of the joint capsule allowing fluid to collect within the anterior recess. Palpate the greater trochanter. The femoral neck should follow an imaginary line from the greater trochanter towards a point on the abdomen just above the pubic symphysis.

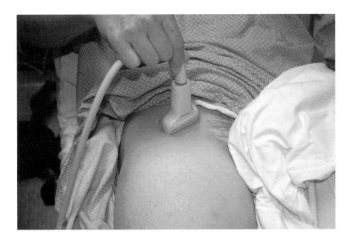

Figure 13.35. Placement of the transducer for hip ultrasound.

Place the transducer on this imaginary line with the transducer indicator pointing superomedially as seen in Figure 13.35. The femoral head can be seen as a large curved hyperechoic structure (Fig. 13.36). There should also be a thin hypoechoic stripe over the articular portion of the femoral head. This is the articular cartilage. The joint capsule is a thick hyperechoic band that runs from the acetabular rim to the distal femoral neck, running over the femoral head and proximal portions of the neck. The area just distal to the femoral head and anterior to the femoral neck is the anterior recess. While several criteria exist for the diagnosis of joint effusion, most sources cite an effusion of more than 5 to 6 mm or a 2-mm difference when compared with the contralateral side to be clinically significant (45,48,50).

PROCEDURE

Once the anterior recess has been identified, the anterior thigh and groin area should be prepped using povidone-iodine or chlorhexidine and a sterile sleeve placed over the transducer. Local anesthesia should be used for patient comfort. Insertion of the needle can be done freehand or through the use of a needle guide attached to the transducer. An 18- or 20-gauge spinal needle is visualized as it advances through the soft tissue and into the joint capsule.

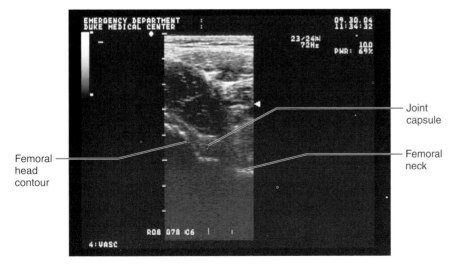

Figure 13.36. Ultrasound of the hip along the long axis of the femoral neck. Note the femoral head on the left side of the picture and the femoral neck on the right, as well as the hyperechoic joint capsule just superficial.

PITFALLS

Several pitfalls exist in ultrasound-guided hip arthrocentesis. The articular cartilage is seen as a thin hypoechoic stripe over the femoral head that can be mistaken for an effusion. It is important to make sure the effusion is noted to extend along the entire length of the femoral head and neck. Doppler ultrasound of the femoral vessels may be useful to locate and identify them to avoid injury during the procedure.

KNEE ARTHROCENTESIS

ANATOMY AND LANDMARKS

Several approaches can be used for the sonographic evaluation of the knee. The posterior approach is used for diagnostic ultrasound of pathology within the popliteal fossa such as a Baker's cyst, but should not be used for arthrocentesis given the number of important blood vessels and nerves that run in this area (48). The anterior approach is used for arthrocentesis. Begin by having the patient lay supine with a rolled towel placed behind the knee to flex it slightly. Start by palpating the patella and placing the transducer longitudinally on the proximal edge in the midline of the patella, with the orientation marker pointing cephalad (Fig. 13.37). It is important to apply gentle pressure to avoid compressing the bursa and thereby masking a small effusion. The suprapatellar bursa lies just deep to the quadriceps tendon. It is important to point out that the suprapatellar bursa is a synovial bursa and is in direct communication with the knee joint, therefore fluid within this space implies a knee effusion. The suprapatellar bursa is normally seen as a thin hypoechoic line outlined by fat pads on either side. If this line is greater than 2 mm it is considered abnormal. Figures 13.38 and 13.39 show the ultrasound findings of a normal knee and a large effusion. The prepatellar bursa is different in that it has no communication with the joint. Sliding the transducer to the medial and lateral sides of the patella will often provide the best picture and help locate the largest fluid collection (48,51).

PROCEDURE

Locate the largest fluid collection on either side of the patella. In general, the needle should be aimed at the posterior surface of the patella and the femoral intercondylar notch. A small amount of local anesthetic can be applied to minimize patient discomfort. There are two

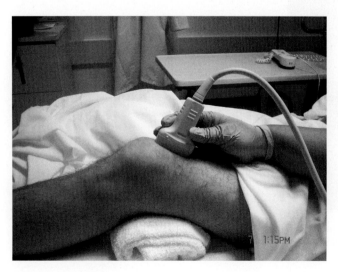

Figure 13.37. Placement of the transducer for knee ultrasound using the suprapatellar approach.

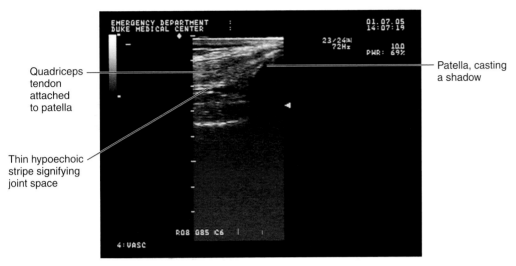

Figure 13.38. Ultrasound of a suprapatellar view of a normal knee. The thin hypoechoic stripe below the quadriceps tendon should be no thicker than 2mm.

ways the joint can be accessed. One method involves prepping the joint with povidone-iodine, using a sterile sleeve over the transducer, and performing the arthrocentesis under ultrasound guidance. The other option is to find the landmarks with the transducer, mark where the needle will be placed with four tic marks, and then prep the site and perform the arthrocentesis as if the landmarks were found by palpation alone.

PITFALLS

There are several sites that can be chosen for knee arthrocentesis. Going superior to the joint and angling behind the patella and toward the femoral intercondylar notch is the most common and safest approach. Moving the insertion point more caudad increases the likelihood of injury to the medial or lateral meniscus. It is also important to avoid damaging the delicate and highly innervated cartilaginous surfaces of the knee.

Finally, fluid adjacent to the suprapatellar region without demonstrable fluid within the joint may signify a muscle rupture and aspiration should not be attempted (48).

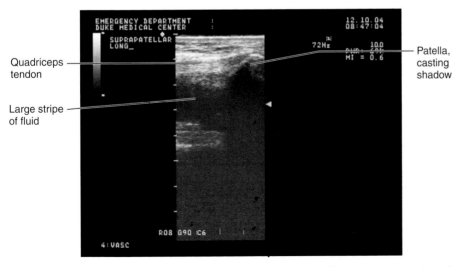

Figure 13.39. Ultrasound of a suprapatellar view of large knee effusion. Note the enlarged hypoechoic stripe beneath the quadriceps tendon. The hypoechoic stripe of the effusion is interrupted by the acoustic shadow cast by the patella on the right side of the image.

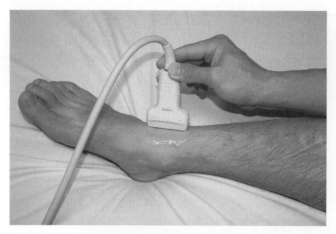

Figure 13.40. Transducer placement for ultrasound of the ankle. The patient is plantar flexed to help open the anterior joint space.

ANKLE ARTHROCENTESIS

ANATOMY AND LANDMARKS

The ankle joint can be assessed from an anterior or a posterior approach but, like the knee, only the anterior approach is amenable to arthrocentesis. With the patient lying supine, plantar flex the foot. Scan the anterior surface of the tibia in a longitudinal plane with the transducer indicator pointing cephalad (Fig. 13.40). Center the transducer over the tibia and move distally. The distal articular portion of the tibia will be seen going deep into the ankle, and the articular surface of the talus will come into view (Fig. 13.41). These two surfaces will form a hypoechoic triangular or v-shaped recess which represents the synovial fluid within the tibiotalar joint (52). There is commonly fluid within this tibiotalar recess and its presence or amount does not always suggest pathology (48,51,53).

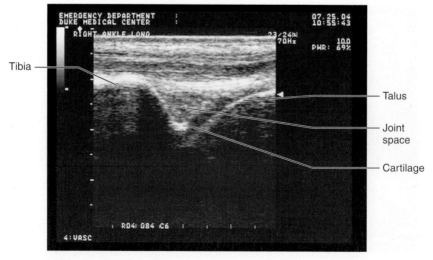

Tibia —

Talus

Joint space

Cartilage

Figure 13.41. Ultrasound of the anterior ankle. The distal tibia is more square while the talus is more rounded with a thin hypoechoic stripe representing cartilage. There is a small amount of fluid in this normal ankle.

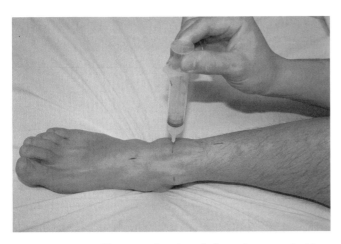

Figure 13.42. Ankle prepped and ready for arthrocentesis. Note the tic marks to identify the puncture site as well as the plantar flexion.

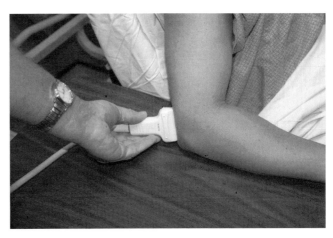

Figure 13.43. Patient positioning and transducer placement for elbow ultrasound. Note that the hand is prone and the elbow bent.

PROCEDURE

Scanning medially and laterally through the tibiotalar joint will allow for the location and amount of fluid to be identified. Once the transducer is centered over the largest fluid collection, mark the location using four tic marks in a superior/inferior and medial/lateral distribution. The transducer is then removed and the ankle is prepped with povidone-iodine. Local anesthetic should be injected to minimize patient discomfort. Maintain plantar flexion to help open the joint. The arthrocentesis can then be performed using the tic marks to guide needle insertion as if the landmarks had been found by palpation alone (Fig. 13.42).

PITFALLS

As with other approaches to arthrocentesis, care should be taken to avoid damaging the articular cartilage of the joint during insertion of the needle. Doppler ultrasound of the anterior portion of the joint should also be done to locate the dorsalis pedis artery and veins. It should also be noted that the deep peroneal nerve runs in proximity to the dorsalis pedis vessels therefore, this area should be avoided. The superficial peroneal nerve runs on the anterolateral aspect of the ankle and should be avoided as well. Lastly, care should be taken to avoid damage to the tibialis anterior tendon anteromedially, extensor hallucis longus anteriorly, and extensor digitorum longus, and peroneus tertius tendons laterally.

ELBOW ARTHROCENTESIS

ANATOMY AND LANDMARKS

A posterior approach is used to obtain synovial fluid from the elbow. Have the patient sit upright with the elbow and palm resting on a Mayo stand or another form of support. Place the transducer on the posterior aspect of the humerus just above the olecranon with the transducer indicator toward the shoulder (Fig. 13.43). This will give a longitudinal view of the humerus. As the transducer is moved distally, the cortex of the humerus will be visualized, followed by the olecranon fossa, and then the cortex of the olecranon will come into view (Fig. 13.44). A fluid collection here will be seen as a hypoechoic area against the distal humerus within the olecranon fossa (48,51).

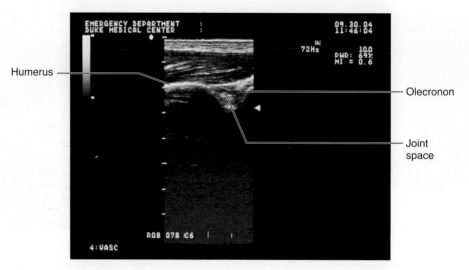

Figure 13.44. Ultrasound of the elbow. The distal humerus in seen on the left side of the screen, and part of the olecranon is on the far right. The v-shaped joint space is seen between these two structures.

PROCEDURE

Locate the fluid collection as described above and place tic marks on the skin that identify the tip of the olecranon and the humerus. Because the ulnar nerve courses over the medial epicondyle and runs medial to the trochlea and olecranon, needle insertion for arthrocentesis should be performed as far laterally as possible to avoid damage to this nerve. Cleanse the area with povidone-iodine and inject the area where the needle will be inserted with local anesthetic. Advance the needle for arthrocentesis into the joint space just over the olecranon, being careful to keep the syringe in a line parallel to the radius and ulna.

PITFALLS

The most significant pitfall in performing this procedure is inserting the needle too far medially and subsequently damaging the ulnar nerve. It is also important to use gentle pressure when placing the ultrasound transducer to avoid compressing the bursa and masking an effusion.

SHOULDER ARTHROCENTESIS

ANATOMY AND LANDMARKS

Ultrasound of the shoulder can be done from an anterior approach or a posterior approach. Fluid typically collects in the posterior aspect of the glenohumeral joint first, but the anterior approach is most commonly used for arthrocentesis (45). Both approaches will be described here.

For a posterior approach, the patient should be seated comfortably with the ipsilateral hand positioned on the contralateral shoulder to help open up the joint space. Place the transducer in a transverse orientation over the approximate area of the infraspinatus tendon just below the angle of the acromion. The curved echogenic cortex of the humeral head will be seen against the more flat glenoid rim. There should be a relatively thick hypoechoic stripe just below the skin, with a hyperechoic stripe just under this. These are the deltoid and infraspinatus tendons, respectively. Fluid within the joint will appear as an anechoic

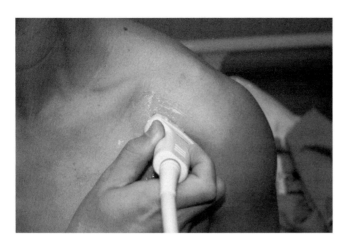

Figure 13.45. Transducer placement for anterior shoulder ultrasound. The transducer is placed to get a longitudinal view of the glenohumeral joint.

or hypoechoic area just below the infraspinatus tendon. A significant effusion is noted if the infraspinatus tendon is elevated more than 2 mm from the glenoid labrum (48).

The anterior approach is done while the patient is sitting upright with the arm down by the side and the palm of the hand resting comfortably in the lap. Palpate the coracoid process and place the transducer just inferior and lateral to the tip of the coracoid (Fig. 13.45). Images should be obtained in longitudinal and transverse orientations. The transducer indicator should be directed cephalad and to the patient's right side. The curved echogenic cortex of the humeral head will be seen against the more flat anterior portion of the glenoid, with a hypoechoic region between the two representing fluid within the joint space (Fig. 13.46). Internal and external rotation of the humeral head may help confirm the sonographic anatomy, as the head of the humerus will be seen to move while the glenoid remains still. An alternative approach is to perform the procedure with the patient lying supine. The arm is still placed at the patient's side, but the hand is now rested on the chest.

PROCEDURE

Locate the joint space as described in the previous section. Mark the location with tic marks and prep the joint with povidone-iodine. Inject a small amount of local anesthetic and then insert the needle in the center of the marks, directing it just lateral to the glenoid rim. The

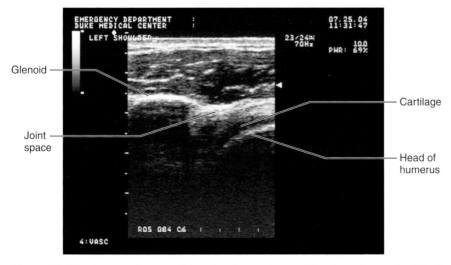

Figure 13.46. Ultrasound image of the glenohumeral joint. The glenoid is on the left of the screen, and the head of the humerus on the right. Internal and external rotation of the joint helps confirm the anatomy.

procedure can also be performed under ultrasound guidance by prepping the site with povidone-iodine and using a sterile sleeve on the transducer. Locate the joint space and insert the needle just lateral to the glenoid rim.

PITFALLS

With the arm abducted, the majority of major nerves and blood vessels course well inferior to the glenohumeral joint and are unlikely to be injured. Adduction of the shoulder pulls these structures superiorly and increases the chance of damage. The acromial branch of the thoracoacromial artery travels superior to the coracoid and then inferior to the acromion, and may be injured if the needle is inserted too far superiorly. This is another area where gentle pressure is necessary to avoid compressing the bursa and masking an effusion.

THORACENTESIS

CLINICAL APPLICATIONS

The presence of fluid in the pleural space is a common clinical entity. Ultrasound is ideal for identifying pleural effusions as well as facilitating fluid removal for diagnostic and therapeutic purposes. Thoracentesis performed under ultrasound guidance has a lower complication rate than thoracentesis performed blindly. Two recent studies found pneumothorax rates as low as 1.3% to 2.5% in patients who had ultrasound-guided thoracentesis (54,55). In contrast, studies of patients who have undergone traditional thoracentesis without ultrasound guidance have demonstrated a 4% to 30% incidence of pneumothorax (56–59). In addition to identifying fluid, ultrasound can identify other abnormalities accounting for findings on chest radiographs such as atelectasis, consolidation, masses, or an elevated hemidiaphragm.

IMAGE ACQUISITION

Pleural effusions are frequently detected on images obtained during abdominal scanning. The fluid appears as an echofree space cephalad to the hyperechoic line of the diaphragm when scanning from the mid- or posterior axillary line in the right and left upper quadrants. In this position, the liver and spleen act as excellent acoustic windows, so the fluid can usually be seen easily. Interestingly, it is also possible for ultrasound to detect subpulmonic effusions that may not be detected on plain chest radiographs (60). Occasionally the character of the fluid may appear differently from other forms of free fluid. For instance, internal echoes may be present in the effusion. This echogenicity may be homogeneous, which occurs with proteinaceous or highly cellular effusions, or heterogeneous as is the case with septate effusions or pleural metastases. When looking for pleural fluid, it is important to appreciate dynamic changes associated with the patient's respiratory cycle such as alterations in the shape of the echofree fluid with inspiration and expiration, compressed lung, and swirling of fluid with the patient's breathing.

PROCEDURE

Technique with patient sitting upright

The patient should be directed to sit upright facing away from the physician performing the procedure. Place a 3.5-MHz transducer on the patient's posterior hemithorax in the transverse orientation in between the ribs (Fig. 13.47). The pleural effusion will appear as a dependent hypoechoic fluid collection above the diaphragm (Fig. 13.48). Scan the relevant hemithorax from the paravertebral region to the anterior axillary line observing the fluid collection during normal breathing. Once the fluid collection is identified and

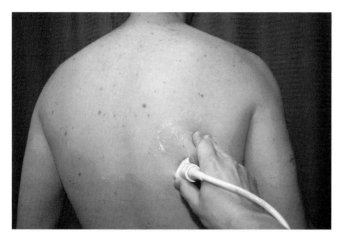

Figure 13.47. Transducer placement for thoracentesis with patient sitting upright.

well delineated, mark the area on the chest and note how deeply you will need to insert the needle in order to reach the fluid. This spot is typically located along the midscapular line. Once the area has been identified, prepare the patient using standard aseptic technique for a thoracentesis. Proceed with the procedure after removing the ultrasound transducer.

Technique with patient in a lateral decubitus position

Begin with the patient lying on the side facing away from the person performing the procedure. The hemithorax with the pleural effusion should be positioned down against the patient's bed. With the patient in this position, the effusion can be seen layering out in a dependent position in the horizontal plane parallel to the bed. Scan the midportion of the dependent hemithorax from the midscapular line to the edge of the bed to assess the size of the effusion. Once the fluid collection is identified and well delineated, mark the area on the chest wall where the fluid will be aspirated. This should generally be done no lower than the level of the 8th rib interspace. Remember to use caution to avoid the diaphragm as well as the intercostal vessels when aspirating fluid.

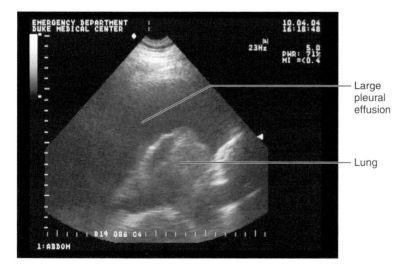

Large pleural effusion

Lung

Figure 13.48. Large right hypoechoic pleural effusion with lung floating in the far field.

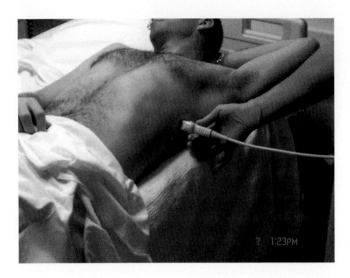

Figure 13.49. Transducer placement for thoracentesis with patient in supine position.

Technique with patient in a supine position

Have the patient lie flat on the back with the affected hemithorax facing the physician performing the procedure and close to the edge of the bed. The ipsilateral arm should be abducted and flexed at the elbow and positioned either over or under the patient's head (Fig. 13.49). Scan the patient's anterior and lateral chest from the midclavicular line to posterior axillary line looking for hypoechoic fluid (Fig. 13.50). Once the fluid collection is identified and well delineated, mark the area on the chest wall where the fluid will be aspirated. Special care must be used when performing the procedure on the left hemithorax to identify the heart and stay clear from this area.

Real-time ultrasound guidance

If you choose to perform the procedure using continuous real-time ultrasound guidance, position the patient and identify the effusion with ultrasound, then prepare the transducer with a sterile glove or sheath. Remember to place conductive gel on the inside and outside of the sterile covering. Insert the needle immediately above a rib in the area where the fluid has been identified. The needle can be seen as a hyperechoic streak on the ultrasound screen.

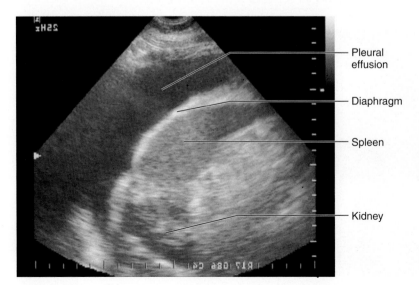

Figure 13.50. Large left pleural effusion with hypoechoic fluid above the diaphragm, spleen, and kidney.

PITFALLS

When selecting the optimal insertion site, it is important to avoid vital structures. By choosing an entry site with a clear path to the effusion, the lungs are typically avoided because the ultrasound image is obscured when there is underlying air. One must be careful not to enter the chest wall too low and damage intraperitoneal organs such as the liver or spleen. One must also be careful to avoid the neurovascular bundle which runs along the inferior edge of each rib. Occasionally, despite good visualization it is possible to cause an iatrogenic pneumothorax. Although possible, it is probably much less likely to cause a vascular injury.

PARACENTESIS

CLINICAL APPLICATIONS

There are two general reasons for performing a paracentesis — therapeutic and diagnostic. In the ED, a paracentesis is frequently performed as a therapeutic modality to relieve abdominal distension due to ascites when alcoholic, cancer, or liver-failure patients present with cardiopulmonary distress or abdominal pain. Paracentesis can also be performed for diagnostic purposes in a patient presenting with new onset ascites or to rule out infection in a patient with known ascites.

IMAGE ACQUISITION

Ascitic fluid may not always be apparent on physical examination, but it is generally easily recognizable with the aid of abdominal ultrasound (61). The fluid within the peritoneal cavity will outline the intra-abdominal organs making them easily identifiable on ultrasound. The bowel can be seen floating freely within the abdominal cavity (Fig. 13.51) but one must not mistake a bowel obstruction with fluid seen filling the bowel for free intraperitoneal fluid. As well, the location of the bladder should be noted. Although typically the patient is encouraged to void or a Foley catheter is placed to avoid injuring the bladder during a blind paracentesis, this is probably not absolutely necessary when using ultrasound guidance, because the physician can see the bladder and avoid it when inserting the needle. Sonography should be performed with a 3.5-MHz transducer. Before prepping the skin with povidone-iodine, the ultrasound transducer should be placed on the lower abdomen to localize a large pocket of fluid.

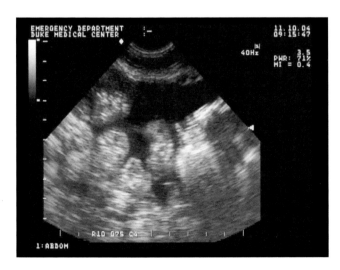

Figure 13.51. Loops of bowel floating in hypoechoic ascites. Note that this is a good site for insertion given bowel and other organs are not located in the near field closest to skin and needle insertion.

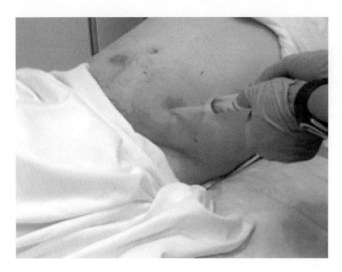

Figure 13.52. Paracentesis using left lower quadrant approach. The best ascites pocket is located using ultrasound and marked. Without moving the patient, the area is prepped in usual sterile fashion (no drape for illustration purposes).

PROCEDURE

The ascites should be confirmed and the largest pocket of fluid identified and marked for paracentesis (Fig. 13.52). The paracentesis should then be performed using sterile technique as one would typically do, but using the marked area as the location where the needle is inserted. If one prefers, the entire procedure can be performed under direct ultrasound visualization using aseptic technique with the transducer covered with a sterile sheath. It is important to note that the continuous visualization of the procedure generally requires two people (one to hold the transducer and the other to perform the procedure) but sonographers with significant experience may be able to accomplish this task alone or with the help of commercially available needle guides. Once a pocket of fluid is identified, a needle is inserted immediately adjacent to the midportion of the transducer directed perpendicular to the skin (Fig. 13.53A). The needle tip can be seen tenting the skin before penetrating the internal aspect of the abdominal wall and then again as a hyperechoic shadow once it enters the anechoic fluid-filled abdominal cavity (Fig. 13.53B). Once the ascitic fluid has been aspirated, the transducer can be set aside and the procedure can be continued in usual fashion.

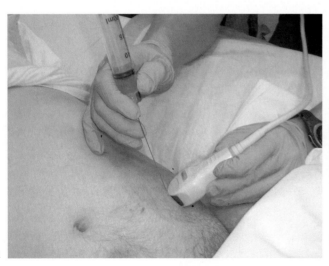

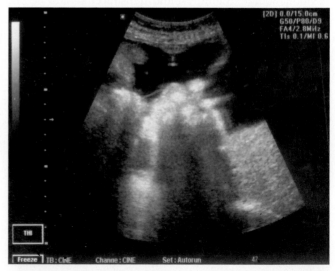

A   B

Figure 13.53. Paracentesis using real-time ultrasound guidance. Sterile transducer sleeve and drape excluded for illustration purposes in **A**. In **B**, an echogenic signal is seen where the needle enters the abdomen in a patient undergoing paracentesis for ascites.

PITFALLS

When a paracentesis is performed, one must take special care to avoid iatrogenic injury to intra-abdominal contents. The most common cause of nontraumatic ascites is cirrhosis and alcoholic liver disease. Some of these patients may have hepatomegaly. Ultrasound is particularly useful in this patient population to avoid damaging the enlarged liver. The use of ultrasound provides additional safety to minimize the chance of bowel and bladder perforation because these structures can be well-visualized with ultrasound (62). Another local complication of paracentesis is ascites fluid leaking from the puncture site. Tracking the needle horizontally under the skin before puncturing the peritoneal cavity can minimize the possibility of a fluid leak. If there is a persistent leak, it can be corrected with a suture at the site.

PERICARDIOCENTESIS

CLINICAL APPLICATIONS

In the ED, patients with pericardial effusions exhibiting tamponade or impending hemodynamic instability have been traditionally managed by blind percutaneous puncture of the pericardium for the removal of fluid. The usual method is the insertion of a needle via the subxiphoid approach. This blind technique has been associated with morbidity and mortality rates as high as 50% and 19%, respectively (63–68). Complications include right ventricular puncture, pneumothorax, pneumopericardium, liver puncture, and puncture of the coronary arteries. Despite the safeguards of electrocardiographic needle monitoring and fluoroscopic guidance, complication rates persist (63,67,68). Some authors have advocated the complete abandonment of the blind pericardial puncture technique because of the associated risks (69).

Two-dimensional (2-D) echocardiography has been routinely used to diagnose and evaluate pericardial effusions since the 1970s. The natural progression of its use has extended to the guidance of pericardiocentesis. Since 1980, the Mayo Clinic has described and developed 2-D–echoguided percutaneous pericardiocentesis (70–73). The procedure can be performed rapidly under emergent conditions and has been described in the emergency medicine literature (74). This method combines the simplicity of percutaneous puncture with the safety of direct visualization and is considered the gold standard for the management of pericardial effusion and cardiac tamponade (71,75–77).

IMAGE ACQUISITION

An ultrasound system equipped with a 2.5–5-MHz transducer is used to perform the examination. A small footprint phased array transducer is ideal due to its ability to scan between rib spaces but is not required. The curvilinear array transducer used for general abdominal imaging can be used as well. The patient is placed supine with the head of the bed at 30 degrees. The pericardial effusion should be assessed first with the standard views (described in Chapter 5) before the ideal entry site for needle insertion is chosen.

ANATOMY AND LANDMARKS

Parasternal approach
The parasternal long axis view provides a cross section of the longitudinal axis of the heart. The transducer is placed obliquely on the left sternal border between the 4th and 5th ribs with the transducer indicator aimed at the right shoulder (Fig. 13.54). Normal ultrasound anatomy and pericardial effusion is shown in Figures 13.55 and 13.56. This transducer position reveals a 3-chamber view of the heart and the best approach to visualize posterior effusions.

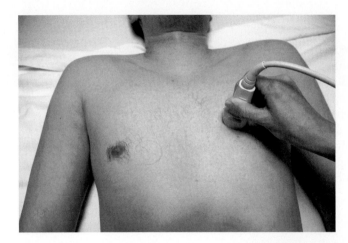

Figure 13.54. Transducer placement for parasternal long axis view of heart.

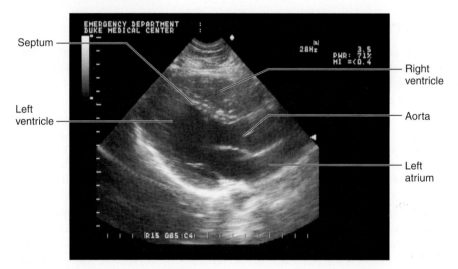

Figure 13.55. Corresponding ultrasound of a normal heart in parasternal long axis orientation. Note that this is a 3-chamber view of the heart. The right ventricle is closest to the transducer in the near field. Counterclockwise is the septum, left ventricle, mitral valve with anterior and posterior leaflets, left atrium, and aorta outflow tract.

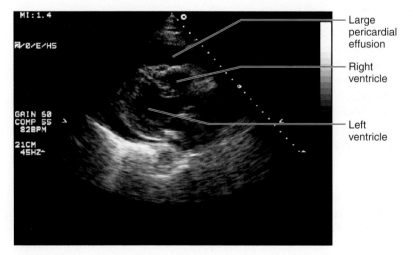

Figure 13.56. Corresponding ultrasound of a large circumferential pericardial effusion in parasternal long axis orientation.

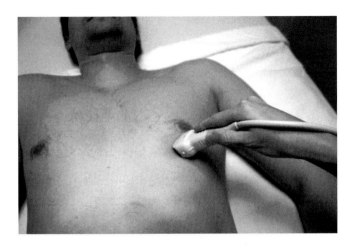

Figure 13.57. Transducer placement for apical view of the heart.

Apical approach

The apical view provides a coronal cross section down the long axis of the heart and visualization of all four chambers. The transducer is placed at the patient's point of maximal impulse (PMI) and aimed at the patient's right shoulder (Fig. 13.57). The normal 4-chamber view and a pericardial effusion are depicted in Figures 13.58 and 13.59.

Subxiphoid approach

This approach uses the liver as an acoustic window to provide a 4-chamber view of the heart. The transducer is placed just inferior to xiphoid process and left costal margin with the beam aimed at the left shoulder (Fig. 13.60). This view can be physically difficult to obtain in obese patients. Normal ultrasound anatomy is depicted in Figure 13.61.

PROCEDURE

Once the pericardial effusion is evaluated thoroughly with all standard echocardiographic views, the ideal needle insertion site is determined. This is the point where the effusion is closest to the transducer, fluid accumulation is maximal, and the track of the needle will most effectively avoid any vital structures, such as the lung (72,73). Note that the ultrasound transducer is not used for real-time guidance of needle insertion in this procedure.

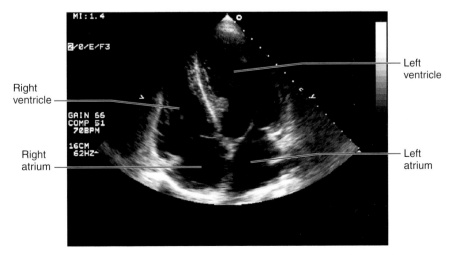

Figure 13.58. Corresponding ultrasound of a normal heart in apical view. This is a 4-chamber view of the heart. Note the bright hyperechoic pericardium without fluid.

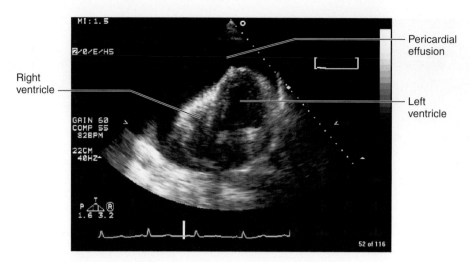

Figure 13.59. Corresponding ultrasound of a pericardial effusion in apical view. There is a large amount of anechoic fluid surrounding the heart. Note the right ventricle is collapsed during diastole, an echocardiographic sign of cardiac tamponade.

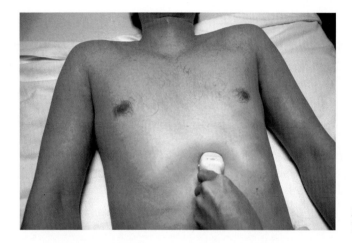

Figure 13.60. Transducer placement for subxiphoid view of the heart.

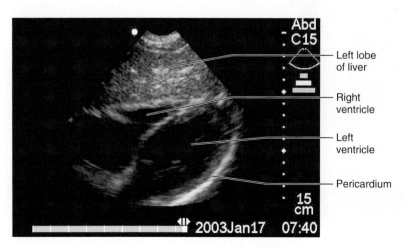

Figure 13.61. Corresponding ultrasound of a normal heart in subcostal view. In the near field is the left lobe of the liver. Adjacent to the liver is the right ventricle and in the far field, the left ventricle.

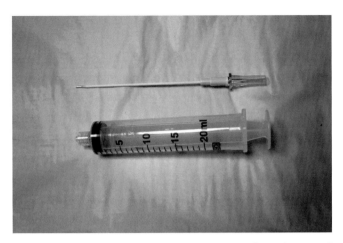

Figure 13.62. Pericardiocentesis over-the-needle catheter and 20-cc syringe.

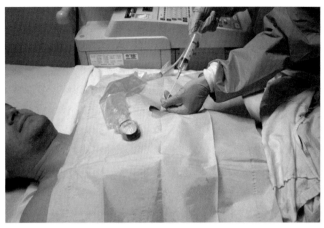

Figure 13.63. Pericardiocentesis using the apical approach. Optimal insertion site and trajectory determined using an ultrasound transducer with sterile sleeve.

Once the site has been chosen, mark the skin with a pen. The trajectory of needle insertion is determined by the trajectory of the transducer used to obtain the best image of the effusion. The depth of insertion is also assessed using the centimeter marks on the ultrasound screen. The patient is kept in the exact same position while the area is prepped with povidone-iodine and sterile drape is placed. The ultrasound transducer is also prepared with a sterile sleeve. Once the patient's skin and the ultrasound transducer are prepared in a sterile fashion, confirm the optimal insertion site and needle trajectory repeatedly until it is visualized in the operator's mind. Local anesthetic is applied to the skin and needle path. A 16–18-gauge needle (8.25 cm in length) with plastic "angiocath" sheath is attached to a saline-filled syringe (Fig. 13.62). Figure 13.63 shows how the needle is inserted at the pre-determined site and trajectory. As the needle is advanced gentle aspiration is applied until there is a flash of fluid. Once flash occurs, insert the needle 2 to 3 mm and advance the plastic sheath into the pericardial space. The needle is withdrawn, leaving only the plastic sheath within the pericardial space. Placement can be confirmed with direct sonographic visualization of the plastic sheath within the pericardial effusion or with color flow detection of agitated saline administered through the sheath. The agitated saline is prepared by using two syringes connected to a three-way stopcock. One syringe has 5 mL of saline and the other syringe is empty. The saline is agitated by rapidly injecting the saline back and forth between the two syringes. The ultrasound transducer is placed so that the pericardial effusion is well-visualized. The saline is then quickly injected into the pericardiocentesis sheath (attached to the third port of the three-way stopcock). Color flow ultrasound is used to visualize the dynamic injection of saline in the pericardial sac. This confirms proper placement allowing for the safe continuation of the procedure in which the pericardial fluid is aspirated into a syringe. Once clinical improvement is achieved, the indwelling sheath can be withdrawn or replaced with a pigtail catheter over a guidewire.

PITFALLS

When selecting the optimal insertion site, it is important to avoid vital structures. By choosing an entry site with a clear path to the pericardial effusion, the lungs are typically avoided because the ultrasound image is obscured when there is underlying air. One must be careful to avoid the left internal mammary artery which travels in a cephalad-caudal direction 3 to 5 cm lateral to the left sternal border (78). Though extremely rare, damage to this artery can result in significant bleeding and cardiac tamponade. One must also be careful to avoid the neurovascular bundle which runs along the inferior edge of each rib.

Use in Decision Making

In the ED, a pericardial effusion can present with a spectrum of clinical presentations from the asymptomatic to the classic Beck's triad associated with cardiac tamponade. The emergency physician is likely to perform bedside pericardiocentesis in an emergent situation when the patient is hemodynamically unstable, in respiratory extremis, or in pulseless electrical activity. 2-D echocardiography can still be used in these situations (76). An abbreviated 2-D scan of the heart is done to localize the pericardial fluid, choose the ideal insertion site, and determine the trajectory of needle insertion.

Transvenous Pacemaker Placement and Capture

Clinical Applications

When placing a transvenous cardiac pacemaker it is important that it be placed in the apex of the right ventricle for capture. Unfortunately, in the ED it can be difficult to get real-time localization of the pacer wires, therefore they are often passed blindly while watching a monitor for capture. Ultrasound can be used for direct visualization of correct positioning of the catheter in the heart while also confirming electrical and mechanical capture (79–84).

Image Acquisition and Anatomy

Several approaches can be used to confirm placement of the pacemaker electrode, but the subcostal position is relatively easy to perform and provides visualization of all four chambers of the heart. In some instances, other views such as the parasternal long axis or the apical approach may also be useful.

For the subcostal view the transducer is placed in the subxiphoid area with the transducer indicator toward the patient's left shoulder. The liver provides an acoustic window that allows good visualization of the heart. The liver is the structure closest to the transducer at the top of the screen. The right ventricle is seen just beyond the liver and has a somewhat triangular shape projected on the left side of the ultrasound monitor. The right atrium can also be visualized as a more rounded structure adjacent to the right ventricle. The left ventricle and atria are seen deep to the right atria and ventricle. A properly placed pacemaker lead should be seen longitudinally as it enters the right atria and, as it is inserted further, the right ventricle. Proper insertion into the apex of the right ventricle is seen in Figure 13.64.

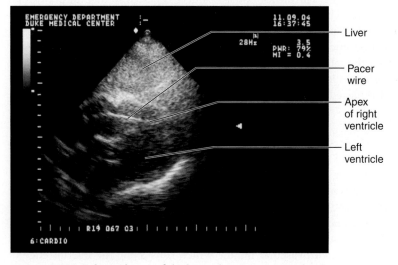

Figure 13.64. Subcostal view of the heart showing a pacemaker lead inserted into the apex of the right ventricle.

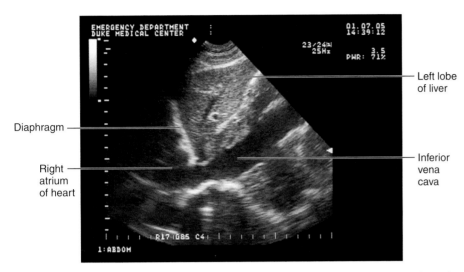

Figure 13.65. Subcostal longitudinal view of the inferior vena cava emptying into the right atrium. In the near field is the left lobe of the liver which is an acoustic window to obtain the image.

The parasternal long axis and apical views are described in Chapter 5. Both allow for excellent visualization of the right ventricle and can be used as additional views to confirm correct placement of the pacemaker lead.

It may also be helpful to visualize the inferior vena cava (IVC) because a pacemaker lead can occasionally traverse the right atrium and enter the IVC. This is best done through a subcostal approach with the transducer oriented in the sagittal plane. Figure 13.65 shows the IVC emptying into the right atria.

PROCEDURE

The standard procedure for insertion of a transvenous pacemaker should be followed. Ultrasound can be used to follow the pacemaker lead through the right atrium and into the right ventricle with ultimate placement in the apex. It can also be used after insertion to confirm placement and capture.

PITFALLS

The pitfalls associated with this procedure are the same pitfalls seen with transvenous pacemaker implantation without ultrasound guidance.

LUMBAR PUNCTURE

CLINICAL APPLICATIONS

Lumbar puncture for cerebrospinal fluid sampling is a commonly performed procedure in the ED that is usually performed with the aid of visual and tactile landmarks. While physicians are generally able to identify the appropriate spinal interspace and insert a needle to obtain fluid for diagnostic and therapeutic purposes, in certain cases this is difficult. In these instances imaging is necessary to successfully accomplish the procedure. Although ultrasound may not be the first choice of an imaging modality for locating the epidural space, it has been described in both the radiology and anesthesia, and to a lesser extent, the emergency medicine literature (85–88).

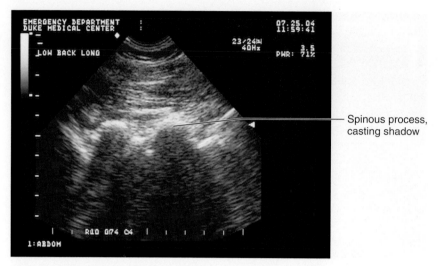

Figure 13.66. Ultrasound of lumbar spine in longitudinal cross section. Two hyperechoic spinous processes are visualized.

IMAGE ACQUISITION

For most ultrasound applications bone is an obstacle to be avoided, but the goal of ultrasound-guided lumbar puncture is to identify the spinous processes of the lumbar vertebrae. The appropriate transducer for this procedure depends on the patient's body habitus. In an obese patient, a 3.5-MHz transducer that allows interrogation of deeper tissues is recommended. On rare occasions, a higher-frequency transducer may be used if the skin and the interspinous space are in close proximity. When imaged sonographically, the anterior cortex of bone appears as an echogenic line with an acoustic shadow deep to it.

PROCEDURE

The choice of patient positioning is less important for lumbar puncture than with other ultrasound-guided procedures, so either the lateral decubitus or sitting position is satisfactory. With the transducer positioned in the longitudinal orientation, the spinous processes above and below the desired interspace can be located and marked (Fig. 13.66). The procedure can then be performed in usual fashion, using the marked point as the location for placing the spinal needle. Real-time guidance of needle insertion is rarely necessary and, in fact, may make this procedure more technically demanding. Ultrasound is also useful in the infant's spine because of incompletely ossified posterior elements that allow the thecal sac and cord structures to be visualized (89).

PITFALLS

Probably the most frustrating pitfall with lumbar punctures is a "dry tap." This is often the result of lateral displacement of the needle, but can result from not positioning the needle deep enough into the back. One may need to use a longer needle, especially in obese patients. Other potential complications following a lumbar puncture include headache, vascular injury, infection, and herniation.

PEDIATRIC CENTRAL VENOUS ACCESS

CLINICAL APPLICATIONS

Central venous access is challenging in the pediatric patient, in particular those patients younger than 2 years old (90). Factors that contribute to this include smaller, less-distinct anatomical landmarks; smaller-caliber vessels; the procedure is less frequently performed by nonpediatric specialists; greater proximity of important anatomical structures; and there is less patient cooperation from pediatric patients than adults (91). Three randomized controlled trials comparing real-time ultrasound guidance versus the landmark technique for internal jugular vein cannulation have shown that ultrasound can result in superior success rates, shorter mean times to successful cannulation, lower mean number of attempts, and lower complication rates (91–93).

A critical analysis of these three studies resulted in the National Institute of Clinical Excellence (NICE) recommendation for ultrasound guidance in pediatric CVC placement. Overall relative risk reduction for internal jugular vein CVC placement failure and for complications is 85% and 73%, respectively (33). It is important to mention the limitations of these recommendations. First is the small number of patients (180) included in these trials. Second, all procedures were performed in the operating room under ideal conditions with patients under general anesthesia. Third, all CVC insertions were performed using ultrasound transducers with needle guide attachments. The freehand method has not been studied. Finally, subsequent to the NICE recommendations, a randomized controlled trial demonstrated that ultrasound guidance was inferior to the traditional landmark technique in terms of success rates and carotid artery punctures (94). These factors make it difficult, at the current time, to generalize success of ultrasound guidance in adults to the pediatric ED population.

Image Acquisition

A 7.5–10-MHz linear array transducer is used to obtain the ultrasound images. A needle guide attachment placed on the ultrasound transducer is recommended but not mandatory. The needle guide is recommended based on the fact that all published studies that have found ultrasound to be helpful have utilized needle guide attachments. If a needle guide is not used, the operator should be very familiar with the freehand technique.

Anatomy and Landmarks

Place the patient in the Trendelenburg position with the head kept in the midline position. A brief nonsterile ultrasound scan is performed to affirm normal anatomic relationships, ensure absence of thrombosis, and determine the optimal segment of the target vein for catheterization. The transducer is placed superior to the clavicle between the two heads of the sternocleidomastoid muscles (Fig. 13.67). Figure 13.68 shows normal short axis views of the right internal jugular vein and carotid artery of a 12-month-old. The vein is less pulsatile, more irregularly shaped, and should be easily compressible with gentle transducer pressure. Once the ideal site of entry is determined, prepare the ultrasound transducer with a sterile sleeve and attach the appropriate depth needle attachment.

Procedure

The ultrasound transducer should be held in the nondominant hand while the needle and syringe are held in the other. Once the target vessel is identified, center it on the ultrasound screen. Apply local anesthetic to the skin and proposed needle path. Introduce the finder needle using the appropriate depth needle guide attachment. The needle guide is angulated so that as the needle advances the tip will intersect the segment of the vein that is directly under the transducer. This will allow visualization of needle entry into the vessel. Once the needle enters subcutaneous tissue, apply gentle aspiration. As the needle is slowly advanced, look at the ultrasound screen, being careful not to slide the hand holding the ultrasound transducer. The needle may appear as a small brightly echogenic dot; however, the needle is not typically visualized on the ultrasound screen. Instead, secondary markers of needle location are used. These include ring down artifact, acoustic shadowing, and

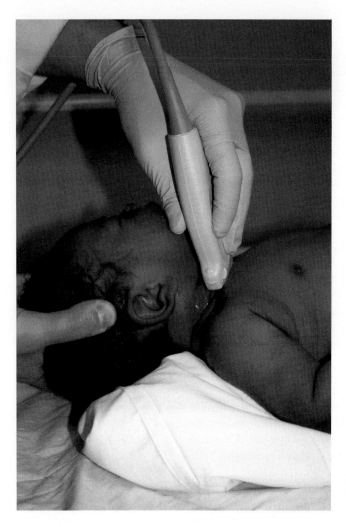

Figure 13.67. Transducer placement for internal jugular vein in pediatric patient. Note the roll under the shoulders to allow room for the neck to extend.

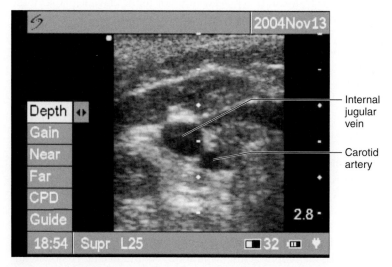

Figure 13.68. Short axis view of right internal jugular vein and carotid artery in a 4-week-old neonate.

buckling of the vein contour correlating with needle entering the vessel (Figs. 13.24–13.26). If the acoustic shadow or ring down artifact is off-center of the vessel, slowly withdraw the needle and adjust the transducer appropriately until the target vessel is centered on the monitor. Free return of venous blood confirms vessel entry. Frequently the needle tip will traverse both the anterior and posterior walls of the vessel as the needle hits and buckles the vein. When this happens, little or no blood flash will occur. Using continued gentle aspiration, slowly withdraw the needle until the tip is pulled back into the lumen of the vessel, resulting in venous blood return. With free return of blood, the needle is released from needle guide attachment and the ultrasound transducer is placed aside onto the sterile drape. Continue central line placement with usual standard Seldinger technique.

PITFALLS

One of the primary difficulties of placing a CVC in a pediatric patient is the inability of the child to cooperate with the procedure. Many children who need central venous access are critically ill or neurologically compromised, and may be less likely to move during the procedure. However, when alert pediatric patients need a CVC, procedural sedation is strongly recommended. The optimal medication for procedural sedation will depend on the clinical scenario and whether peripheral intravenous access has already been established.

SUPRAPUBIC BLADDER ASPIRATION

CLINICAL APPLICATIONS

Obtaining a sterile urine specimen can be critical in diagnosing infection in certain populations. While most adults and older children are able to provide a reasonably sterile clean-catch specimen or cooperate with a urethral catheterization, some patients may require a suprapubic catheterization. Neonates and young children are the most frequent groups that require a suprapubic bladder aspiration, but some older children and adults, such as those with phimosis or severe urethral strictures, may also require this procedure. Suprapubic bladder aspiration is a relatively safe and benign procedure, however ultrasound offers several benefits. Ultrasound can be used to detect the approximate volume of the bladder as well as the best location for aspiration, reducing the chance of a dry tap and reducing the need for multiple needlesticks. Ultrasound has been used to assist suprapubic urinary bladder catheterization for more than 30 years (95). Several studies have been done that show an increase in the success rate of suprapubic aspiration with ultrasound guidance versus without, along with the need for fewer attempts and fewer complications (96–98).

IMAGE ACQUISITION

There are two ways ultrasound can be used to assist in suprapubic aspiration. First, it can be used to determine the size of the bladder and confirm the presence of urine prior to a blind aspiration attempt. Second, the aspiration can be done under direct ultrasound guidance. Both methods rely on visualization of the bladder. The bladder is best imaged with a 5–7.5-MHz convex transducer. Larger patients may require the lower frequency transducer to allow for deeper tissue penetration. Depth markers on the side of the display may be useful for determining how deep the needle will need to go, and for estimating the actual volume of urine within the bladder. For male patients, compression of the penis during image acquisition may help prevent bladder emptying during the procedure. Another option is to be prepared to collect the spontaneously voided specimen.

ANATOMY AND LANDMARKS

Visualization of the bladder is accomplished by placing the transducer immediately above the pubic symphysis in a sagittal plane with the orientation marker pointing superiorly or in a transverse plane with the marker pointing to the patient's right (Fig. 13.69). The bladder is seen as a well-demarcated anechoic structure beneath the abdominal musculature (Fig. 13.70). Scanning left to right may help find the greatest depth because structures deep to the bladder may distort the posterior border of the bladder. In children the bladder tends to be high in the abdominal cavity, above the pubic symphysis. With age the bladder moves lower into the pelvis. Tilting the transducer cephalad or caudad may help locate the best place for aspiration.

PROCEDURE

Perform an initial scan of the bladder to make sure there is enough urine. Only the transverse diameter has been shown to be useful in predicting the volume of urine needed for successful aspiration. One study found higher success rates with a transverse diameter of greater than 3.5 cm compared to transverse diameters less than 2 cm (99). If the bladder does not appear adequately full, wait 30 minutes and rescan after fluid resuscitating the patient. Prep the area with povidone-iodine and slide a sterile sleeve over the transducer. A small amount of local anesthetic may make the procedure more comfortable for the patient and allow a larger needle (such as a 21-gauge or larger) to be used. Connect the needle to a syringe. A stopcock may be helpful if the bladder needs to be drained because of urinary retention or obstruction. Find the area with the largest collection of urine and insert the needle under direct observation into this area, while maintaining constant aspiration on the syringe (100–101).

PITFALLS

The most frequent complication after suprapubic aspiration is microhematuria. This usually clears very rapidly and is relatively benign. The needle may inadvertently puncture bowel, which is also typically a benign occurrence and requires only observation. Developing a significant infection from needle puncturing bowel is extremely rare.

It is very important to confirm that the fluid collection seen is contained within the bladder and not some other intra-abdominal fluid collection. Scanning the bladder in

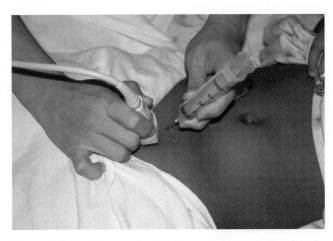

Figure 13.69. Ultrasound-guided suprapubic aspiration (sterile drape not included for illustration purposes).

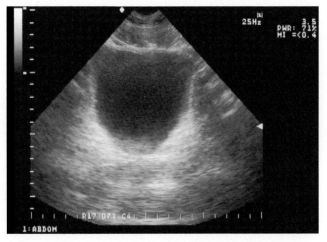

Figure 13.70. Corresponding ultrasound of a bladder in transverse cross section. The bladder is full with anechoic urine.

sagittal and transverse planes may be helpful in distinguishing bladder from other fluid-filled structures. As well, fluid contained within the bladder is mostly anechoic, whereas bowel will demonstrate peristalsis and have areas of fluid and shadows caused by air intermixed within the lumen.

REFERENCES

1. Sznajder JI, Zveibil FR, Bitterman H, et al. Central vein catheterization. Failure and complication rates by three percutaneous approaches. *Arch Intern Med.* 1986;146:259–261.
2. Mansfield PF, Hohn DC, Fornage BD, et al. Complications and failures of subclavian-vein catheterization. *N Engl J Med.* 1994;331:1735–1738.
3. McGee DC, Gould MK. Preventing complications of central venous catheterization. *N Engl J Med.* 2003;348:1123–1133.
4. Steele R, Irvin CB. Central line mechanical complication rate in emergency medicine patients. *Acad Emerg Med.* 2001;8:204–207.
5. Merrer J, De Jonghe B, Golliot F, et al. Complications of femoral and subclavian venous catheterization in critically ill patients: a randomized controlled trial. *JAMA.* 2001;286:700–707.
6. Polderman KH, Girbes AJ. Central venous catheter use. Part 1: mechanical complications. *Intensive Care Med.* 2002;28:1–17.
7. Droll KP, Lossing AG. Carotid-jugular arteriovenous fistula: case report of an iatrogenic complication following internal jugular vein catheterization. *J Clin Anesth.* 2004;16:127–129.
8. Schummer W, Schummer C, Hoffman E. Chylothorax after central venous catheterization. Considerations to anatomy, differential diagnosis and therapy. *Anaesthetist.* 2003;52:919–924.
9. Yoshida S. A lethal complication of central venous catheterization. *Lancet.* 2003;362:569.
10. Shields LB, Hunsaker DM, Hunsaker JC 3rd. Iatrogenic catheter-related cardiac tamponade: a case report of fatal hydropericardium following subcutaneous implantation of a chemotherapeutic injection port. *J Forensic Sci.* 2003;48:414–418.
11. Fangio P, Mourgeon E, Romelaer A, et al. Aortic injury and cardiac tamponade as a complication of subclavian venous catheterization. *Anesthesiology.* 2002;96:1520–1522.
12. Reddy G, Coombes A, Hubbard AD. Horner's syndrome following internal jugular vein cannulation. *Intensive Care Med.* 1998;24:194–196.
13. Denys BG, Uretsky BF. Anatomical variations of the internal jugular vein location: impact on central venous access. *Crit Care Med.* 1991;19:1516–1519.
14. Lin BS, Kong CW, Tarng DC, et al. Anatomical variation of the internal jugular vein and its impact on temporary haemodialysis vascular access: an ultrasonographic survey in uraemic patients. *Nephrol Dial Transplant.* 1998;13:134–138.
15. Gordon AC, Saliken JC, Johns D, et al. US-guided puncture of the internal jugular vein: complications and anatomic considerations. *J Vasc Interv Radiol.* 1998;9:333–338.
16. Lichtenstein D, Saifi R, Augarde R, et al. The Internal jugular veins are asymmetric. Usefulness of ultrasound before catheterization. *Intensive Care Med.* 2001;27:301–305.
17. Forauer AR, Glockner JF. Importance of US findings in access planning during jugular vein hemodialysis catheter placements. *J Vasc Interv Radiol.* 2000;11:233–238.
18. Scherhag A, Klein A, Jantzen JP. Cannulation of the internal jugular vein using 2 ultrasonic technics. A comparative controlled study. *Anaesthetist.* 1989;38:633–638.
19. Mallory DL, McGee WT, Shawker TH, et al. Ultrasound guidance improves the success rate of internal jugular vein cannulation. A prospective, randomized trial. *Chest.* 1990;98:157–160.
20. Troianos CA, Jobes DR, Ellison N. Ultrasound-guided cannulation of the internal jugular vein. A prospective, randomized study. *Anesth Analg.* 1991;72:823–826.
21. Denys BG, Uretsky BF, Reddy PS. Ultrasound-assisted cannulation of the internal jugular vein. A prospective comparison to the external landmark-guided technique. *Circulation.* 1993;87:1557–1562.
22. Gualtieri E, Deppe S, Sipperly ME, et al. Subclavian venous catheterization: greater success rate for less experienced operators using ultrasound guidance. *Crit Care Med.* 1995;23:692–697.
23. Hilty WM, Hudson PA, Levitt MA, et al. Real-time ultrasound-guided femoral vein catheterization during cardiopulmonary resuscitation. *Ann Emerg Med.* 1997;29:331–336.
24. Teichgraber UK, Benter T, Gebel M, et al. A sonographically guided technique for central venous access. *AJR Am J Roentgenol.* 1997;169:731–733.
25. Slama M, Novara A, Safavian A, et al. Improvement of internal jugular vein cannulation using an ultrasound-guided technique. *Intensive Care Med.* 1997;23:916–919.

26. Miller AH, Roth BA, Mills TJ, et al. Ultrasound guidance versus the landmark technique for the placement of central venous catheters in the emergency department. *Acad Emerg Med.* 2002;9:800–805.

27. Kwon TH, Kim YL, Cho DK. Ultrasound-guided cannulation of the femoral vein for acute haemodialysis access. *Nephrol Dial Transplant.* 1997;12:1009–012.

28. Sulek CA, Blas ML, Lobato EB. A randomized study of left versus right internal jugular vein cannulation in adults. *J Clinical Anesth.* 2000;12:142–145.

29. Randolph AG, Cook DJ, Gonzales CA, et al. Ultrasound guidance for placement of central venous catheters: a meta-analysis of the literature. *Crit Care Med.* 1996;24:2053–2058.

30. Keenan SP. Use of ultrasound to place central lines. *J Crit Care.* 2002;17:126–137.

31. Hind D, Calvert N, McWilliams R, et al. Ultrasonic locating devices for central venous cannulation: meta-analysis. *BMJ.* 2003;327:361.

32. Rothschild JM. Ultrasound Guidance of Central Vein Catheterization. In: Markowitz AJ, ed. *Making Health Care Safer: A Critical Analysis of Patient Safety Practices.* Evidence Report/Technology. Rockville, MD, US Dept of Health and Human Services; 2001. Assessment No. 43, AHRQ Publication No. 01-E058.

33. National Institute for Clinical Excellence. Guidance on the use of ultrasound locating devices for placing central venous catheters. *Technology Appraisal Guidance No. 49,* September 2002, www.nice.org.uk.

34. Blaivas M, Brannam L, Fernandez E. Short-axis versus long-axis approaches for teaching ultrasound-guided vascular access on a new inanimate model. *Acad Emerg Med.* 2003;10: 1307–1311.

35. Sofocleous CT, Schur I, Cooper SG, et al. Sonographically guided placement of peripherally inserted central venous catheters: review of 355 procedures. *AJR Am J Roentgenol.* 1998;170: 1613–1616.

36. Parkinson R, Gandhi M, Harper J, et al. Establishing an ultrasound guided peripherally inserted central catheter (PICC) insertion service. *Clin Radiol.* 1998;53:33–36.

37. Chrisman HB, Omary RA, Nemcek AA, et al. Peripherally inserted central venous catheters: guidance with the use of US versus venography in 2,650 patients. *J Vasc Interv Radiol.* 1999;10:473–475.

38. Donaldson JS, Morello FP, Junewick JJ, et al. Peripherally inserted central venous catheters: US-guided vascular access in pediatric patients. *Radiology.* 1995;197:542–544.

39. LaRue GD. Efficacy of ultrasonography in peripheral venous cannulation. *J Intraven Nurs.* 2000;23:29–34.

40. Moureau NL. Using ultrasound to guide PICC insertion. *Nursing.* 2003;33:20.

41. McMahon DD. Evaluating new technology to improve patient outcomes: a quality improvement approach. *J Infus Nurs.* 2002;25:250–255.

42. Keyes LE, Frazee BW, Snoey ER, et al. Ultrasound-guided brachial and basilic vein cannulation in emergency department patients with difficult intravenous access. *Ann Emerg Med.* 1999;34:711–714.

43. Sandhu NP, Sidhu DS. Mid-arm approach to basilic and cephalic vein cannulation using ultrasound guidance. *Br J Anaesth.* 2004;93:292–294.

44. Smith SW. Emergency physician-performed ultrasonography-guided hip arthrocentesis. *Acad Emerg Med.* 1999;6:84–86.

45. Cardinal E, Chhem RK, Beauregard CG. Ultrasound-guided interventional procedures in the musculoskeletal system. *Radiol Clin North Am.* 1998;36:597–604.

46. Mayekawa DS, Ralls PW, Kerr RM, et al. Sonographically guided arthrocentesis of the hip. *J Ultrasound Med.* 1989;8:665–667.

47. Zawin JK, Hoffer FA, Rand FF, et al. Joint effusion in children with an irritable hip: US diagnosis and aspiration. *Radiology.* 1993;187:459–463.

48. Valley VT, Stahmer SA. Targeted musculoarticular sonography in the detection of joint effusions. *Acad Emerg Med.* 2001;8:361–367.

49. Wilson DJ, Green DJ, MacLarnon JC. Arthrosonography of the painful hip. *Clin Radiol.* 1984;35:17–19.

50. Zieger MM, Dorr U, Schultz RD. Ultrasonography of hip joint effusions. *Skeletal Radiol.* 1987;16: 607–611.

51. Dewitz A, Frazee BW. Soft Tissue Applications. In: Ma OJ, Mateer JR, eds. *Emergency Ultrasound.* New York: McGraw-Hill; 2003:361–390.

52. Roy S, Dewitz A, Paul I. Ultrasound-assisted ankle arthrocentesis. *Am J Emerg Med.* 1999;17: 300–301.

53. Schweitzer ME, van Leersum M, Ehrlich SS, et al. Fluid in normal and abnormal ankle joints: amount and distribution as seen on MR images. *AJR Am J Roentgenol.* 1994;162:111–114.
54. Jones PW, Moyers JP, Rogers JT, et al. Ultrasound-guided thoracentesis: is it a safer method? *Chest.* 2003;123:418–423.
55. Mayo PH, Goltz HR, Tafreshi M, et al. Safety of ultrasound-guided thoracentesis in patients receiving mechanical ventilation. *Chest.* 2004;125:1059–1062.
56. Grogan DR, Irwin RS, Channick R, et al. Complications associated with thoracentesis: A prospective, randomized study comparing three different methods. *Arch Intern Med.* 1990:150:873–877.
57. Sennef MG, Corwin RW, Gold LH, et al. Complications associated with thoracentesis. *Chest.* 1986;90:97–100.
58. Collins TR, Sahn SA. Thoracocentesis. Clinical value, complications, technical problems, and patient experience. *Chest.* 1987;9:817–822.
59. Bartter T, Mayo PD, Pratter MR, et al. Lower risk and higher yield for thoracentesis when performed by experienced operators. *Chest.* 1993;103:1873–1876.
60. Heller M, Jehle D. Ultrasound in Emergency Medicine. Philadelphia: WB Saunders; 1995:160–162.
61. Cattau E, Benjamin SB, Knuff TE, et al. The accuracy of the physical examination in the diagnosis of suspected ascites. *JAMA.* 1982;247:1164–1166.
62. Bard C, Lafortune M, Breton G. Ascites: ultrasound guidance or blind paracentesis? *CMAJ.* 1986;135:209–210.
63. Wong B, Murphy J, Chang CJ, et al. The risk of pericardiocentesis. *Am J Cardiol.* 1979;44:1110–1114.
64. Krikorian JG, Hancock EW. Pericardiocentesis. *Am J Med.* 1978;65:808–814.
65. Morin JE, Hollomby D, Gonda A, et al. Management of uremic pericarditis: a report of 11 patients with cardiac tamponade and a review of the literature. *Ann Thorac Surg.* 1976;22:588–592.
66. Kwasnik EM, Koster K, Lazarus JM, et al. Conservative management of uremic pericardial effusions. *J Thorac Cardiovasc Surg.* 1978;76:629–632.
67. Ball JB, Morrison WL. Cardiac tamponade. *Postgrad Med J* 1997;73:141–145.
68. Bishop LH Jr, Estes EH Jr, McIntosh HD. Electrocardiogram as a safeguard in pericardiocentesis. *JAMA.* 1956;162:264–265.
69. Guberman BA, Fowler NO, Engel PJ, et al. Cardiac tamponade in medical patients. *Circulation.* 198;64:633–640.
70. Callahan JA, Seward JB, Tajik AJ, et al. Pericardiocentesis assisted by two-dimensional echocardiography. *J Thorac Cardiovasc Surg.* 1983;85:877–879.
71. Callahan JA, Seward JB, Nishimura RA, et al. Two-dimensional echocardiographically guided pericardiocentesis: experience in 117 consecutive patients. *Am J Cardiol.* 1985;55:476–479.
72. Callahan JA, Seward JB, Tajik AJ. Cardiac tamponade: pericardiocentesis directed by two-dimensional echocardiography. *Mayo Clin Proc.* 1985;60:344–347.
73. Tsang TS, Freeman WK, Sinak LJ, et al. Echocardiographically guided pericardiocentesis: evolution and state-of-the-art technique. *Mayo Clin Proc.* 1998;73:647–652.
74. Mazurek B, Jehle D, Martin M. Emergency department echocardiography in the diagnosis and therapy of cardiac tamponade. *J Emerg Med.* 1991;9:27–31.
75. Spodick D. Pericardial Diseases. In: Braunwald E, ed. *Heart Disease: A Textbook of Cardiovascular Medicine. 6th ed.* New York: WB Saunders; 2001:1847–1848.
76. Tsang TSM, Oh JK, Seward JB. Review: Diagnosis and management of cardiac tamponade in the era of echocardiography. *Clin Cardiol.* 1999;22:446–452.
77. Salem K, Mulji A, Lonn E. Echocardiographically guided pericardiocentesis-the gold standard for the management of pericardial effusion and cardiac tamponade. *Can J Cardiol.* 1999;15:1251–1255.
78. Kronzon I, Glassman LR, Tunick PA. Avoiding the left internal mammary artery during anterior pericardiocentesis. *Echocardiography.* 2003;20:533–534.
79. Tam MM. Ultrasound for primary confirmation of mechanical capture in emergency transcutaneous pacing. *Emerg Med (Fremantle).* 2003;15:192–194.
80. Macedo W Jr, Sturmann K, Kim JM, et al. Ultrasonographic guidance of transvenous pacemaker insertion in the emergency department: a report of three cases. *J Emerg Med.* 1999;17:491–496.
81. Aguilera PA, Durham BA, Riley DA. Emergency transvenous cardiac pacing placement using ultrasound guidance. *Ann Emerg Med.* 2000;36:224–227.
82. Tobin AM, Grodman RS, Fisherkeller M, et al. Two-dimensional echocardiographic localization of a malpositioned pacing catheter. *Pacing Clin Electrophysiol.* 1983;6:291–299.

83. Meier B, Felner JM. Two-dimensional echocardiographic evaluation of intracardiac transvenous pacemaker leads. *J Clin Ultrasound*. 1982;10:421–425.
84. Gondi B, Nanda NC. Real-time, two-dimensional echocardiographic features of pacemaker perforation. *Circulation*. 1981;64:97–106.
85. Cork RC, Kryc JJ, Vaughan RW. Ultrasonic localization of the lumbar epidural space. *Anesthesiology*. 1980;52:513–516.
86. Currie JM. Measurement of the depth to the extradural space using ultrasound. *BrJ Anaesth*. 1984;56:345–347.
87. Wallace DH, Currie JM, Gilstrap LC, et al. Indirect sonographic guidance for epidural anesthesia in obese pregnant patients. *Reg Anesth*. 1992;17:233–236.
88. Sandoval M, Shestek W, Sturman K, et al. Optimal patient position for lumbar puncture, measured by ultrasonography. *Emerg Radiol*. 2004;10:179–181.
89. Coley BD, Shiels WE 2nd, Hogan MJ. Diagnostic and interventional ultrasonography in neonatal and infant lumbar puncture. *Pediatr Radiol*. 2001;31:399–402.
90. Nicolson SC, Sweeney MF, Moore RA, et al. Comparison of internal and external jugular cannulation of the central circulation in the pediatric patient. *Crit Care Med*. 1985;13:747–749.
91. Alderson PJ, Burrows FA, Stemp LI, et al. Use of ultrasound to evaluate internal jugular vein anatomy and to facilitate central venous cannulation in paediatric patients. *Br J Anaesth*. 1993;70:145–148.
92. Verghese ST, McGill WA, Patel RI, et al. Ultrasound-guided internal jugular venous cannulation in infants: a prospective comparison with the traditional palpation method. *Anesthesiology*. 1999;91:71–77.
93. Verghese ST, McGill WA, Patel RI, et al. Comparison of three techniques for internal jugular vein cannulation in infants. *Paediatr Anaesth*. 2000;10:505–511.
94. Grebenik CR, Boyce A, Sinclair ME, et al. NICE guidelines for central venous catheterization in children. Is the evidence base sufficient? *Br J Anaesth*. 2004;92:827–830.
95. Goldberg BB, Meyer H. Ultrasonically guided suprapubic urinary bladder aspiration. *Pediatrics*. 1973;51:70–74.
96. Kiernan SC, Pinckert TL, Keszler M. Ultrasound guidance of suprapubic bladder aspiration in neonates. *J Pediatr*. 1993;123:789–791.
97. Gochman RF, Karasic RB, Heller MB. Use of portable ultrasound to assist urine collection by suprapubic aspiration. *Ann Emerg Med*. 1991;20:631–635.
98. Özkan B, Kaya O, Akdağ R, et al. Suprapubic bladder aspiration with or without ultrasound guidance. *Clin Pediatr (Phila)*. 2000;39:625–626.
99. Garcia-Nieto V, Navarro JF, Sanchez-Almeida E, et al. Standards for ultrasound guidance of suprapubic bladder aspiration. *Pediatr Nephrol*. 1997;11:607–609.
100. Sagi EF, Alpan G, Eyal FG, et al. Ultrasonic guidance of suprapubic aspiration in infants. *J Clin Ultrasound*. 1983;11:347–348.
101. Chu RW, Wong YC, Luk SH, et al. Comparing suprapubic urine aspiration under real-time ultrasound guidance with conventional blind aspiration. *Acta Pædiatr*. 2002;91:512–516.

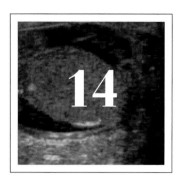

SOFT TISSUE

Bradley W. Frazee
Douglas A.E. White

INTRODUCTION

Skin and soft tissue infections and foreign bodies are encountered on a daily basis by emergency physicians. Ultrasound, unlike plain x-ray, can provide detailed images of the immediate subcutaneous and submucosal tissue and has therefore emerged as an extremely useful tool in the rapid assessment of these common problems. This chapter is divided into the following three sections that cover the major soft tissue scanning applications: skin and soft tissue infection, peritonsillar abscess, and soft tissue foreign body.

SKIN AND SOFT TISSUE INFECTIONS

CLINICAL APPLICATIONS

Correctly differentiating occult abscess from simple cellulitis on the basis of clinical exam alone can be difficult. Faced with an undifferentiated skin and soft tissue infection, ultrasound can be used to do the following: confirm the presence of cellulitis; detect an occult or deep abscess; localize the abscess pocket for accurate aspiration or incision; and detect fluid adjacent to fascial planes, indicative of necrotizing fasciitis.

IMAGE ACQUISITION

Sonographic evaluation of skin and soft tissue infections is usually best accomplished with a 5–to 7.5-MHz linear array transducer. A 3.5-MHz convex array transducer may be preferable in the case of deep collections, such as an intramuscular buttock abscess. Fluid collections should be interrogated in two planes to define their shape. Depth is estimated using the depth markers at the side of the display. It is helpful to compare the area of interest to the contralateral side to define the normal depth of subcutaneous tissue, fascial planes, and muscle. In the case of superficial infections, particularly of the hand, use of a standoff pad is recommended to optimize image quality where small anatomic structures and bones are located near the skin surface. (Standoff pads are discussed further below in the foreign body section.)

ULTRASOUND ANATOMY AND LANDMARKS

Normal subcutaneous tissue is composed primarily of fat, which appears hypoechoic, and is traversed by irregular strands of hyperechoic connective tissue. Fascial planes are brightly hyperechoic and of regular thickness, while muscle has a characteristic striated

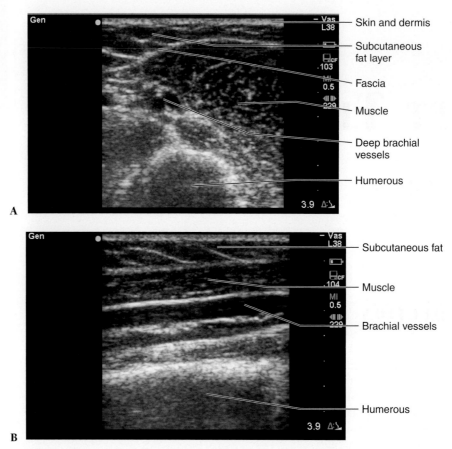

Figure 14.1. Normal sonographic appearance of the subcutaneous structures of the arm, showing skin, subcutaneous fat, fascial planes, muscle, deep brachial vessels and humerous bone. (**A**) Transverse view. (**B**) Longitudinal view.

appearance when scanned in long axis. Vascular structures are anechoic. Arteries usually are pulsatile while veins compress with gentle transducer pressure. Lymph nodes are seen as irregular, circular, echogenic structures, often with hypoechoic rims. Bones, with their brightly echogenic cortices and dense acoustic shadows, can often be seen in the far field of the image, providing useful landmarks and depth perspective. Figure 14.1 demonstrates normal sonographic appearance of the subcutaneous structures of the arm.

PATHOLOGY

Faced with an undifferentiated soft tissue infection where there is suspicion of an occult abscess, cellulitis becomes a diagnosis of exclusion. It is therefore important to be familiar with the sonographic appearance of cellulitis. Because most of the findings associated with cellulitis arise from edema formation, they are nonspecific. Swelling is reflected in an increased distance between the skin and underlying fascial planes or bone (Fig. 14.2). The echogenicity of the subcutaneous tissue is diffusely increased, and often is traversed by a lattice of broad hypoechoic bands giving rise to a cobblestonelike appearance (Figs. 14.3, 14.4). Differentiating interconnected bands of edema fluid from an irregular pus collection can be difficult.

Although subcutaneous abscesses most commonly appear as hypoechoic roughly spherical masses (Fig. 14.5), it is important to realize that their sonographic appearance is quite variable (1). The contour may be lobulated or interdigitate with surrounding edema and tissue planes (Fig. 14.6). The interior may contain hyperechoic sediment (Fig. 14.5), septae, or gas and may be isoechoic or hyperechoic compared to surrounding tissue (Fig. 14.7). In

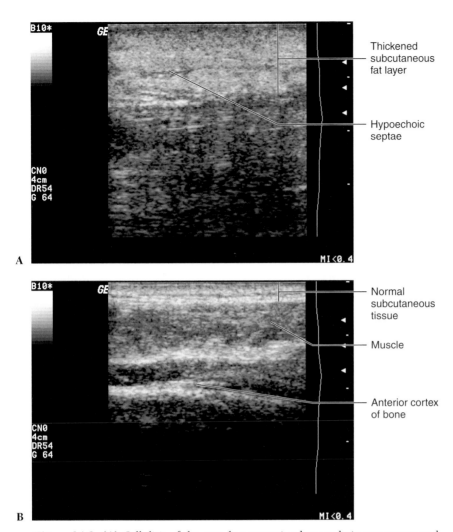

Figure 14.2. (A) Cellulitis of the arm demonstrating hyperechoic appearance and diffuse thickening of the subcutaneous fat due to edema, few hypoechoic septae, and poor resolution of farfield tissues. (B) Contralateral normal arm showing thin dermal layer and well resolved muscle and bone in the far field.

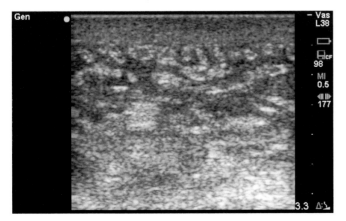

Figure 14.3. Cellulitis of the forearm demonstrating prominent hypoechoic septae in the subcutaneous fat layer, giving rise to a cobblestone or lattice appearance.

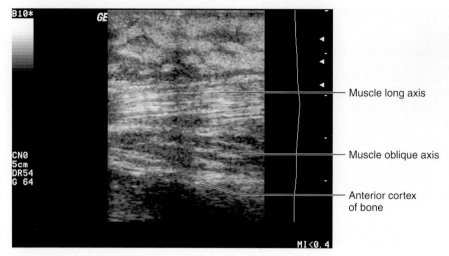

Figure 14.4. Cellulitis. Underlying muscle layer and bone are seen.

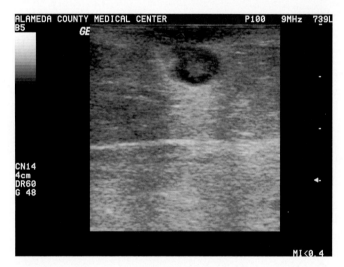

Figure 14.5. Typical abscess. Spherical abscess cavity containing hyperechoic debris. Note far field acoustic enhancement.

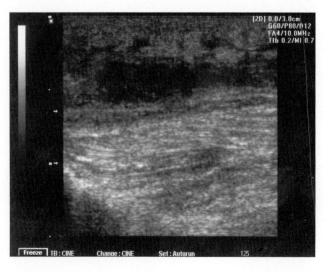

Figure 14.6. Atypical appearing subcutaneous abscess. A broad irregular anechoic fluid collection is seen deep and adjacent to what appears to be cellulitis in the near field.

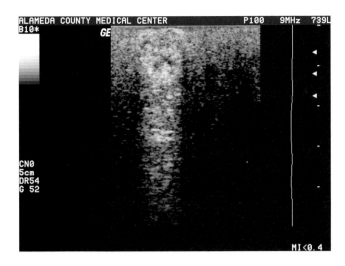

Figure 14.7. Isohyperechoic abscess cavity giving rise to prominent far field acoustic enhancement.

the latter case, the finding of posterior acoustic enhancement (Fig. 14.5, 14.7) and the ability to induce motion of the material with palpation provide clues to the presence of liquefied pus. Figure 14.8 demonstrates the typical appearance of a deep intramuscular abscess. In Figure 14.9, a standoff pad was used to gain a clear image of a fingertip felon.

The sonographic appearance of necrotizing fasciitis has been characterized by one group in Taiwan (1). The main findings are marked thickening of the subcutaneous layer (as seen in cellulitis) combined with a layer of anechoic fluid, measuring greater than 4 mm, adjacent to the deep fascia (Fig. 14.10). Subcutaneous gas, which may give rise to acoustic shadowing and reverberation artifact, is present in some cases (Fig. 14.11).

ARTIFACTS AND PITFALLS

Potential pitfalls in the ultrasound assessment of soft tissue infections include the following.

1. Failure to recognize an isoechoic abscess cavity (evident by the presence of far field acoustic enhancement).
2. Failure to consider, in a case of abscess versus cellulitis, that irregular hypoechoic areas may represent pus collections rather than simply edema.
3. Failure to use a standoff pad to interrogate superficial infections, particularly in the hand.

COMPARISON WITH OTHER IMAGING MODALITIES

Computed tomography (CT) has been used extensively to evaluate soft tissue infections, and may be considered the gold standard for imaging of abscesses. Its advantages are that it reveals deep fluid collections well, can delineate the extent of inflammation (in relation to fascia, vessels, and bone), and is well accepted by surgeons. Disadvantages compared to ultrasound are its high cost, that it is time-consuming, and that it cannot be employed at the bedside to directly guide aspiration or incision.

For the evaluation of possible necrotizing soft tissue infection, the gold standard remains operative findings. Plain films reveal the characteristic soft tissue gas in as few as 39% of cases (2). CT scan and magnetic resonance imaging (MRI) may demonstrate edema adjacent to fascial planes or small amounts of soft tissue gas, but these imaging modalities are time-consuming and may present an additional risk to an unstable patient (3). Ultrasound is an attractive alternative in this setting because it can be performed rapidly at the bedside. While one study has reported favorable results with screening emergency department (ED) ultrasound for suspected necrotizing fasciitis, published clinical experience from other centers is lacking, as is data comparing it to more accepted imaging modalities such as CT or MRI (1).

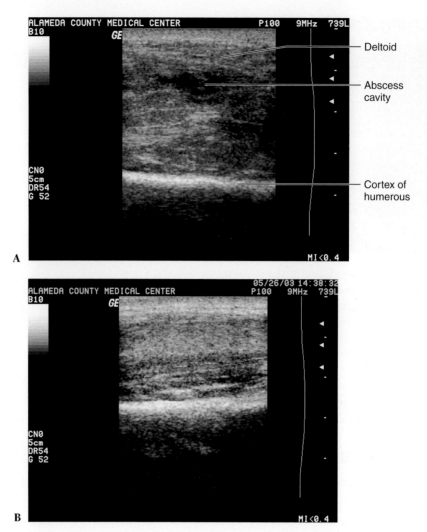

Deltoid

Abscess cavity

Cortex of humerous

Figure 14.8. (A) Intramuscular deltoid abscess. (B) Contralateral normal deltoid muscle.

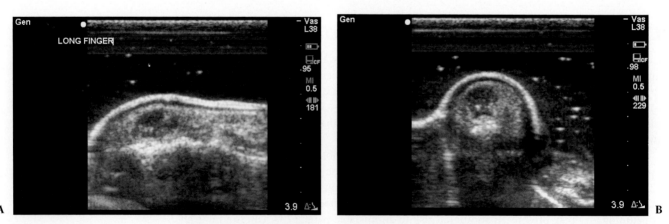

Figure 14.9. Fingertip felon. A water-filled latex glove was used as a standoff pad. (A) Longitudinal view. (B) Transverse view.

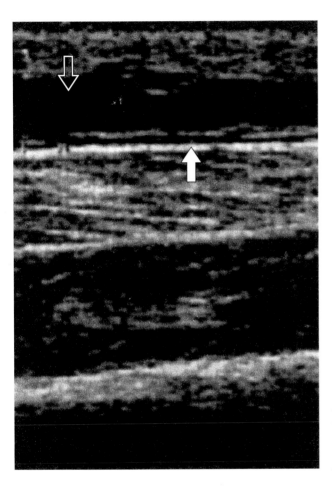

Figure 14.10. Typical sonographic findings in necrotizing fasciitis, demonstrating a fluid layer (open arrow) of greater than 4 mm adjacent to fascia (solid arrow). (By permission from Yen Z, et al. Ultrasonographic Screening of Clinically-Suspected Necrotizing Fasciitis. *Acad Emerg Med.* 2002;9: 1448–1451.)

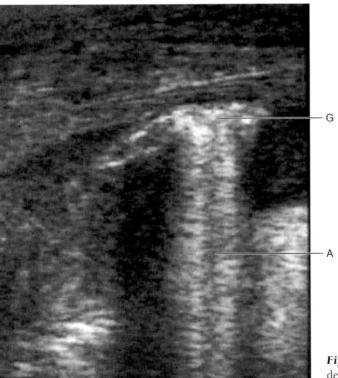

Figure 14.11. Necrotizing fasciitis of the proximal forearm, demonstrating the sonographic appearance of gas (*G*) in the deep tissues giving rise to artifact (*A*) in the far field.

USE IN CLINICAL DECISION MAKING

Although CT scanning is known to reliably identify soft tissue fluid collections, bedside ultrasound may reveal the correct diagnosis much more rapidly and at less cost, and provides real-time localization at the bedside (2). A general approach to skin and soft tissue infections that incorporates bedside ultrasound is presented in Figure 14.12. In many cases the diagnosis of abscess is obvious based on the finding of fluctuance or drainage. On the other hand, when cellulitis seems likely the provider should be careful to consider the possibility of an occult or early abscess, or necrotizing soft tissue infection. When doubt exists about the possibility of an abscess, ultrasound is used to search below the surface for a subcutaneous or intramuscular fluid collection. In addition, ultrasound can be used to define the best location for aspiration or incision, where the collection is largest and closest to the skin surface.

The utility of such an approach in the ED setting has been investigated in 2 studies involving a total of 135 patients (4, 5). Addition of bedside ultrasound to the history and physical resulted in a change in clinical impression in up to 66% of cases, and lead to successful abscess drainage in 11 cases in which it otherwise would not have been attempted. Ultrasound may be particularly useful in abscesses occurring around the head and neck and in the groin, where vascular structures are numerous, and in sites where prior infections and surgical scars can alter the surface presentation of an underlying pus pocket (6–8). (See Case One at end of chapter.)

Necrotizing soft tissue infections can be fatal rapidly without prompt recognition and definitive surgical debridement. Yet accurate diagnosis remains notoriously difficult. Plain x-rays are insensitive whereas CT and MRI may be impractical in an unstable patient. Although the role of bedside ultrasound remains to be defined, findings of marked subcutaneous edema and fluid adjacent to fascia support the diagnosis and may be sufficient confirmatory evidence to proceed to surgery. With the possible exception of MRI, no imaging modality is considered sensitive enough to exclude the diagnosis of necrotizing soft tissue infection once it is suspected on clinical grounds. A low threshold for surgical exploration should be maintained regardless of the results of imaging.

PERITONSILLAR ABSCESS

CLINICAL APPLICATIONS

Successful drainage of a suspected peritonsillar abscess often presents a significant challenge. Ultrasound can be used in this setting to accomplish the following: differentiate abscess from peritonsillar cellulitis; localize the abscess for aspiration; and rescue a failed blind aspiration.

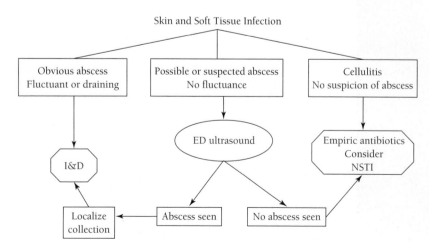

Figure 14.12. Approach to skin and soft tissue infections incorporating ultrasound. (NSTI: necrotizing soft tissue infection.)

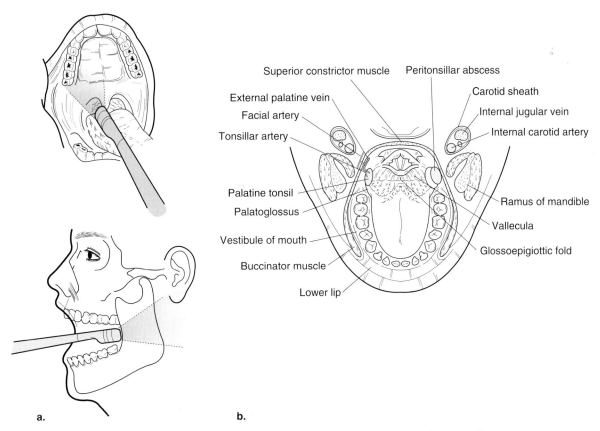

Figure 14.13. Scanning approach for suspected peritonsillar abscess (**A**). Anatomy of peritonsillar area, noting proximity to the internal jugular vein and carotid artery (**B**).

IMAGE ACQUISITION

Sonographic evaluation of suspected peritonsillar abscess is usually performed with a 5-to10-MHz curved array intracavitary transducer, as is used for transvaginal sonography. A small dollop of gel is applied to the transducer, followed by a protective sheath such as a condom. While anesthesia does not appear to be necessary, topical anesthetic spray is recommended prior to the exam in part to reduce gagging. The scanning approach is shown in Figure 14.13. The soft palate is interrogated in both the sagittal and transverse planes with the goal of identifying the superior and inferior extent of the abscess cavity, its depth, and its relation to the carotid artery. The inferior portion of the pharynx should be scanned carefully because pus accumulates adjacent to the mid and lower pole of the tonsil in up to 40% of cases (which correlates with false negative needle aspiration) (9). Comparison to the contralateral side and use of color Doppler may be helpful (Figs. 14.14, 14.15). A percutaneous approach has been described using a 5-MHz linear transducer to scan the pharynx. The transducer is placed inferior and adjacent to the angle of the mandible (10). Although not routinely available in the ED setting, a transducer-mounted biopsy guide can facilitate real-time ultrasound-guided drainage (11).

ULTRASOUND ANATOMY AND LANDMARKS

It is unrealistic to expect to identify all the structures in the peritonsillar region that are seen with ultrasound. These include the palatine tonsil, the margin of the bony hard palate and styloid process of the temporal bone, the medial pterygoid muscle, and various fascial planes. However it is important to locate the internal carotid artery, which courses anterior to the jugular vein in the carotid sheath, and is usually located posterolateral to the tonsil within 5 mm to 25 mm of a peritonsillar abscess (11).

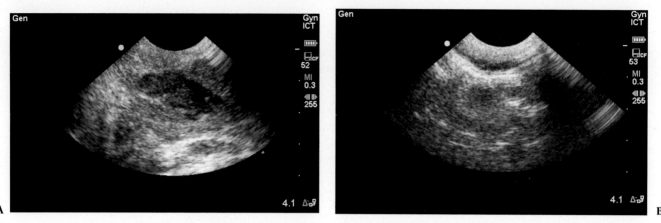

Figure 14.14. (A) Peritonsillar abscess, sagital view. (B) Contralateral normal pharynx. Note that in the right side of both images there is loss of contact between the inferior surface of the transducer and the pharynx.

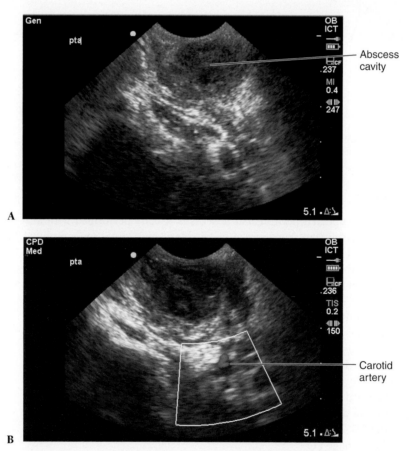

Figure 14.15. (A) Ultrasound of a peritonsillar abscess, taken in transverse plane. (B) With color Doppler, revealing location of the internal carotid artery. (See color insert.)

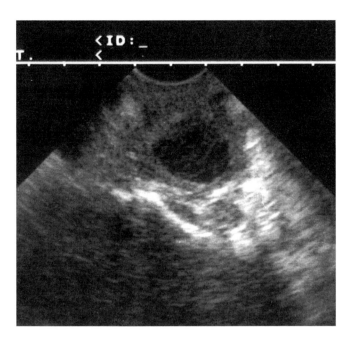

Figure 14.16. Peritonsillar abscess, demonstrating prominent posterior acoustic enhancement.

PATHOLOGY

On ultrasound a peritonsillar abscess usually appears as a hypoechoic, heterogeneous mass, but like all abscesses, the appearance is variable. The abscess may be isoechoic compared with the surrounding tissue in one-third of cases, however posterior acoustic enhancement is a consistent finding (12) (Figure 14.16). Figure 14.15B demonstrates the proximity of a peritonsillar abscess to the carotid artery with color flow.

ARTIFACTS AND PITFALLS

There are numerous potential difficulties inherent in the ultrasound assessment of peritonsillar abscesses.

1. Patients may have trismus or have difficulty cooperating with the exam.
2. Technical difficulties include a degraded image caused by air bubbles between the condom and transducer face, or by poor contact with the pharyngeal wall. Failure to adjust the depth to magnify the near field may cause superficial abscesses to be missed.
3. Inferiorly located abscesses can be missed by failure to scan in the sagittal plane.
4. Isoechoic abscesses can be missed if the sign of increased posterior acoustic enhancement is not recognized.
5. Because the anatomy includes numerous structures and tissue planes of varying acoustic impedance, failure to compare to the contralateral side can lead to either false positive or false negative results.

COMPARISON WITH OTHER IMAGING MODALITIES

CT scan is considered the gold standard for imaging a peritonsillar abscess (9). Ultrasound has emerged as an excellent alternative because it is rapid, noninvasive, and can be used at the bedside to directly guide aspiration and drainage. Use of intraoral ultrasound for diagnosis and localization of peritonsillar abscess was first described in 1993 and since then numerous reports have appeared in the otolaryngology and emergency medicine literature documenting its utility (9,10,12–15). Compared to CT, its sensitivity and specificity are 89% to 90% and 83% to100% (9,13).

Use in Clinical Decision Making

It is often difficult in clinical practice to distinguish peritonsillar cellulitis, which can be treated with antibiotics alone, from peritonsillar abscess, which requires drainage. The traditional approach to diagnosis has been blind needle aspiration of the peritonsillar swelling, but this unnecessarily subjects patients with cellulitis to discomfort and risk, and carries a 10% false negative rate (14). Obtaining a CT scan for this problem is too time-consuming and expensive for routine emergency medicine practice (9).

When the diagnosis of peritonsillar cellulitis versus abscess is in question, ultrasound can be used as the first step in determining management. If no pus pocket is visualized, antibiotics and close follow-up are prescribed. If an abscess is seen, the optimal site for aspiration can be identified. When an abscess seems obvious on physical exam, blind aspiration is often undertaken, but may fail to locate the pus pocket. Ultrasound can be invaluable in this setting, either by locating the abscess and rescuing an initially failed aspiration attempt, or by confirming that no abscess exists (15).

Soft Tissue Foreign Body

Clinical Applications

Retained foreign bodies can complicate skin and soft tissue injuries. Despite their usual superficial location, foreign bodies are difficult to detect by history and physical exam alone and are frequently overlooked. In a retrospective review of 200 patients referred for evaluation of retained hand foreign bodies, 38% were misdiagnosed on their index visit (16). Missed foreign bodies are also one of the most common causes of malpractice claims against emergency physicians (17,18). In the case of a suspected soft tissue foreign body, ultrasound can be used to accomplish the following: detect radiolucent foreign bodies not visible on plain radiographs; localize and characterize foreign bodies and surrounding structures; and facilitate foreign body removal.

Image Acquisition

High-frequency (7.5–10 MHz) linear array transducers are recommended for imaging small superficially located foreign bodies because of their excellent resolution and shallow focal zone. Deeper objects may require a lower-frequency transducer that affords greater tissue penetration. Foreign bodies are difficult to locate—a slow methodical scanning approach is mandatory. Foreign bodies are best visualized when the plane of scanning is either directly parallel to the long axis of the object or directly perpendicular to it (19,20). Scanning must occur in multiple planes because conventional transverse and longitudinal orientations may miss small, obliquely oriented foreign bodies. Sterile technique has been recommended when scanning open wounds or performing ultrasound-guided procedures but the necessity of this practice is doubtful, provided the wound is later irrigated.

Near field acoustic dead space, which occurs immediately adjacent to the transducer surface and is broader when scanning with lower frequencies, can impede the identification of very superficial objects. To compensate, "standoff pads" may be necessary. Standoff pads are made of a low acoustic impedance material and elevate the transducer from the skin surface, eliminating the near field dead space and bringing superficial objects into the transducer's focal zone. Standoff pads range from commercially manufactured models to water-filled latex gloves or small bags of saline (250 cc to 500 cc). In many cases, however, a liberal amount of acoustic gel will suffice. Commercial pads can be trimmed to various sizes and are less prone to slipping, which makes them useful for scanning small, awkward surfaces such as fingers, toes, and web spaces. A water-bath technique, in which the extremity is scanned while submerged in a bath of water, represents an alternative to the standoff pad. Compared to direct contact with gel, the water-bath technique was easy to perform and provided superior images of tendons and foreign bodies (21,22).

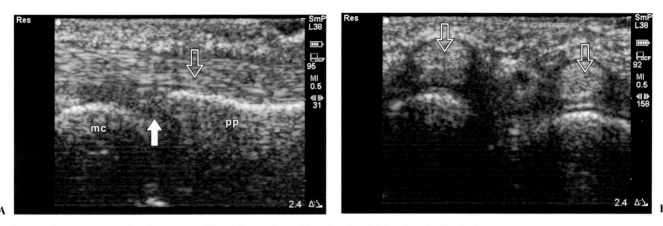

Figure 14.17. Normal hand anatomy. (A) Volar surface of hand at MCP joint, longitudinal view. (B) Volar surface of hand at MCP joint, transverse view. (mc,metacarpal; pp, proximal phalanx; *arrowhead*, MCP joint; *open arrow*, flexor tendon)

ULTRASOUND ANATOMY AND LANDMARKS

Foreign bodies frequently lodge in hands and feet in close proximity to sensitive structures with complex anatomy, which makes sonography difficult. Familiarity with the normal ultrasonographic anatomy is therefore essential (Fig. 14.17). The skin surface is the most proximal echogenic structure. Muscle tissue is readily identified by its uniform hypoechoic texture and internal striations. Fascia appear as thin, brightly echogenic structures. Tendons have a characteristic internal fibrillar pattern and appear as echogenic, ovoid, or linear structures, depending on whether scanned in transverse or longitudinal planes. Interestingly, tendons appear hypoechoic when imaged obliquely (23). The anterior surface of bone is brightly echogenic with far-field anechoic acoustic shadowing. Blood vessels are anechoic and can be further identified using color flow Doppler. With transducer pressure veins compress whereas arteries remain pulsatile.

PATHOLOGY

The most common soft tissue foreign bodies are glass, wood, and metal (16,24,25). All foreign bodies appear hyperechoic and, depending upon their composition and proximity to certain anatomic structures, will display variable degrees of acoustic shadowing or reverberation artifact (19,20,26–29). Gravel and wood cast a characteristic acoustic shadow similar to that of a gallstone (Fig. 14.18) (19,28,29). A large wood fragment with its brightly echogenic anterior surface can easily be mistaken for bone (Fig. 14.19). Metallic objects frequently display a "comet tail," or a reverberation artifact in which bright, regularly spaced parallel lines are seen distal to the foreign body (Fig. 14.20) (20,28,30). The acoustic profile of glass is less consistent—acoustic shadows, comet-tail artifacts, and diffuse beam scattering can be seen (Fig. 14.21) (19,28,31,32). Foreign bodies retained for longer than 24 to 48 hours are frequently surrounded by an echolucent halo, resulting from reactive hyperemia, edema, abscess, or granulation tissue, which may aid in their identification (Fig. 14.22) (19,20,26,29,33).

REMOVAL TECHNIQUES

Numerous techniques for ultrasound-assisted foreign body removal have been described. The simplest of them is ultrasound-guided incision. The transducer is centered over the foreign body and the skin is marked with a pen to identify the incision site for exploration (20,27,34,35). Several reports advocate using real-time ultrasound to guide placement of forceps or a hemostat next to the foreign body (20,35–37). This technique is said to work

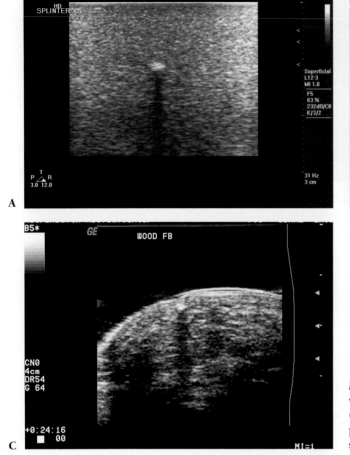

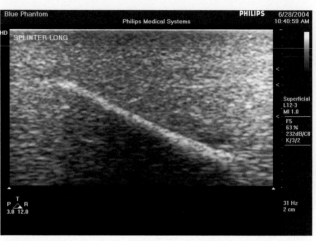

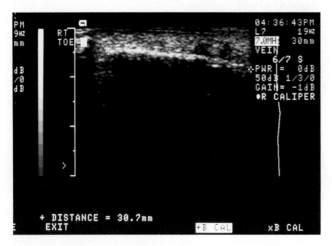

Figure 14.18. Wood foreign bodies. Tissue model containing a wood splinter demonstrating acoustic shadows, short (**A**) and long (**B**) axis views (Courtesy of Brian Keegan). Wood splinter in the plantar aspect of the heel (**C**). Short axis view, using commercial standoff pad. Note shadowing (Courtesy of Robert Jones, DO).

particularly well with linear foreign bodies. It is outlined in Figure 14.23. After making a lateral skin incision, advance the forceps toward the foreign body while scanning both objects in their longitudinal axis. If extraction is unsuccessful, attempt removal after rotating the transducer 90 degrees, thereby imaging both the tip of the foreign body and the mouth of the hemostat transversely. Alligator forceps may be more maneuverable under the skin and cause less tissue injury than the instruments found in standard suture kits (38).

Figure 14.19. Wood foreign body in toe, long axis view (Courtesy of Tim Gibbs, RDMS).

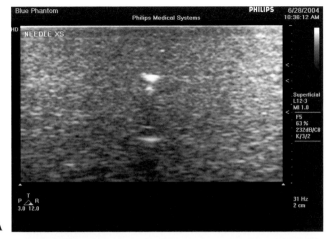

A

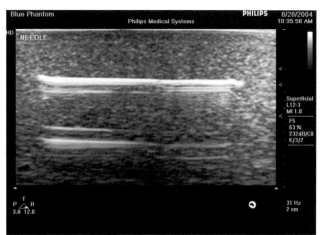

B

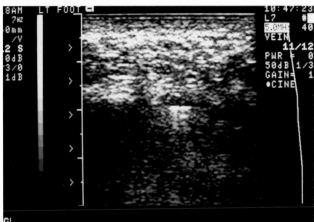

C

Figure 14.20. Metallic foreign bodies. Tissue model containing a sewing needle demonstrating reverberation artifact, short (**A**) and long (**B**) axis views (Courtesy of Brian Keegan). Copper wire in the foot with reverberation artifact (**C**) (Courtesy of Tim Gibbs, RDMS).

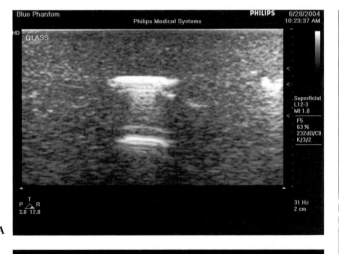

A

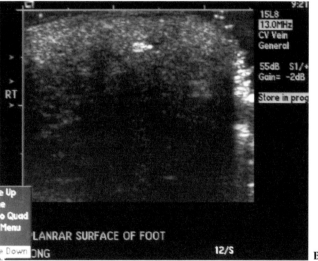

B

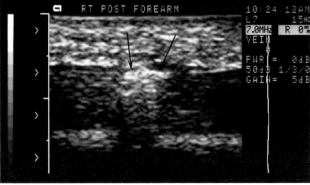

C

Figure 14.21. Glass foreign bodies. (**A**) Model containing a glass foreign body demonstrating reverberation artifact (Courtesy of Brian Keegan). (**B**) Glass foreign body in the foot without artifact (Courtesy of Tim Gibbs, RDMS). (**C**) Glass foreign body (*arrows*) in the forearm with reverberation artifact (Courtesy of Tim Gibbs, RDMS).

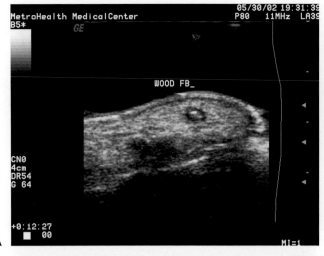

A

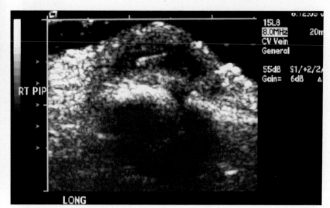

B

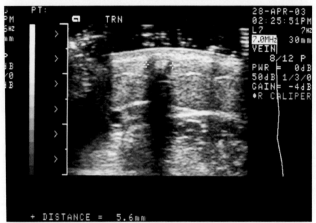

C

Figure 14.22. Wood foreign bodies with surrounding halos. (**A**) Wood foreign body with surrounding fluid in volar pad of distal phalanx, long axis view (Courtesy of Robert Jones, DO). (**B**) Wood foreign body with surrounding fluid overlying the PIP joint, long axis view. (**C**) Bee stinger in leg with surrounding inflammatory capsule (Courtesy of Tim Gibbs, RDMS).

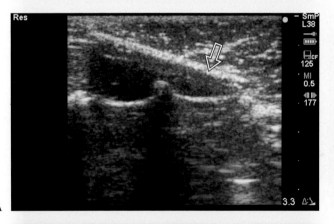

A

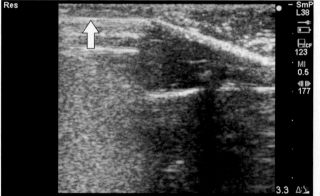

B

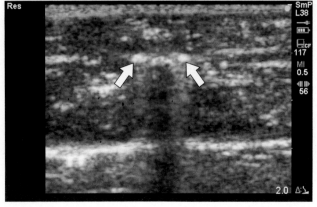

C

Figure 14.23. Ultrasound-guided removal of a subcutaneous toothpick with forceps in a chicken breast model. (**A**) Preoperative ultrasound revealing toothpick (*open arrow*) in long axis. (**B**) Long axis view of toothpick with approaching forceps (*solid arrow*)—note reverberation artifact. (**C**) Short axis view of toothpick and forceps—toothpick is centered between mouth of open forceps (*solid arrows*).

A third, well-described technique is ultrasound-guided needle localization (20,35,37–40). This technique is outlined in Figure 14.24. It is ideal for irregularly shaped and deeply embedded foreign bodies. It is less suitable for superficial foreign bodies of the hand and feet, where sensitive structures such as tendons and bone can easily become interposed. Using ultrasound guidance, a single operator directs one or more sterile finder needles under the base of a foreign body. Placing two needles at 90 degree angles to one another has been recommended (40). The needles are left in place and serve as landmarks during open retrieval. Local infiltration followed by incision and dissection down to the tip or intersection of the needles should lead directly to the foreign body.

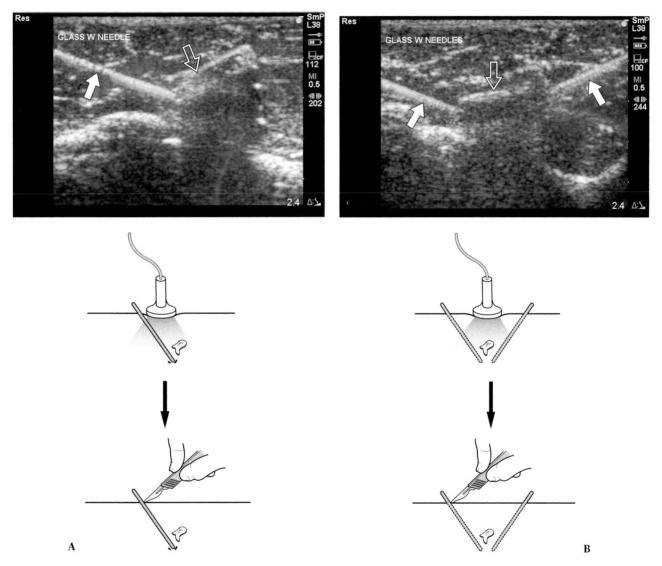

Figure 14.24. Ultrasound-guided localization of a glass foreign body in a chicken breast model. Needle localization technique. (**A**) Single-needle technique. (**B**) Two needles at right angle technique. (*open arrow* = glass; *solid arrow* = needle).

ARTIFACTS AND PITFALLS

Both detection and retrieval of foreign bodies using ultrasound is technically very challenging. The relatively large linear transducers available in EDs make scanning in areas such as the fingers and toes tricky. Contact may be limited to a small portion of the transducer surface, creating a small field of view and peripheral artifacts. Moreover, certain anatomic areas are almost impossible to scan, such as the web spaces between digits, which can lead to missed foreign bodies (19). Makeshift standoff pads are cumbersome and frequently slip off the area being scanned. Attempts at maintaining sterility may be futile. Ultrasound detection of foreign bodies is time-consuming. In one report, exam times by radiologists averaged 10 minutes and extended up to 30 minutes (19). Likewise, ultrasound-guided foreign body removal is often a lengthy procedure (20,29).

Though most foreign bodies can be identified by ultrasound, false-negative results can occur. Superficial foreign bodies may be overlooked when low-frequency transducers are used and acoustic dead space is not overcome by standoff pads. Small objects may simply exceed the limit of a transducer's resolution. Foreign bodies may be mistaken for hyperechoic anatomic structures such as bone or tendon. Overlying bone or trapped air can hide foreign bodies (20,27). Air is usually present under large skin defects or introduced during anesthetic infiltration, probing, or dissection. Steady transducer pressure over open wounds may displace air and help minimize artifact. False-positive results can arise from vascular and tissue calcifications, sesamoid bones, ossified cartilage, scar tissue, hemorrhage, entrapped air, and keratin plugs (25,27,34,35,41). Comparison to the contralateral extremity is an invaluable internal control, helping to distinguish a foreign body from normal anatomy.

COMPARISON WITH OTHER IMAGING MODALITIES

No single imaging technique will identify all foreign bodies. The majority of retained foreign bodies will be identified by standard, two-view radiography (16,24). X-rays are 100% sensitive for metallic objects and nearly 100% sensitive for glass particles, regardless of composition (24,42). Gravel particles are also visible (43). However, x-ray does not readily identify radiolucent foreign bodies such as wood, plastic, and organic compounds like thorns and cactus spines. Plain x-rays identify only 15% of retained wooden particles (16). If clinical suspicion for a foreign body remains high despite negative x-rays, the diagnosis must be pursued with additional imaging modalities, such as ultrasound.

Ultrasound has emerged as the imaging modality of choice for foreign bodies that are radiolucent on plain films. Though CT and MRI have shown efficacy in detecting soft tissue foreign bodies, their use is limited by cost, availability, and radiation exposure. Moreover, ultrasound was found to be more sensitive and accurate than CT in several studies. One study comparing ultrasound and CT demonstrated accuracies of 90% and 70% for radiolucent foreign body detection, respectively (44). Other studies report the sensitivity of CT for the detection of soft tissue foreign bodies to be poor, ranging from 0% to 60% (32,45,46).

Ultrasound can accurately detect small foreign bodies in a variety of tissue models, including beef cubes, chicken thighs, and human cadaver extremities (41,47–52). More importantly, ultrasound has been shown to be an accurate and sensitive modality for foreign body detection when used in the clinical setting (19,20,25,27,29,34,35,37,44). In 50 ED patients who were referred for sonography, radiologist-performed ultrasound was 95.4% sensitive and 89.2% specific in the detection of radiolucent foreign bodies (19). In a prospective analysis of 31 patients with suspected radiolucent foreign bodies who eventually underwent operative exploration, ultrasound by nonemergency physicians successfully identified 18 of 20 foreign bodies (44).

The literature on emergency physician-performed ultrasound for foreign body detection is limited to in vitro experiments and observational case series (51,53,54). One report demonstrated that emergency physicians with limited ultrasound experience could

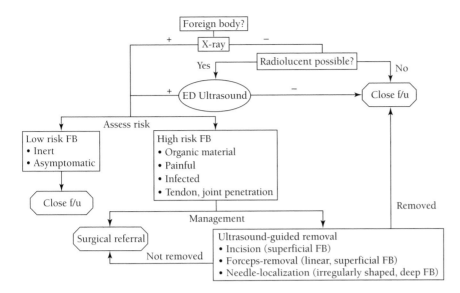

Figure 14.25. Approach to a suspected foreign body.

accurately detect radiolucent foreign bodies embedded in chicken thighs (51). In another, four cases were described in which ultrasound was successfully used by emergency physicians to detect and remove radiolucent foreign bodies (53). Lastly, other authors described a case of emergency physician-directed ultrasound localization of a wood foreign body using a 7.5-MHz intracavitary probe and a standoff pad fashioned from a water-filled latex glove (54).

USE IN CLINICAL DECISION MAKING

The clinical approach to a suspected retained foreign body is outlined in Figure 14.25. The savvy clinician maintains a low threshold for ruling out foreign body in the face of a suspicious mechanism of injury or exam findings. Begin with plain x-rays. If radiographs are negative and a radiolucent foreign body is a possibility, proceed to ultrasound. If a foreign body is detected, one of three treatment strategies is chosen: expectant management, bedside extraction, or referral to a specialist.

Not all foreign bodies need to be extracted (55). Asymptomatic, inert, and nonreactive foreign bodies, such as superficial shotgun pellets, may be left in place (55). Organic and reactive materials, such as wood, thorns, and cactus spines generally should be removed because they cause inflammation and infection (55). Infected foreign bodies and those that that cause pain, compromise function, or penetrate joints should also be removed (55). Consider specialty consultation and referral when a foreign body is deeply embedded or in close proximity to an anatomically sensitive area, such as a joint (16).

Before attempting an extraction procedure, ultrasound should be used to precisely locate the foreign body. Unlike standard x-rays, ultrasound can accurately determine an object's size, depth, course, three-dimensional orientation, and relationship with surrounding structures. This information is used to guide removal, allowing smaller incision sizes and leading to less tissue dissection (20).

CASE ONE

A 55-year-old man presented to the ED complaining of abdominal wall pain. On the previous day he was diagnosed with abdominal wall cellulitis and oral antibiotics were prescribed, but erythema and pain had worsened and fever developed. There was a history of diabetes and renal failure currently treated with hemodialysis, but previously treated with peritoneal dialysis. Surgical history included peritoneal dialysis catheter placement, incision and drainage of a prior abdominal wall abscess, and appendectomy. The temperature was 38.2°C and the abdominal wall had multiple old scars and was diffusely erythematous

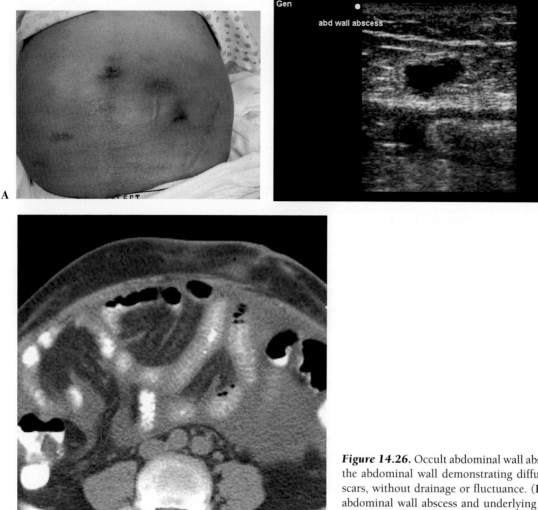

A
B
C

Figure 14.26. Occult abdominal wall abscess. (A) Physical exam of the abdominal wall demonstrating diffuse erythema and multiple scars, without drainage or fluctuance. (B) ED ultrasound showing abdominal wall abscess and underlying peritoneum. (C) CT scan showing abscess with surrounding inflammatory changes.

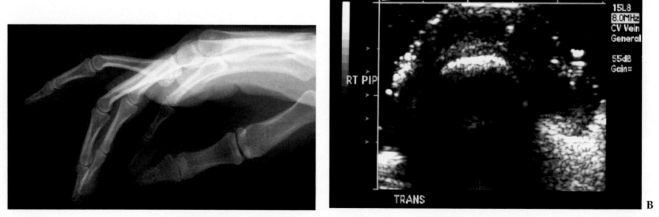

A
B

Figure 14.27. Wooden thorn in finger. (A) X-ray shows overlying soft tissue swelling but fails to demonstrate the foreign body. (B) Transverse ultrasound over PIP reveals a hyperechoic foreign body in short axis (Courtesy of Tim Gibbs, RDMS).

and tender (Fig. 14.26A). ED ultrasound revealed a hypoechoic spherical mass 1.5 cm below the skin in the abdominal wall (Fig. 14.26B). CT scan confirmed presence of an abdominal wall abscess (Fig. 14.26C). The patient was admitted to the surgical service and the following day underwent an uncomplicated incision and drainage procedure in the operating room.

CASE TWO

A 45-year-old man presented to the ED with the chief complaint of finger pain and swelling one day after being punctured by a thorn while gardening. Physical exam revealed a tender, soft tissue swelling over the proximal interphalangeal joint of the right index finger. No fluctuance, erythema, warmth, or visible foreign body was identified. Plain radiographs did not identify a foreign body and the patient was discharged home and told to return for worsening symptoms (Fig. 14.27A). The patient returned to the ED 48 hours later. His finger was erythematous, warm, and swollen. Using bedside ultrasound, the emergency physician identified a small echogenic mass surrounded by an anechoic halo consistent with a subcutaneous foreign body and surrounding edema or pus (Fig. 14.27B). Following digital block anesthesia, an incision was made and alligator forceps were directed beneath the foreign body by ultrasound guidance. The foreign body, a thorn, was then removed without difficulty. The patient was placed on antibiotics and did well at follow-up.

REFERENCES

1. Yen ZS, Wang HP, Ma HM, et al. Ultrasonographic screening of clinically-suspected necrotizing fasciitis. *Acad Emerg Med.* 2002;9:1448–1451.
2. Wall DB, de Virgilio C, Black S, et al. Objective criteria may assist in distinguishing necrotizing fasciitis from nonnecrotizing soft tissue infection. *Am J Surg.* 2000;179:17–21.
3. Cardinal E, Bureau NJ, Aubin B, et al. Role of ultrasound in musculoskeletal infections. *Radiol Clin North Am.* 2001;39:191–201. Review.
4. Page-Wills C, Simon B, Christy D. Utility of ultrasound on emergency department management of suspected cutaneous abscess. *Acad Emerg Med.* 2000;7:493.
5. Squire B, Fox CJ, Zlidenny A, et al. ABSCESS: applied bedside sonography for convenient evaluation of superficial soft tissue infections. In: California Chapter, Amercian College of Emergency Physicians, Scientific Assembly, Squaw Valley, May 29th, 2004.
6. Sandler MA, Alpern MB, Madrazo BL, et al. Inflammatory lesions of the groin: ultrasonic evaluation. *Radiology.* 1984;151:747–750.
7. Yusa H, Yoshida H, Ueno E, et al. Ultrasound-guided surgical drainage of face and neck abscesses. *Int J Oral Maxillofac Surg.* 2002;31:327–329.
8. Blaivas M. Ultrasound-guided breast abscess aspiration in a difficult case. *Acad Emerg Med.* 2001;8:398–401.
9. Scott PM, Loftus WK, Kew J, et al. Diagnosis of peritonsillar infections: a prospective study of ultrasound, computerized tomography and clinical diagnosis. *J Laryngol Otol.* 1999;113:229–232.
10. Miziara ID, Koishi HU, Zonato AI, et al. The use of ultrasound evaluation in the diagnosis of peritonsillar abscess. *Rev Laryngol Otol Rhinol (Bord).* 2001;122:201–203.
11. Haeggstrom A, Gustafsson O, Engquist S, et al. Intraoral ultrasonography in the diagnosis of peritonsillar abscess. *Arch Otolaryngol Head Neck Surg.* 1993;108:243–247.
12. O'Brien E, Valley VT, Summers RL. Intraoral sonography of peritonsillar abscesses: feasibility and sonographic appearance. *Ann Emerg Med.* 1999;34:S26.
13. Strong EB, Woodward PJ, Johnson LP. Intraoral ultrasound evaluation of peritonsillar abscess. *Laryngoscope.* 1995;105(8 Pt 1):779–782.
14. Kew J, Ahuja A, Loftus WK, et al. Peritonsillar abscess appearance on intra-oral ultrasonography. *Clin Radiol.* 1998;53:143–146.
15. Blaivas M, Theodoro D, Duggal S. Ultrasound-guided drainage of peritonsillar abscess by the emergency physician. *Am J Emerg Med.* 2003;21:155–158.
16. Anderson MA, Newmeyer WL 3rd, Kilgore ES Jr. Diagnosis and treatment of retained foreign bodies in the hand. *Am J Surg.* 1982;144:63–67.

17. Trautlein JJ, Lambert RL, Miller J. Malpractice in the emergency department—review of 200 cases. *Ann Emerg Med*. 1984;13(9 Pt 1):709–711.
18. Roberts J. Soft tissue foreign bodies. *Emerg Med Amb Care News*. 1988;10(2):2–6.
19. Gilbert FJ, Campbell RS, Bayliss AP. The role of ultrasound in the detection of non-radiopaque foreign bodies. *Clin Radiol*. 1990;41:109–112.
20. Shiels WE 2nd, Babcock DS, Wilson JL, et al. Localization and guided removal of soft-tissue foreign bodies with sonography. *AJR Am J Roentgenol*. 1990;155:1277–1281.
21. Leech SJ, Gukhool JU, Blaivas M. ED ultrasound evaluation of the index flexor tendon: a comparison of water-bath evaluation technique (WET) versus direct contact ultrasound. *Acad Emerg Med*. 2003;10:573.
22. Leech SJ, Blaivas M, Gukhool J. Water-bath vs direct contact ultrasound: a randomized, controlled, blinded image review. *Acad Emerg Med*. 2003;10:573–574.
23. Fornage BD. The hypoechoic normal tendon. A pitfall. *J Ultrasound Med*. 1987;6:19–22.
24. Morgan WJ, Leopold T, Evans R. Foreign bodies in the hand. *J Hand Surg [Br]*. 1984;9:194–196.
25. Gooding GA, Hardiman T, Sumers M, et al. Sonography of the hand and foot in foreign body detection. *J Ultrasound Med*. 1987;6:441–447.
26. Fornage BD, Schernberg FL, Rifkin MD. Ultrasound examination of the hand. *Radiology*. 1985;155:785–788.
27. Banerjee B, Das RK. Sonographic detection of foreign bodies of the extremities. *Br J Radiol*. 1991;64:107–112.
28. Horton LK, Jacobson JA, Powell A, et al. Sonography and radiography of soft-tissue foreign bodies. *AJR Am J Roentgenol*. 2001;176:1155–1159.
29. Rockett MS, Gentile SC, Gudas CJ, et al. The use of ultrasonography for the detection of retained wooden foreign bodies in the foot. *J Foot Ankle Surg*. 1995;34:478–484; discussion 510–511.
30. Scanlan KA. Sonographic artifacts and their origins. *AJR Am J Roentgenol*. 1991;156:1267–1272.
31. Donaldson JS. Radiographic imaging of foreign bodies in the hand. *Hand Clin*. 1991;7:125–134.
32. Oikarinen KS, Nieminen TM, Makarainen H, et al. Visibility of foreign bodies in soft tissue in plain radiographs, computed tomography, magnetic resonance imaging, and ultrasound. An in vitro study. *Int J Oral Maxillofac Surg*. 1993;22:119–124.
33. Davae KC, Sofka CM, DiCarlo E, et al. Value of power Doppler imaging and the hypoechoic halo in the sonographic detection of foreign bodies: correlation with histopathologic findings. *J Ultrasound Med*. 2003;22:1309–1313; quiz 1314–1316.
34. Crawford R, Matheson AB. Clinical value of ultrasonography in the detection and removal of radiolucent foreign bodies. *Injury*. 1989;20:341–343.
35. Blankstein A, Cohen I, Heiman Z, et al. Ultrasonography as a diagnostic modality and therapeutic adjuvant in the management of soft tissue foreign bodies in the lower extremities. *Isr Med Assoc J*. 2001;3:411–413.
36. Bradley M, Kadzombe E, Simms P, et al. Percutaneous ultrasound guided extraction of non-palpable soft tissue foreign bodies. *Arch Emerg Med*. 1992;9:181–184.
37. Blankstein A, Cohen I, Heiman Z, et al. Localization, detection and guided removal of soft tissue in the hands using sonography. *Arch Orthop Trauma Surg*. 2000;120:514–517.
38. Jones RA. Ultrasound-guided procedures. *Critical Decisions in Emergency Medicine* 2004; 18:11–17.
39. Yiengpruksawan A, Mariadason J, Ganepola GA, et al. Localization and retrieval of bullets under ultrasound guidance. *Arch Surg*. 1987;122:1082–1084.
40. Teisen HG, Torfing KF, Skjodt T. [Ultrasound pinpointing of foreign bodies. An in vitro study]. *Ultraschall Med* 1988;9:135–137.
41. Jacobson JA, Powell A, Craig JG, et al. Wooden foreign bodies in soft tissue: detection at US. *Radiology*. 1998;206:45–48.
42. Tandberg D. Glass in the hand and foot. Will an X-ray film show it? *JAMA*. 1982;248:1872–1874.
43. Chisholm CD, Wood CO, Chua G, et al. Radiographic detection of gravel in soft tissue. *Ann Emerg Med*. 1997;29:725–730.
44. Al-Zahrani S, Kremli M, Saadeddin M, Ikram A. Ultrasonography detection of radiolucent foreign bodies in soft tissues compared to computed tomography scan. *Ann Saudi Med*. 1995; 15:110–112.
45. Bodne D, Quinn SF, Cochran CF. Imaging foreign glass and wooden bodies of the extremities with CT and MR. *J Comput Assist Tomogr*. 1988;12:608–611.
46. Ginsburg MJ, Ellis GL, Flom LL. Detection of soft-tissue foreign bodies by plain radiography, xerography, computed tomography, and ultrasonography. *Ann Emerg Med*. 1990;19:701–703.
47. Bray PW, Mahoney JL, Campbell JP. Sensitivity and specificity of ultrasound in the diagnosis of foreign bodies in the hand. *J Hand Surg [Am]*. 1995;20:661–666.

48. Blyme PJ, Lind T, Schantz K, et al. Ultrasonographic detection of foreign bodies in soft tissue. A human cadaver study. *Arch Orthop Trauma Surg.* 1990;110:24–25.

49. Turner J, Wilde CH, Hughes KC, et al. Ultrasound-guided retrieval of small foreign objects in subcutaneous tissue. *Ann Emerg Med.* 1997;29:731–734.

50. Hill R, Conron R, Greissinger P, et al. Ultrasound for the detection of foreign bodies in human tissue. *Ann Emerg Med.* 1997;29:353–356.

51. Orlinsky M, Knittel P, Feit T, et al. The comparative accuracy of radiolucent foreign body detection using ultrasonography. *Am J Emerg Med* 2000;18:401–403.

52. Schlager D, Sanders AB, Wiggins D, et al. Ultrasound for the detection of foreign bodies. *Ann Emerg Med.* 1991;20:189–191.

53. Graham DD Jr. Ultrasound in the emergency department: detection of wooden foreign bodies in the soft tissues. *J Emerg Med.* 2002;22:75–79.

54. Dean AJ, Gronczewski CA, Costantino TG. Technique for emergency medicine bedside ultrasound identification of a radiolucent foreign body. *J Emerg Med.* 2003;24:303–308.

55. Lammers RL, Magill T. Detection and management of foreign bodies in soft tissue. *Emerg Med Clin North Am.* 1992;10:767–781.

INDEX